# CLINICAL PROCEDURES FOR
# OCULAR EXA

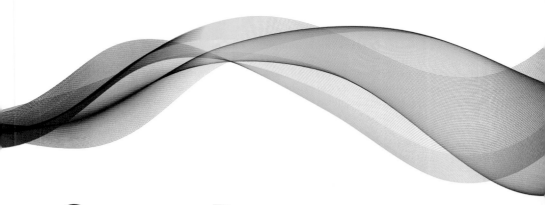

# CLINICAL PROCEDURES FOR OCULAR EXAMINATION

*Fifth Edition*

**JENNIFER REILLY, OD, MSC, FAAO**

Assistant Professor of Optometry
New England College of Optometry
Boston, Massachusetts

**HILARY GAISER, OD, MSC**

Assistant Professor of Optometry
New England College of Optometry
Boston, Massachusetts

**BENJAMIN YOUNG, OD, FAAO**

Assistant Professor of Optometry
New England College of Optometry
Boston, Massachusetts

New York    Chicago    San Francisco    Athens    London    Madrid    Mexico City
Milan    New Delhi    Singapore    Sydney    Toronto

**Clinical Procedures for Ocular Examination, Fifth Edition**

Previous editions copyright © 2016 by McGraw-Hill Education; 2004 by The McGraw-Hill Companies, Inc.; 1996 and 1991 by Appleton & Lange.

1 2 3 4 5 6 7 8 9 DSS 28 27 26 25 24 23

ISBN 978-1-264-27743-8
MHID 1-264-27743-1 ●

This book was set in Minion Pro by MPS Limited.
The editors were Sydney Keen Vitale and Kim J. Davis.
The production supervisor was Catherine Saggesse.
Project management was provided by Pradhiba Kannaiyan, MPS Limited.

This book is printed on acid-free paper.

**Library of Congress Cataloging-in-Publication Data**

Names: Reilly, Jennifer (Professor of optometry) editor. | Gaiser, Hilary, editor. |
  Young, Benjamin (Professor of optometry) editor.
Title: Clinical procedures for ocular examination / [edited by] Jennifer
  Reilly, Hilary Gaiser, Benjamin Young.
Description: Fifth edition. | New York : McGraw Hill, [2023] | Includes
  bibliographical references and index. | Summary: "This edition will
  expand upon the foundation developed by the previous authors and reflect
  the increasing scope of optometric practice while staying true to their
  primary mission: to describe how to perform a wide variety of useful
  tests without a large body of theory"—Provided by publisher.
Identifiers: LCCN 2022035754 (print) | LCCN 2022035755 (ebook) |
  ISBN 9781264277438 (paperback ; alk. paper) | ISBN 9781264277445 (ebook)
Subjects: MESH: Eye Diseases—diagnosis | Vision Tests—methods |
  Optometry—methods | Optometry—instrumentation
Classification: LCC RE75  (print) | LCC RE75  (ebook) | NLM WW 141 |
  DDC 617.7/15—dc23/eng/20221109
LC record available at https://lccn.loc.gov/2022035754
LC ebook record available at https://lccn.loc.gov/2022035755

# Contents

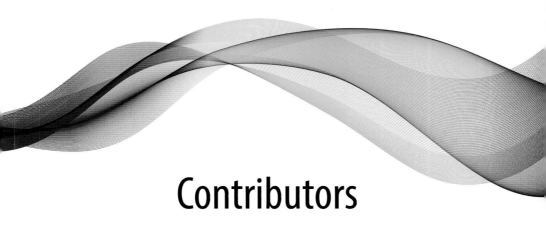

# Contributors

**Elena Z. Biffi, OD, MSc, FAAO**
Associate Professor of Optometry
New England College of Optometry
Boston, Massachusetts

**Anita Gulmiri, OD, FAAO**
Assistant Professor of Clinical Optometry
New England College of Optometry
Boston, Massachusetts

**Maureen Hanley, OD**
Associate Professor of Biomedical Sciences and Disease
New England College of Optometry
Boston, Massachusetts

**Lance McNaughton, OD, PhD**
Associate Professor of Optometry
New England College of Optometry
Boston, Massachusetts

**Bina Patel, OD, FAAO**
Professor of Biomedical Sciences and Disease
New England College of Optometry
Boston, Massachusetts

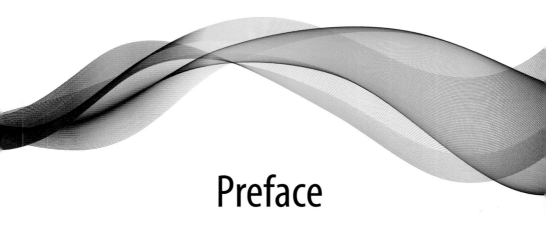

# Preface

It has been over 30 years since the publication of the first edition of *Clinical Procedures for Ocular Examination* and 7 years since the publication of the fourth edition. This fifth edition marks the first time that the text was edited by someone other than one of the first four founding authors of the original publication. The goal of this new edition was to expand upon the foundation developed by the previous authors and incorporate newer technology and advanced procedures while staying true to their primary mission: to describe how to perform a wide variety of useful tests without a large body of theory.

Technology in healthcare continues to rapidly evolve and instrumentation for ocular imaging has become common place in optometric practice. The fifth edition includes this advanced instrumentation due to its expanding role in comprehensive eye care. While the general procedures for ocular imaging are outlined, it is always recommended that the manufacturer instructions are followed when using this highly technical instrumentation.

Increasing access to eye care has been the underlying common goal of expanding the scope of optometric practice in many states across the country. Optometrists who are appropriately trained and certified are now performing anterior segment laser and microsurgical techniques in several states. Two new chapters have been added to this text to incorporate diagnostic ocular imaging and advanced therapeutic ophthalmic procedures, respectively.

Reviewing peer-reviewed literature, evidence-based medicine, and modern trends in eye care were key drivers to the rewrite of this text. It was intentional to include several techniques that pertain to myopia management such as ocular biometry and fit and assessment of orthokeratology (ortho-k) lenses, as the need for such management is on the rise. This text also includes two new sections on best practices for patient privacy and infection control.

One of the key motivations for the 1990 first edition of this book was the lack of standardization for many clinical procedures. Books such as this one attempt to alleviate the problem to some degree. Nevertheless, it remains true now as it did at the time of the first four editions: there is still more than one acceptable way to perform many of the procedures included in this text. In some of these instances, we have added variations in the step-by-step procedures, clearly indicating that there is a valid, alternate way to perform that step or procedure.

The movement to standardize optometry on a national level continues. The intellectual foundations of optometric practice have been strengthened by an ever-growing body of scientific literature. Consequently, we have updated the reference sections with recent citations and added or modified procedures in accordance with contemporary concepts and knowledge.

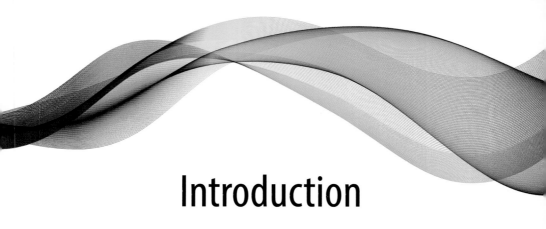

# Introduction

The purpose of *Clinical Procedures for Ocular Examination* is to provide students and practitioners with detailed step-by-step procedures for a comprehensive battery of techniques used in the examination of the eye. These procedures include tests for assessing refractive error, accommodative function, binocular coordination, the health of the eyes, the fit and condition of contact lenses, screening tests for neurological and systemic health conditions, ocular imaging, and advanced procedures. The book contains detailed, step-by-step instructions on how to perform each technique. For each procedure, the reader is provided with comprehensive information on the purpose of the test, what equipment is needed, how to setup the equipment and the patient properly, and how to record the findings. Expected findings are listed for most tests. The text includes diagrams and photographs to reinforce the descriptions of the techniques.

The emphasis in this book is technical. It provides little in the way of the theory of the test and limited management following the procedure. Removal of the theoretical discussion leaves a pure, concise description of the techniques and allows the reader to concentrate on the psychomotor mechanics of the procedures. Mastery of the techniques and interpretation and management of the findings, however, cannot be obtained solely through the use of this book, but requires supervised clinical practice as well as a thorough understanding of the theoretical basis for each technique. Included in the References section at the end of the book are the cited sources that will provide the reader with more information on the necessary theory and background for each of the procedures.

The first chapter of the book deals with patient communication, clearly the most important aspect of patient care. Good communication improves patient outcomes and makes the encounter more enjoyable for both the patient and the doctor. The first time the patient and doctor meet is usually during the case history, a critical phase of the examination. In addition to establishing rapport with the patient and setting the tone for the exam, the history marks the beginning of the doctor's diagnostic thought process. Knowing the patient's concerns, the examiner can now begin to develop their examination strategy and differential diagnosis. Based on the patient's chief complaints and routine background information gathered in the case history, the examiner can decide which phases of the examination to concentrate on and which problem-specific testing should be done. Good communication techniques should be utilized throughout the duration of the exam. Specifically, the examiner should also explain what they are about to do and why they are doing it before they perform any of the procedures contained in this text. Professional communication with other healthcare providers regarding patient information is outlined in the verbal presentation and written communication procedures. A new section has been added outlining best practices for patient privacy as this should be considered when transmitting any patient information whether verbal, written, or electronic.

The second chapter describes the entrance tests. These techniques are the first procedures performed following the case history. They are relatively simple procedures that use minimal, primarily handheld equipment. These tests often require patient contact with exam equipment or with the examiner and so a section on infection control has been added to highlight some best practices in patient care. The entrance tests screen for problems in each of the three major problem areas: refraction, visual function, and health. Most of the entrance tests screen for problems in more than one of these three areas. Thoughtful interpretation of the results of the entrance tests can greatly increase the efficiency of the examination. Augmented by the information gathered in the case history, entrance test data aid the examiner in pinpointing the patient's problem areas and appropriately directing the examination strategy.

Chapters 3, 4, and 5 correspond to the problem areas of refraction, visual function, and ocular health, respectively. The tests chosen by the examiner to assess each of these areas will depend upon the patient's age, symptoms, screening results from the entrance tests, and physical mobility. Many states, health insurance companies, and optometric organizations will set recommendations or requirements for procedures to be included in a comprehensive eye exam. It is then up to the examiner to determine which additional procedures will help confirm or rule out suspected diagnoses developed during the course of the history and exam. There also may be times when sound professional judgment dictates the need to omit certain tests from the routine examination. Each of these three chapters include common, essential tests used in the majority of comprehensive eye care encounters such as the distance subjective refraction, slit lamp biomicroscopy, and dilated binocular indirect ophthalmoscopy, to name a few. Also described in these chapters is a variety of problem-specific tests, by which the examiner explores a specific area of concern in detail. These tests are not done on a routine basis but are selected based on the patient's case history and the results of other testing. Problem-specific tests are not placed in a separate chapter. They are included in the chapter corresponding to their problem area.

Included within Chapters 3, 4, and 5 are flowcharts that illustrate how tests might be grouped or sequenced in order to promote examination efficiency. These charts do not represent the only appropriate sequencing of the techniques, but they do illustrate one sequence for efficiently combining the procedures. Separate flowcharts are presented for the most commonly applied core entrance tests, refractive tests, and ocular health assessment tests. Since functional testing and problem-specific testing are almost always customized to the patient and depend strongly on the individual patient's problem or complaint, there is no standard flowchart for these parts of the ocular examination.

Individual flowcharts could not possibly work for all patients. Rather, they are intended to provide a standard sequence of testing for the majority of patients seen in most examiners' practices. This standard test order can be compared to the itinerary of a trip. The traveler plans the trip from start to finish along a standard pathway, or "main route." Similarly, the flowcharts depict a standard itinerary of ocular tests that lead from the beginning to the end of the routine exam.

However, many patients need problem-specific tests, which can be compared to points of interest along the main route. When indicated, the examiner takes a "side trip." That is, they perform certain tests that are supplemental to the main route. The flowcharts and text show when side trips are indicated. Once the necessary side trip is completed, the examiner should usually return to the main route and continue the examination from there. For the sake of examination efficiency, however, some side trips may be postponed.

Chapter 6 concentrates on the procedures necessary for basic fitting and monitoring of contact lenses. It is possible to quickly and efficiently incorporate these procedures into a comprehensive ocular examination as shown in the flow chart at the beginning of Chapter 6. This chapter includes soft lenses, rigid corneal and scleral lenses, and a new section describing the fit and assessment of orthokeratology (ortho-k) lenses. Fit and assessment of the multifocal contact lenses wearer and monovision patient are also discussed.

Chapter 7 deals with procedures used to screen a patient's systemic health. The eye care professional may be the patient's entry point into the health care system. Therefore, they have the responsibility to evaluate the overall health of the patient. The examiner may select to perform certain procedures based on the patient's age, medical history, or presenting symptoms or as the result of information gathered during the comprehensive examination. Alternately, the examiner may prefer to perform some of these screening procedures routinely on all patients. Patients with abnormal results should be referred to the appropriate health care provider for more thorough evaluation, diagnosis, and management.

Chapter 8 concentrates on procedures used to assess the cranial nerves when screening for neurological disorders. These techniques are rarely used for routine screening, but they are particularly helpful when a problem is suspected on the basis of the patient's case history or ocular examination findings. Many of these screening procedures should be performed as side trips from corresponding entrance tests.

Chapter 9 outlines commonly used ocular imaging techniques. Imaging technology has proven to be a useful tool in disease diagnosis, documentation, monitoring, and patient education. Many of these instruments are now key components of the ocular examination and should be employed when indicated based on patient symptoms and ocular examination findings. The use of imaging technology highlights the importance of the examiner's analytical abilities and critical thinking. Used intelligently and critically, imaging will enhance an examiner's capabilities.

Chapter 10 addresses advanced ocular procedures which are to be used on a problem-specific or as needed basis. These techniques are generally therapeutic for anterior segment maladies. Several of the procedures outlined in this chapter may require additional licensure and certification in order to perform them in the patient care setting and restrictions may be in place in certain states and jurisdictions. The examiner should consult with regional authorities to ensure the proper training and credentials are obtained before performing these procedures in patient care.

Throughout the text, the singular "they/them" is used as a generic third-person singular pronoun when referring to the patient during a procedure. This form is intentionally used for the purpose of simplicity as well as eliminating assumptions or implications regarding the gender of the patient referenced in the procedure.

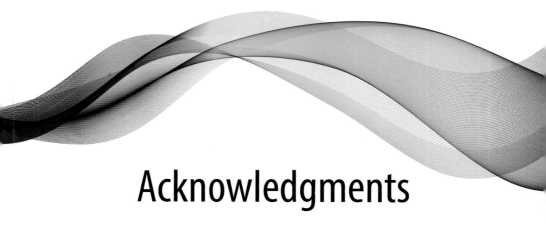

# Acknowledgments

First and foremost, we wish to thank the authors of the previous editions of this text, **Nancy Carlson, OD**, and **Daniel Kurtz, OD, PhD**. Their diligent work and revisions of the text have made *Clinical Procedures for Ocular Examination* a staple in optometric education both domestically and internationally. We thank them for all that they have contributed to the field of optometry and optometric education. We also appreciate and recognize the prior contributions of David Heath, OD, EdM, Catherine Hines, OD, Robert Capone, OD, Marion Hau, OD, and Ronald Watanabe, OD, to the prior editions of this text.

We wish to thank Amy Moy, OD, for her assistance with the sections on "Patient Privacy" and "Infection Control." We acknowledge Rudolf Mireles, PharmD, for help with prior preparation of the section on "Writing a Prescription for Medication." Thank you to Nicole Ross, OD, MS, for her help with "Trial Frame Refraction." We wish to thank Fuensanta Vera-Diaz, OD, PhD, for her help with preparation of "Ocular Biometry." Thank you to John J. Lee, MD, MPH, Vinny Keshav, MD, and Alexander Martin, OD, for their help developing "Chalazion Removal" and "Suturing, Excision, and Biopsy" and Jason Brenner, MD, for his help with "Anterior Segment Lasers." We wish to thank Aurora Denial, OD, for her mentorship.

"It takes a village" rings true, and we'd like to thank our New England College of Optometry colleagues who are part of our village. Thank you to our library staff, Heather Edmonds, MLIS, and Heather Pierce-Lopez for endless assistance, resources, and review. Finally, we wish to thank our students who have helped shape us as educators. It is our hope that you benefit from this text and never stop learning.

Thank you to those who sat for photos including, William Amuah, Nikita Aneja, OD, Purva Atreay, Niki BayatFard, Kristen Col, Lauren Butler, OD, Brittany Darnley, OD, Ricardo Delgado, Pip Dorling, Mia Gheduzzi, Raviv Katz, Anastasia Logotheti, Jim Mertz, OD, PhD, Emely MininoSoto, Greta Pucci, Twinkle Sehgal, Jessica Tarka, Marilyn Tran, Samuel White, and Darick Wright. Thank you, Jonathon Jimmerson, OD, and the Charles River Community Health Center for assistance with photos, as well as Timothy Bossie, OD, and the NECO Center for Eye Care for various graphics.

We would also like to acknowledge the sacrifices, support, and contributions of our families and mentors: Dylan and Anya Reilly, Scott, JoAnn and Sarah Williams, David and Sandy Young, Bruce Moore, OD, Stacy Lyons, OD, Caleb and Leon Gaiser. Dr. Gaiser would also like to dedicate her contributions to the text in loving memory to Susan Gaiser.

# 1

# Patient Communication

Jennifer Reilly, OD, MSc, FAAO

## 1.1 INTRODUCTION TO PATIENT COMMUNICATION

Communicating with patients and other healthcare providers is the most important aspect of patient care. Communication is a skill that can be learned and improved over time with practice. Good patient communication facilitates the examination process, improves the accuracy of diagnosis, improves patient compliance, decreases patient complaints and malpractice claims, and makes every patient encounter more enjoyable for the clinician as well as for the patient.

There are many opportunities to demonstrate good patient communication throughout the patient care process, and it starts when the patient first calls to schedule an appointment. All staff need to know that the patient is the most important person in the care process, and they must be treated with dignity and respect. Early demonstration of good communication skills is important and should be continued throughout the examination process until the patient leaves the office.

This chapter starts by highlighting the importance of patient privacy and how it should be respected throughout all patient care communications. Other communication opportunities presented in this chapter include acquiring the case history, presenting the findings to the patient at the end of the examination, presenting the case to colleagues or to an attending doctor, developing an assessment and plan, writing consultation and/or referral letters, reporting abuse, and writing a prescription for medication.

Case history is the most important procedure in the entire repertoire of examination procedures, and it is one of the most difficult to learn. History taking can be mastered only after the acquisition of a broad base of knowledge and after years of clinical experience. An experienced and knowledgeable clinician often can determine the diagnosis from the history alone. Conversely, the novice is frequently overwhelmed by the information gathered in the case history and is rarely able to effectively gather and use the relevant information in the diagnostic process. It is beyond the scope of this book to provide sufficient information for a novice clinician to conduct a proficient, comprehensive case history. Rather, the components of the case history are presented to illustrate the main parts of a history for a typical primary care examination and for a typical follow-up examination.

The case history is usually conducted at the beginning of the examination and is the time for the clinician and patient to become acquainted. The clinician must present themselves to the patient as a caring and empathetic individual if they expect the patient to be forthcoming about their problems and to comply with advice given. At the same time, the clinician begins the diagnostic thought process by asking the patient appropriate questions to determine the potential causes for each of the patient's symptoms. The information is then used in deciding which procedures the clinician will use to confirm or rule out each potential diagnosis. During the case history, the clinician also has an opportunity to begin educating the patient about their visual function and about their ocular and general health.

The case history for a typical primary care examination is divided into several parts: the Chief Complaint or History of the Present Illness (HPI), Past Medical and Ocular History including medications and allergies, Review of Systems, Family History, Social History, and the Summary. In the beginning of the history, the clinician asks open-ended questions to assess the patient's reason for seeking care (the chief complaint/history of the present illness) and to ascertain the visual needs of the patient's daily life. If the patient does not initially volunteer a complaint, it is wise to ask key, probing questions about their vision, visual function, and visual efficiency.

The Past Medical and Ocular History portion of the history consists of a series of questions to determine if the patient is at risk for any of a variety of ocular, systemic, or neurological disorders. The clinician asks about the patient's previous ocular history, medical history, and about their family's ocular and medical history. The clinician also gives the patient a list of symptoms of common eye problems to find out if the patient has ever experienced any of them. Some clinicians gather this information in a written questionnaire that the patient fills out prior to the examination. Although this is an efficient method of data collection, it must be followed by a conversation between the clinician and the patient to establish a doctor-patient relationship and to be certain that all relevant information was gathered.

Finally, the case history concludes with a brief recapitulation, or summary, of the patient's chief complaint or complaints, but this time in the clinician's words. This summary ensures for both the clinician and the patient that the clinician understands the patient's concerns and gives the patient an opportunity to add anything that may have been missed. It also gives the clinician an opportunity to start the process of patient education that will be concluded at the end of the examination.

The case history can be modified for a problem-focused examination for an established patient by omitting the information that has been gathered in the previous primary care examination and by asking only the questions that are relevant to the patient's reason for the visit. A problem-focused case history should include the patient's reason for the visit, questions about the symptoms that will help the clinician in the differential diagnosis process, and a summary of the patient's complaints in the clinician's words.

Another hallmark of good communication in healthcare is explaining to the patient what you are about to do before you do it. The examiner should develop a clear and concise explanation for each of the clinical procedures in the subsequent chapters of this text. Furthermore, many countries, states, or jurisdictions require that healthcare be provided in the preferred language of the patient. Be sure to consult with your regional guidelines when providing care.

After the examination is completed, the clinician must summarize the findings of the examination for the patient along with recommendations for appropriate care, referrals, and follow-up care. It is important to relate the examination findings back to the patient's reason for visit or chief complaint, as it helps the patient to see the value in the information extracted from the exam and to confirm that the patient understands everything about their diagnosis and treatment plan.

Documentation of all patient communication in the patient's record is essential. As the old adage goes, "if you didn't document it, you didn't do it." Examination documentation must be clear such that other providers participating in current or future care of the patient can easily understand the examination findings and treatment plan. Many electronic health record systems have special tabs or locations for patient communication documentation outside of the typical examination notes. These communication notes may include phone conversations, verbal encounters, or copies of letters sent to the patient or to other healthcare providers involved in that patient's care.

## 1.2 PATIENT PRIVACY

### Purpose
The aim of this procedure is to protect patient information and respect the patient's right to privacy. Failure to do so may result in unfavorable outcomes for the patient, and legal and financial consequences for the clinic site and providers involved.

*Note:* This outline reflects the rules and regulations as outlined by the Health Insurance Portability and Accountability Act of 1996 (HIPAA). This is a federal regulation; be sure to consult with regional and national guidelines when it comes to protecting patient information at your office. Regular and routine HIPAA training for providers and staff is an integral part of healthcare compliance and patient protection.

### Indications
Appropriate efforts to safeguard patient information should be made across all parts of patient workflows, including clinical encounters, communications, and orders. Protected health information (PHI) includes, but is not limited to, patient name, birthdate, medical record number, address, phone number, email or other contact information, social security number, credit card number, admission or discharge date (except the year), medical exam findings and diagnoses, insurance information, names of relatives, facial photos, biometric identifiers, and license or vehicle numbers to name a few. PHI can occur in verbal or spoken, written, or electronic form. Each of these forms is included and are to be protected under the regulations of HIPAA. Healthcare practices and practitioners must take the required privacy and security measures to protect against threats to PHI.

### Procedure
While there is no "step-by-step" procedure for protecting patient information, the following is a list of guidelines to ensure the protection of PHI.

*Minimum Necessary Rule*

The cardinal rule of HIPAA's Privacy Rule is the "Minimum Necessary Rule." This rule states that disclosing PHI must be limited only to the minimum necessary for the stated purpose. If it is not someone's role to know PHI, then the information should not be disclosed.

## Verbal Communications

- When patient information is spoken, such as in a case presentation (see Procedure 1.5), ensure that you are presenting in a private area and not in a communal space. Speak in a clear and reasonable volume.
- Identify and verify a caller before releasing any patient information. When disclosing patient information, make sure it is the minimum amount necessary.

## Written Communications

- Patient information is often kept on billing sheets and patient intake forms. Be sure that these documents are always kept out of the line of sight of other patients and in secure areas.
- Dispose of confidential information according to the proper procedure, such as a paper shredder or secure and locked shredder container.

## Electronic Communications

- Most patient information is kept electronically, therefore computers, tablets, and other electronic devices should be password protected and locked when not in use.
- Computer screens should face away from common areas so that private information cannot be viewed.
- Electronic health records should have individual account logins with usernames and passwords specific to that person. Passwords should never be shared.
- If patient information is being shared over fax or secure email, the receiving contact information should be verified before sending the transmission.
- Personal health information should never be posted on social media. This includes identifiable pictures of a patient or comments about a specific patient.

## General Office Practices

- Clinical offices should designate a privacy officer and a designated person to receive and manage privacy complaints.
- Breaches to confidentiality are serious and must be addressed promptly and decisively. Depending on the number of patients affected and whether a data breach has been discovered, the Department of Health and Human Services must be notified. Thus, the role of a designated privacy officer in the clinic is vital to the organization.
- A Notice of Privacy Practices must be developed, maintained, and distributed as appropriate.
- Office policies and procedures should be well documented and regular patient privacy training should take place for all of those participating in any aspect of patient care, even if not in "patient-facing" roles.
- Typical permissible reasons for disclosure of PHI include coordinating treatment, payment, or healthcare operations. All other reasons for disclosure require written consent from the patient. *Disclaimer:* always use caution when disclosing PHI. Ensure the proper safeguards are in place and only provide the minimum information necessary. Consult your clinic/hospital, regional, and federal laws and regulations when it comes to patient privacy and information disclosure.
- Patients must sign authorizations when requesting their PHI to be released to another entity. Through HIPAA, patients have the right to obtain a copy of their health records and request corrections of errors within 30 days.

## Notes

The guidelines listed above are some of the "best practices" to ensure patient privacy and are not meant to act as legal guidance. The list is not all encompassing, and therefore regional and federal rules and regulations should be carefully observed and obeyed when participating in any form of patient care. There are hefty fines for providers and clinics in violation of HIPAA regulations. It is important that all healthcare providers do their part to ensure patient privacy and security.

## 1.3 CASE HISTORY

### Purpose

The aim of this procedure is to establish a caring relationship with the patient, showing compassion, empathy, and respect for the patient. Also, to gather information about the patient's chief complaint, visual function, ocular and systemic health, risk factors, and lifestyle. Acquiring the case history allows the examiner to begin the process of developing their differential diagnosis, and to begin the process of patient education.

### Indications

A case history should be performed for all patient examination encounters.

### Setup

- Prior to starting the formal case history, the doctor should welcome the patient, show the patient where to put their coat and belongings during the examination, introduce themself to the patient, and exchange a few pleasantries with the patient (e.g., "How about the Patriots/Bruins/Celtics/Red Sox?" "What do you think about the weather we've been having?").
- Be sure that the patient is comfortable where they are seated and that the overhead light is not shining in the patient's eyes.
- The doctor should be seated at the same height as the patient, in a position that makes it easy to maintain eye contact with the patient and to facilitate conversation. When using electronic health records, a tablet may facilitate good communication and positioning, as shown in **Figure 1-1**.
- Although the case history is usually done at the beginning of the examination, data may be added to it as information is gathered during testing. Patients sometimes reveal more information as they become more comfortable with the doctor.

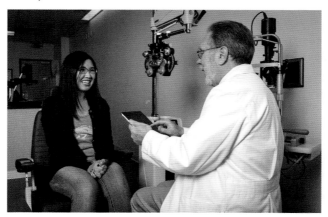

**FIGURE 1-1** | The examiner takes the case history and records it on a tablet, enhancing their ability to maintain eye contact with the patient.

## Case History Components for an Adult Primary Care Examination

*History of the Present Illness (HPI)*

The HPI includes the patient's chief complaint and elaboration of the chief complaint as outlined below.

1. **Chief Complaint (or Chief Concern)**

   a. Initiation: Ask the patient about the reason for their visit with an open-ended question such as:

   "What brought you in today?"

   "What problems are you having with your eyes?"

   "How can I help you today?"

   "What is the main reason for today's eye examination?"

   b. Elaboration of the chief complaint (FOLDARQ).

   For each complaint the patient presents, ask for additional information using any of the following qualifiers that will help you in your differential diagnosis of each complaint:

   **Frequency:** "How often does this occur? Have you had anything similar in the past or is this the first time?"

   **Onset:** "When did the problem begin?"

   **Location:** "Where is the problem located?" (e.g., OD [oculus dexter; right eye], OS [oculus sinister; left eye]? At distance, at near?)

   **Duration:** "How long do your symptoms last?"

   **Associated factors:** "What other symptoms do you experience with this problem? Does the symptom occur with your glasses or only when you do not wear them? Does this happen only when you wear your contact lenses or also when you are not wearing your contact lenses?"

   **Relief:** "What seems to make your symptoms go away?"

   **Quality:** "On a scale of 1 to 10, with 10 being the worst, how would you rate the severity of your symptoms?"

   c. Visual function and visual efficiency, if not already covered in the chief complaint.

   Ask, "Can you see clearly and comfortably both far away and up close for all your visual activities?"

   After hearing the patient's description of their complaint(s), summarize for them what you have heard.

*Past Medical History (including past eye history)*

1. **Patient's Ocular History (POHx)**

   a. Last eye examination

   "When was your last eye examination? By whom? What was the outcome of that examination?"

   b. Corrective lenses history

   If the patient wears glasses, ask:

   "How long have you been wearing glasses? Are they for distance, near, or both?" "Can you see clearly and comfortably with them? When were your glasses last changed?"

   If the patient does not currently wear glasses, ask:

   "Have you ever worn glasses? What were they for? When did you wear them?" "When and why did you stop wearing them?"

The examiner should also elicit any history of contact lens use:

"Do you wear or have you ever worn contact lenses?" (For further contact lens history, see Procedure 6.2)

c. Additional pertinent ocular history

"Have you ever had any medical issues with your eyes? Any surgery, injuries, or serious infections?"

"Have you ever worn an eye patch?"

"Have you ever been told that you have an eye turn or a lazy eye?"

"Have you ever used any medication for your eyes?"

"Have you ever been told that you have cataracts, glaucoma, or any other eye disease?"

2. **Symptoms of common eye problems, often referred to as the "pertinent negatives"**

"Have you experienced any of the following: flashes of light, floaters, halos around lights, double vision, frequent or severe headaches, transient vision loss, eye pain, redness, tearing, or a sandy, gritty feeling in your eyes?"

3. **Patient's Medical History (PMHx)**

"How is your general health?"

"When was your last physical examination? By whom?"

"Are you currently under the care of a physician for any health condition?"

"Have you ever been told that you have diabetes, high blood pressure, thyroid disease, heart disease, or any infectious disease?"

"Are you taking any medications? If yes, what medication, how long have you been taking the medication, what is it for, and what is the dosage?"

"Do you have any allergies? If yes, to what, what are your symptoms, and how are your allergies treated?"

4. **Review of Systems (ROS)**

The Review of Systems is a list of organ systems that can help the clinician determine the state of the patient's general health. The examiner should inquire if any symptoms corresponding to the organ system are experienced.  Included in this list are:

| Allergic/Immunological/Lymphatic | Genitourinary |
|---|---|
| Cardiovascular | Musculoskeletal |
| Constitutional | Neurological |
| Endocrine | Psychological |
| Head, eyes, ears, nose, and throat (HEENT) | Respiratory |
| Gastrointestinal | Skin/Integumentary |

Some literature suggests including the corresponding diagnoses in the ROS as well as the symptoms, but in this text, the medical diagnoses are reserved for the PMHx.

*Family Ocular History (FOHx)*

"Has anyone in your family had cataracts, glaucoma, or blindness? Has anyone had an eye turn or lazy eye? If yes, who, when, for how long, and what was the treatment?"

*Family Medical History (FMHx)*

"Has anyone in your family had diabetes, high blood pressure, thyroid disease, heart disease, or any infectious disease? If yes, who, when, for how long, and what was the treatment?"

*Social History*

"What kind of work do you do? Do you use a computer/cellphone/tablet often?"
Be sure to ask about device usage for patients of all ages since screen time is on the rise and may motivate you to perform a dryness assessment.
"What are your hobbies? What do you like to do in your spare time?"
Inquiring about other hobbies is important because a certain hobby may require a specific or different working distance and thus affect the glasses prescription that is considered.
"Do you drive?"
"Do you smoke? Drink alcohol? Use recreational or street drugs?"

*Summary*

"The reason for your visit today is *(restate the chief complaint)* and you have concerns about…?"
"What other concerns about your eyes, your general health, or your family's eyes or health would you like to tell me about?"
"What questions do you have for me at this point in the examination?"

| CASE HISTORY at a glance | |
|---|---|
| **Components** | **Techniques** |
| Introduction | Introduce yourself, make the patient comfortable |
| History of the Present Illness/ Chief Complaint (HPI/CC) | Establish reason for patient's visit and elaborate on their complaint(s) to fully understand them and to begin the process of differential diagnosis |
| Past Medical History (PMHx) and Review of Systems (ROS) | Ask about ocular history, general health, symptoms of common eye problems, medications, allergies, review systems to find out about the patient's health |
| Family History (FHx) | Ask about problems that run in the family (both ocular and systemic) to determine the patient's risk |
| Social History | Inquire about the patient's occupation and hobbies in order to learn more about their visual needs |
| Summary | Summarize in your own words why the patient is here and ask if the patient wants to add anything |

## Case History Components for a Problem-Focused Examination

*Establish the reason for the patient's visit*

Ask, "What is the reason for your visit today?" If you asked the patient to return (doctor-directed follow up), use a declarative statement about what you know is the reason for the patient's visit such as, "I see that you are here for a dilated exam."
Conclude by asking, "Are there any other problems you are having that I can take care of for you today?"

*Probe the patient's symptoms*

1. Use the questions from the History of the Present Illness, above, to elaborate on the patient's reason for this visit.
2. Ask the patient about their medical history, the medications they are currently taking, and any allergies they have, particularly to medications.

*Summary*

Summarize what the patient has told you by saying, "The reason for your visit today is *(restate the chief complaint)* and you have concerns about…?"

### Recording

- Record all collected information in the patient's record, including the pertinent negatives.

## 1.4 PRESENTING EXAMINATION RESULTS TO A PATIENT

### Purpose
The aim of this procedure is to provide a concise verbal summary to the patient of all pertinent information from the examination.

### Indications
Every patient should be given a summary of the results after every examination.

### Setup
- A copy of the patient record or other notes may be helpful references to have at hand. However, you should be sufficiently familiar with the examination findings that you need to consult the record only infrequently.

### Procedure
1. Begin by stating the diagnosis to the patient in language that they can understand. Always relate the diagnosis to the patient's chief complaint or reason for the visit.
2. Summarize the testing that was done to confirm the diagnosis and to rule out other diagnoses.
3. Describe the etiology, prognosis, and expected course of the problem.
4. Inform the patient of your recommended treatment and management of the diagnosis. When there is more than one option for management, inform the patient of the various options with your recommendation for the best option. Include the risks and benefits of each option.
5. If the plan involves a referral to another clinician, inform the patient whom you would like them to see and how urgent it is for the patient to see another practitioner. If the referral is urgent, make the appointment for the patient before they leave your office.
6. Inform the patient of your recommended follow-up interval for the next examination. Let the patient know what and when they should expect changes in their symptoms.
7. Give the patient written or electronic educational materials or resources describing their diagnosis and management when materials are available.
8. Conclude by saying to the patient, "What questions do you have for me?"

### Recording
- Presentations are given verbally to the patient. Details of the diagnoses, management plan, patient education given, referrals, and when you want to see the patient again should be recorded in the patient's record (see Procedure 1.6 for details on writing an assessment and plan).

## EXAMPLES

### Example #1
*Presentation to the Patient*

> **Background, not said to the patient:** Mr. XY is a 43-year-old accountant who presents for a comprehensive eye exam with a chief complaint of difficulty reading, especially at the end of the day or in dim light. He reports that things are easier to see if he holds them further away, but his arms have become too short. Mr. XY's general health is good and further personal and family histories are unremarkable. His dilated ocular exam was otherwise unremarkable.

Say to the patient, "Mr. XY, you have presbyopia, a problem that everyone experiences at some time between the ages of 38 and 45. Presbyopia is caused by the decrease in flexibility of the lens inside your eye that focuses for things close up and is a normal expected change with age. The lens has been losing flexibility since age 15 but catches up to most of us in our early 40s.

"Presbyopia can be corrected with reading glasses. Since you wear glasses all of the time, I recommend progressive addition lenses. These lenses allow you to see at all distances without having to change to a different pair of glasses. Bifocals and separate distance and near glasses are other options that you may consider.

"If you would like to consider contact lenses, I can discuss several contact lens options with you.

"As the lens inside your eye continues to lose flexibility up to age 60, presbyopia will progress over time whether or not it is corrected with glasses. You will notice that the glasses I prescribe for you today will not work as well in a few years as they do now.

"I am going to give you this pamphlet about presbyopia that will summarize the things that I have told you today. Otherwise, your eyes are healthy, and I see no sign of disease today.

"I would like to see you again in 1 year for another comprehensive exam. If you have any questions or problems before that, please call me.

What questions do you have for me?"

*Recording for Patient #1*
Assessment:

1. Presbyopia OU

2. Dilated ocular health unremarkable OU

Plan:

1. Rx PALs, prescription issued today.

   Patient education regarding presbyopia: normal age change that will continue to worsen over time but can be corrected with glasses or contact lenses. Gave patient AOA pamphlet on presbyopia.

   Told the patient to call with questions or concerns, otherwise monitor annually.

2. Patient educated on ocular health assessment today.

   Recommend comprehensive examination in 1 year.

## Example #2

*Presentation to the Patient*

> **Background, not said to the patient:** Ms. BC is a 19-year-old college sophomore who presents for a problem-specific eye exam. She has noticed intermittent vision loss inferiorly in her right eye for the past 3 days since she was hit in the head by a teammate's elbow during basketball practice. BC has also noticed little black specks floating in front of her right eye and occasional flashes of light. She has worn contact lenses since age 12 for moderate myopia and has had yearly examinations since age 10. Ms. BC takes no medications and has no allergies. Her general health is good and further personal or family history is unremarkable. Upon dilated fundus exam, she has a "macula-on" rhegmatogenous retinal detachment in the right eye. After checking the patient's health insurance for in-network options, you call the appropriate retina specialist and make an appointment for Ms. BC.

Say to the patient, "BC, you have a retinal detachment in your right eye. This is when the tissue that lines the inside of your eye has separated from the back of the eye. This most likely occurred when you were hit during basketball practice. Prompt treatment of a retinal detachment is necessary to prevent permanent vision loss. I would like you to see a retina specialist as soon as possible.

"I have called Dr. H and she can see you this afternoon. I made an appointment for you with Dr. H at 2:45 PM today and I will send a copy of your record to her from today. She will examine you and decide on the appropriate treatment for the detachment. Dr. H will let me know when she wants me to see you again.

What questions do you have for me?"

*Recording for Patient #2*
Assessment:

1. Macula-on rhegmatogenous retinal detachment superiorly OD, secondary to blunt trauma

Plan:

1. Refer to retina specialist Dr. H, for appointment today.

   Discussed the importance of prompt follow-up for best visual outcome with the patient.

   Called Dr. H and made appointment for patient for today at 2:45 PM.

   Sent copy of today's record to Dr. H. Gave patient a copy of record to give to Dr. H as well.

   Will call the patient when I have received a report from Dr. H and schedule appropriate follow-up here at that time.

## 1.5 VERBAL PRESENTATION OF YOUR PATIENT TO A COLLEAGUE, PRECEPTOR, OR ATTENDING SUPERVISOR

### Purpose

The aim of this procedure is to provide a concise verbal summary of all pertinent information about a patient to enable your preceptor or supervisor to arrive at an efficient understanding of the case in order to provide efficient, informed care of the patient without wasting their time. This procedure is similar to the procedure for writing a consultancy or referral letter (see Procedure 1.7).

### Indications

A verbal case presentation is indicated when it is necessary to provide a summary of a patient's examination findings to another professional who will become involved in the care of that patient.

### Setup

- A copy of the patient record or other notes may be helpful references to have at hand. However, you should be sufficiently familiar with the examination findings that you need to consult the record only infrequently.

### Procedure

1. Begin with an introduction of the patient, giving name, age, sex, race and/or ethnicity (only if pertinent to the case), and what type of examination you have done (e.g., comprehensive eye examination, problem-specific examination, follow-up examination, contact lens fitting or follow-up).

2. In one sentence, summarize the patient's presenting complaint or reason for seeking care at the present time. Follow this by giving pertinent details about the patient's description of the problem, including things they believe accompanied it.

3. This should be followed by a recitation of all examination data relevant to the patient's presenting complaint. Include the approximate date of the patient's last full eye examination. Avoid providing information that is not relevant to the patient's presenting complaint.

4. The next sentence should provide other information, including pertinent negatives that are relevant.

5. Conclude with a concise statement of your presumed diagnosis and your proposed initial treatment or management strategy. Include the problems that were part of your differential diagnosis that you have ruled out and how you have ruled them out. In this part of the presentation, always include a recall interval and specifically what you propose to assess at the patient's return visit.

| PRESENTING A CASE TO A COLLEAGUE OR ATTENDING at a glance | |
|---|---|
| **Components** | **Details** |
| Introduce patient | State name, age, sex, and type of examination |
| Chief complaint(s) | Give patient's description of their complaint(s) or reason for visit |
| Examination data | Summarize only the examination data relevant to your assessment or diagnosis of the patient's problem(s) |
| Differential diagnosis | Summarize the other possible diagnoses and the examination data that ruled out other possible diagnoses |
| Assessment and plan | Summarize your recommended treatment or management of the patient's problem<br>Give recommended time for the next visit and what should be done at the next visit |

## Recording
- Presentations are given verbally. While they are not recorded, everything that is reported should be part of the patient's official examination record.

## Examples
*Example #1*

1. **Introduce patient:** My patient is a 66-year-old male.

2. **Chief complaint:** He is here for a doctor directed follow up to perform repeat glaucoma testing due to elevated intraocular pressure (IOP) and moderate to large cupping, but is not yet on interventional therapy. He has no ocular or visual complaints.

3. **Examination data:** His best-corrected vision is 20/20 at distance in each eye with a moderate myopic correction. I found his IOP to be 27 in the right eye and 29 in the left eye with average central corneal thickness on pachymetry in both eyes. Cup to disc ratios are 0.50 horizontal and 0.60 vertical right eye and 0.60 horizontal by 0.65 vertical left eye. His anterior chamber angles are open to the ciliary body on gonioscopy with a lightly pigmented trabecular meshwork in both eyes. His automated visual field testing revealed a repeatable early inferior nasal step in the right eye corresponding to superior thinning on optical coherence tomography (OCT) and optic nerve head evaluation, and there was a repeatable early superior nasal step in the left eye corresponding to inferior thinning on OCT and optic nerve head evaluation. His last full eye examination was 2 weeks ago.

4. **Differential diagnosis and other pertinent information**: He is negative for trauma or pseudoexfoliation in either eye and negative for high blood pressure or diabetes. His last physical was 3 months ago and has no known drug allergies. His brother also has a history of glaucoma.

5. **Proposed assessment and plan:** I think he has early stage primary open-angle glaucoma in both eyes. I recommend that we begin treatment with latanoprost eyedrops 0.005% once daily at bedtime in both eyes. He should return in 6 weeks after he begins therapy to recheck his IOP and repeat automated visual field testing.

*Example #2*
1. **Introduce patient:** My patient is a 24-year-old female.

2. **Chief complaint**: She is here because she has noticed that her eyes feel dry after prolonged computer work for the past three weeks. She has no other ocular or visual complaints.

3. **Examination data:** Her best-corrected vision is 20/20 at distance in each eye with a low myopic correction. Her extraocular muscle movements, pupil response, confrontation fields, and ocular alignment are all unremarkable. On slit lamp examination, her eyes were white and quiet, but she did have trace inferior superficial punctate staining (SPK), a reduced tear breakup time of 4 seconds in each eye and a thin lacrimal lake. Her last full eye examination was about 8 months ago here at the health center. Aside from the small eyeglass prescription, no problems were found at that time.

4. **Differential diagnosis and other pertinent information**: She denies any discharge, redness, pain, or light sensitivity. She reports that her systemic health is good; she is not taking any medications other than birth control pills. She was last seen by a physician 7 months ago to renew her birth control prescription.

5. **Proposed assessment and plan:** I believe she has dry eye syndrome due to increased screen time. I have educated her on the "20-20-20 rule," visual hygiene, and instructed her to begin carboxymethylcellulose 0.5% artificial tears, one drop twice a day in both eyes. I plan to see her back in 2 to 4 weeks for a dry eye follow up.

*Notes*
- Best corrected or optimal visual acuity (BCVA) is relevant so often in eye care that you should include it even if you are not sure it is relevant. Unaided VA is rarely relevant but may be helpful if the particular case is addressing a new eyeglass prescription or a problem with the eyeglass prescription.
- Include the patient's medical history: systemic illness(es), medications, recent changes in activities only if relevant to the presentation.
- Include family ocular and medical history only if relevant.
- The key to a good presentation is to concisely report everything that is relevant, but to report nothing that is irrelevant so as not to obfuscate the purpose of the examination or to waste time.
- Knowing what is relevant and what is irrelevant to present is the difficult part, but that is the key to presenting a case effectively and concisely.

## 1.6 WRITING AN ASSESSMENT AND PLAN

**Purpose**
The aim of this procedure is to summarize the examination findings, clearly document any patient education provided, the intended treatment, and the follow up plan.

## Indications

Every patient examination should have a documented assessment and plan in the patient's record.

## Equipment

- A copy of the patient exam record in which the assessment and plan can be documented
- Other notes and images may be helpful references to have at hand

## Procedure

1. Identify all pertinent exam findings to be addressed in the assessment. The assessment must address the reason for the patient's visit (chief complaint) and then any other concerns expressed by the patient, or pertinent examination findings. The assessment should be a list of diagnoses.

   a. For a comprehensive eye examination, the assessment should include a comment on the patient's refractive error and ocular health even if unremarkable. Otherwise, normal findings are not addressed in the assessment and plan. *Note:* Some providers may include a comment on binocular vision function, and some may omit a comment on unremarkable findings.

   b. For a problem-focused examination, the reason for the visit should be addressed first, and then any other secondary concerns or positive findings of the examination.

2. Document each identified assessment in a clear and logical manner. Often, this is a numbered list.

3. The assessment should address the problems or findings identified as diagnoses and to the highest classification possible, e.g., "compound myopic astigmatism OU," "strabismic amblyopia OD," or "diabetes type II with moderate nonproliferative diabetic retinopathy without macular edema OU." *Note:* some healthcare settings may prefer more general diagnoses, e.g., "myopia and astigmatism OU," or "refractive error OU," so be sure to follow site preference.

   a. The assessment should include laterality (OD, OS, or OU), avoid uncommon abbreviations, and be linked to a diagnostic billing code.

   b. In general, recording additional exam findings in the assessment is discouraged, however, it may be appropriate depending upon the exam circumstances or particular clinical finding. For example, the assessment may further quantify or qualify the diagnosis with supportive details such as, "BCVA 20/40 OD" to quantify the reduced vision due to the causative etiology and if that is changed from previous.

4. Each assessment item must have a corresponding plan. This may be two consecutive numbered lists with each assessment number corresponding to the associated plan number, or an assessment item immediately and clearly followed by the associated plan.

5. Each plan item should include:

   a. Patient education provided. It should be clear if any education was provided to the patient, or a parent, guardian, or caregiver as necessary. Any printed or electronic educational materials provided should be referenced. Some providers choose to include the eyeglass prescription in the plan, while others do not.

   b. Any treatment or intervention recommended. Prescription directions should be specific.

   c. Planned correspondence such as a summary letter to a primary care provider (PCP), or specific labs and imaging ordered should be mentioned if relevant.

   d. Recommended follow up interval or referral.

## Recording

- The assessment and plan should be documented in the patient's official examination record.

## Examples

*Example #1*

**Case Background (included to provide context for the assessment and plan below):** A 53-year-old male, new patient presents for a comprehensive eye exam. Chief concern is blur with current bifocals at near OU. The patient has a history of refractive error corrected with bifocals and diabetes type II × 12 years managed with metformin. Personal and family history is unremarkable. His BCVA is 20/20 in each eye with the current distance portion of his glasses and a small update in the add power. Dilated ocular health revealed diabetic eye changes consistent with mild nonproliferative diabetic retinopathy without macular edema OU. All other examination findings were otherwise unremarkable.

Assessment:

1. Simple myopia, and presbyopia OU
2. Diabetes type II × 12 years with mild nonproliferative diabetic retinopathy without macular edema OU

   Last A1c: 7.7%, Last blood sugar: 146 this morning

Plan:

1. Patient educated on today's finding and small change in eyeglass prescription.

   Eyeglass prescription issued today: OD −3.00sph, OS: −3.25sph, Add +1.50.

   Monitor annually at comprehensive eye examination, sooner if changes in vision occur.
2. Patient educated on changes in the eye today associated with diabetes.

   Educated the patient on importance of good blood sugar control, regular visits with their PCP, and potential for other ocular manifestations and complications from diabetes.

   Letter with eye exam findings sent to PCP today.

   Patient directed to return to clinic in 1 year for a dilated eye exam and on the importance of this annual assessment.

*Example #2*

**Case Background (included to provide context for the assessment and plan below):** A 5-year-old female, new patient presents with dad for a comprehensive eye exam. Chief concern is failed vision screening with pediatrician and dad noticing the patient moving closer to see the television. The patient's general health is good, she has met all developmental milestones, and further personal and family history is unremarkable. Upon exam she has refractive error greater in the left eye, and corresponding reduced vision in that same eye. She has no eye turn. Her dilated ocular exam was otherwise unremarkable.

*Assessment and Plan:*

1. Compound hyperopic astigmatism OU

   → Plan: Patient and dad educated on findings and refractive error.

   New glasses prescription issued today with polycarbonate lenses for full time wear:

   OD +1.50 − 1.00 × 180, OS +3.00 −1.00 × 170.

   Monitor vision and refractive error in 3 months at vision check.

2. Refractive amblyopia OS secondary to anisometropic hyperopia

   BCVA: 20/20 OD and 20/40 OS

   → Plan: Patient and dad educated on findings, facts about amblyopia and visual development.

      Educated on the importance of full-time wear of glasses prescription provided today and follow up assessment. Summary letter sent to pediatrician today.

      Instructed to return to clinic in 3 months for a vision check with the new glasses.

3. Dilated ocular health unremarkable OU

   → Plan: Patient and dad educated on good ocular health. Monitor at annual comprehensive eye exam.

   *Note:* For an example of a problem specific assessment and plan, see Procedure 1.4, Example #2.

## 1.7 WRITING A CONSULTANCY, COMMUNICATION, OR REFERRAL LETTER

### Purpose
The aim of this procedure is to provide a written summary of all pertinent information about a patient to enable another practitioner to provide efficient, informed consultation and/or care of the patient without wasting the time of the recipient of the letter.

### Indications
When it is necessary to provide a written summary of a patient's examination findings to another professional who will become involved in the care of the patient or is already involved in the care of the patient.

### Equipment
- Computer
  - Some electronic health record systems allow for referrals to be submitted electronically, or as "messages." The same pertinent information to be included and general principles apply as outlined below.
- Stationery with the letterhead of the referring practice or clinic if sending by mail or fax

### Setup
- A copy of the patient record or other notes may be helpful references to have at hand.

### Procedure
1. Notify the patient that you will be communicating with another provider regarding their care and the purpose of the communication, e.g., referral or communication of ocular examination findings.
2. Begin with standard business-letter format and salutations (e.g., date of the letter, address of the recipient of the letter).
3. Begin the body of the letter with a standard business salutation, such as "Dear Dr. Xyz").
4. List the patient's name, date of birth, chief complaint and/or reason for referral, and date of appointment with the consultant if available.
5. This should be followed by a narrative, such as "(Ms., Mr., Mx., or Mrs.) (patient's full name), a (age)-year-old (male, female, non-binary patient), presented to (my office, the

ABC Health Clinic, etc.) on (date) with a main complaint of (concise statement of the patient's chief complaint for which the consultation is being requested)."

6. The next sentence should then state the purpose of the consultation or referral, "We are referring him/her/them to you to *state the purpose of the referral* (e.g., for consultation concerning his... to rule out..., for treatment of..., for further diagnostic workup..., for further evaluation of...," and so on). Be specific, be concise, identify specific diagnoses about which you are concerned, and state specific tests you wish to have performed (e.g., "for B-scan ocular ultrasound").

7. If the patient already has an appointment to see the consulting doctor, the next sentence should say, "Mx. has an appointment to see you at (indicate the time and date)."

8. Highlight the patient's chief complaint by supplying the following data:
   a. Time of onset (e.g., it began 2 days ago in the evening)
   b. Duration (e.g., it has lasted 2 days)
   c. Description of time-course (e.g., comes and goes, getting steadily worse, etc.)
   d. Accompanying symptoms or signs observed by patient or by you (e.g., quality of the discharge, pain)

9. Provide additional relevant information, including relevant negatives, from the examination and case history, such as:
   a. BCVA. This is relevant so often in eye care that you should include it even if you are not sure it is relevant. If referring to another eye-care provider, include your best refraction along with the VA. Omit the refractive prescription if referring to someone who is not an eye-care specialist. Note: Unaided VA is rarely relevant.
   b. Information obtained from external observation, slit lamp, etc.
   c. Patient's medical history: systemic illness(es), medications, recent changes in activities: only if relevant to the presentation (e.g., you may include that the patient has seasonal allergies if exam findings are positive for allergic conjunctivitis).
   d. Family ocular and medical history only if relevant.

10. Finish with an expression of your appreciation for the consultant's willingness to participate in the care of your patient and request feedback about the results of the further testing or treatment.

11. Sign your name to the letter along with your credentials and preferred contact information. This may be done electronically.

## Recording
• Retain a copy of the letter in the patient's clinic record or file.

## Examples
*Example #1*
**See Figure 1-2.**
*Example #2*
**See Figure 1-3.**

## Notes
• Do include other pertinent information and relevant negatives.
• Do not include information that is irrelevant to this presentation.
• Some practices prefer to receive copies of fax versions of your letter and/or actual patient record or notes. If you are sending copies of your notes, mention this in the

---

*Your Clinic Letterhead, MM Health Center*

September 6, 2022

NR, MD
XXX YYY City Hospital
Street address
City, state, zip code

Re: Ophthalmology referral for cataract evaluation

Patient name: Ms. SS

DOB: April 15th, 1955

Dear Dr. R,

Ms. SS had a comprehensive eye exam today, here at the MM Health Center.

Her best corrected acuity in each eye was 20/30 OD with -1.00sph and 20/60 OS with -1.50-0.50x090. The reduced vision is due to nuclear sclerotic cataract of both eyes and therefore the glasses prescription was deferred today. The patient reports glare at night and difficulty watching TV and is interested in cataract surgery. Pupil function, extraocular muscles, and eye alignment were unremarkable. Anterior ocular health revealed dry eye for which treatment was continued. Intraocular pressures were 16mmHg in each eye. Dilated ocular health was evaluated, revealing nuclear sclerotic cataracts OS>OD, and was otherwise unremarkable OU.

The patient is being referred to your clinic for cataract extraction evaluation OS. Please send completed exam notes to the fax number or address below.

I plan on seeing our patient again in 2-4 weeks for a dry eye follow up. Thank you for taking the time to see this patient.

Please do not hesitate to contact me if you have any further questions.

Sincerely,

Jennifer Reilly, OD, MSc, FAAO

MM Health Center
Street address
City, state, zip code
Tel: 555-555-2020 | Fax: 555-555-2030

---

**FIGURE 1-2** | An example of a referral or consultancy letter.

referral letter. Many clinics now have an electronic means for communication and referrals. Some allow the provider to send an electronic document, while others offer a messaging system. In either case, it is important that the provider ensures that all relevant details of the case are communicated to another provider who may be participating in the patient's care, provided you can confidently comply with HIPAA (see Procedure 1.2).

- The key to a good referral letter is to concisely report everything that is relevant, so the consultant acquires a quick and in-depth understanding of the patient's problem, but to report nothing that is irrelevant so as not to obfuscate the purpose of the referral or to waste the consultant's time trying to find the important information in the midst of irrelevancies.

---

*Your Clinic Letterhead, CC Eye Clinic*

September 5, 2021

MH, MD
XXX YYY Hospital
Street Address
City, state, zip code

Re: Diabetic eye exam findings
Patient name: Mx. BC
DOB: February 26, 1963

Dear Dr. H,

Our mutual patient, Mx. BC, presented to my office at the CC Eye Clinic on September 5, 2021, for their diabetic eye exam.

    The glasses prescription was updated, and the patient is correctable to 20/20 in each eye. Pupil function, extraocular muscles, and eye alignment were unremarkable. Anterior ocular health was also unremarkable. Intraocular pressures were 13mmHg in each eye. Dilated ocular health was evaluated, revealing mild nonproliferative diabetic retinopathy without macular edema in both eyes.

    The patient understands that it is important to return to the eye clinic once a year in order to check if the eyes need treatment for problems related to high blood sugar. They understand that vision problems may be prevented with control of the blood sugar levels.

    I plan on seeing our patient again in 1 year for a dilated eye exam. Please do not hesitate to contact me if you have any further questions.

Sincerely,

Benjamin Young, OD, FAAO

CC Eye Clinic
Street address
City, state, zip code
Tel: 555-555-2040 | Fax: 555-555-2050

---

**FIGURE 1-3** | An example of a professional communication regarding eye examination findings.

- Knowing what is relevant and what is irrelevant is the difficult part, but that is the key to writing an effective and concise referral letter.

## 1.8 REPORTING ABUSE

### Purpose
The aim of this procedure is to protect patients from harm inflicted by others which may be in the form of abuse or neglect.

### Indications
In the United States, laws mandate the reporting of abuse or neglect of vulnerable populations such as children and the elderly. In general, it is required to report even the suspicion of abuse. The optometrist has to be knowledgeable of local and state laws to determine for whom and under what circumstances they are a mandated reporter.

## Equipment

- The specific forms used to report abuse are usually mandated by the relevant jurisdiction. The practitioner should have a supply of such forms readily available in the office or an online account to submit these forms electronically. These forms vary from state to state, e.g., in Massachusetts the form is a 51A.

## Setup

The practitioner is expected to have knowledge of:
- The signs and symptoms of abuse
- The appropriate phone number for their jurisdiction/district
- Access to forms to file the report

## Procedure *(Massachusetts)*

1. Have available all necessary reporting information: the patient's full name, date of birth, address, phone number, as well as the type of abuse you suspect and what you observed in the patient to make you suspicious.
2. Call the relevant hotline for the patient and jurisdiction. In Massachusetts this must be done within 24 hours.
3. Answer all questions and only state the facts of what was observed or witnessed.
4. Obtain and record the name of the person to whom you gave the verbal report.
5. Within 48 hours, a written or electronically documented version of the verbal report must be filed and submitted to the appropriate party or authority.

## Recording

- Your examination record should include all the relevant findings that made you suspect abuse.
- A copy of the actual report does not go into the patient's clinical record, but must be kept in a separate, confidential file.

## Example

- Speaking to the Abuse Hotline in your jurisdiction: "My patient is a 9-year-old male. He came for an eye examination this afternoon at 1 o'clock. He was accompanied by his father. He presented with a round lesion on his left upper eyelid. It was about the diameter of a cigarette. I did not observe other signs of trauma to his face or eyes, but the child was very reticent. I could not figure a way to talk to him separated from his father."

## Notes

- In general, the goal of reporting is to prevent further harm to the patient and to minimize additional risk to the patient.
- Whether or not and how you inform the patient and family members that you have filed a report depends on the circumstances. Above all else, do no harm.

# 1.9 WRITING A PRESCRIPTION FOR MEDICATION

## Purpose

The aim of this procedure is to write a medication prescription that will be recognized, understood, honored, and filled by any licensed pharmacist.

## Indications

When it is necessary to provide a written prescription for medication directly to a patient or through electronic prescribing; usually to prescribe a therapeutic pharmaceutical.

### Equipment
- Prescription form, pad, or computer with electronic prescribing (e-prescribing) abilities
- It is preferred for the prescription to contain the following information, printed at the top:
  - Your name as well as the practice name, if applicable
  - Your license to practice number
  - Your DEA number
  - Your NPI number (optional)
  - Practice address
  - Practice telephone number

If this information is not printed on the prescription form, you must enter it somewhere, such as near your signature. Electronic health record systems or computers with e-prescribing abilities can auto-populate this information.

### Setup
- You must have prescribing authority in your state or jurisdiction for the medication prescribed.
- A copy of the patient's record or other notes may be helpful references to have at hand.

### Procedure
These are the essential elements of the prescription. None may be omitted.
1. Enter the patient's full name.
2. Enter information about the drug being prescribed:
   a. The drug name
   b. The strength in which it is to be dispensed
   c. The form in which the drug is to be dispensed (e.g., solution, ointment, suspension)
   d. The quantity of the drug to be dispensed each time the prescription is filled (e.g., 25 tablets, 5 mL)
3. Enter the directions for use of the drug, including:
   a. The eye or eyes into which the drug will be administered, if relevant
   b. Route of administration (e.g., into the lower cul-de-sac, oral)
   c. Frequency of administration
   d. Duration of the prescribed regimen, usually given in number of days
   e. Dose per administration (e.g., one drop, two drops)
   f. Number of times the prescription may be refilled
4. Enter the date on which the prescription was written.
5. Indicate "do not substitute" or "substitution permitted."
6. Sign with your legible signature.
7. The following elements are optional but frequently included in a prescription:
   a. The patient's address and/or date of birth or age for the purpose of ensuring the identity of the patient
   b. Expiration date or a date after which the prescription is no longer to be honored

### Commonly Used Pharmaceutical Abbreviations
Note: If you are unsure or uncomfortable using an abbreviation, it is always permissible to write out the information longhand.
**See Table 1-1.**

**TABLE 1-1. Common Pharmaceutical Abbreviations**

| Dosage Forms | Ophthalmic usages | Special instructions |
|---|---|---|
| • cap = capsule<br>• cr = cream<br>• gtt(s) = drop(s)<br>• soln = solution<br>• susp = suspension<br>• tab = tablet<br>• ung = ointment | • OD = right eye<br>• OS = left eye<br>• OU = both eyes | • ac = before meals<br>• pc = after meals<br>• atc = around the clock<br>• prn = as needed<br>• ud = as directed |
| **Quantities/units of measure** | **Route of administration** | **Frequency of administration** |
| • mL/cc = milliliter<br>• puff = metered dose inhalation<br>• ss = one-half<br>• T = one<br>• TT = two<br>• TTT = three<br>• tsp = teaspoonful<br>• tbsp = tablespoonful | • Inh = inhalation<br>• IM = intramuscularly<br>• IV = intravenously<br>• PO = orally/by mouth<br>• PR = rectally/per rectum<br>• SL = sublingually<br>• SQ = subc, subq, or<br>• SC = subcutaneously | • qd = daily<br>• bid = twice a day<br>• tid = three times a day<br>• qid = four times a day<br>• qod = every other day<br>• qhs = every night at bedtime<br>• q _ h/hr(s) = every_hour(s) |

## Common Errors to Avoid

- Using illegible writing
- Omitting the form in which the drug is to be dispensed
- Providing unclear directions
- Omitting your full identifying information
- Omitting your signature
- Omitting the date on which the prescription was written
- Failing to use a secure prescription blank
- Failing to match the signature with the name at the top of the Rx

## Recording

- Retain a copy of the prescription in the patient's clinic record or file.

## Example
**See Figure 1-4.**

**ABC Eye Clinic**
930 Commonwealth Ave
Boston, MA 02215                                          (617)262-2020

PATIENT NAME:   Jen Test            DOB:       01/01/2001
ADDRESS:        999 Test Ave        Expires:   03/10/2022
                Boston, MA 99999    Print Date: 03/07/2022

℞    Maxitrol 3.5mg/ml-10,000 Unit/ml-0.1 %

      SIG: Instill 1 drop in right eye four times daily
      for ten days

      ROUTE: OPHTHALMIC
      FORM: Suspension-Opht
      QTY: 3 (three) Milliliters
      DISP:  5 mL dropper bottle

☑ Generic Substitute Allowed    If condition does not improve in 3-5 days or worsens -
☐ Do NOT Substitute             contact provider

Refills:  0

                      Prescriber:    Benjamin Young, OD

LIC#:   99X9                                    DEA#: XX9999999

**FIGURE 1-4** | An example of an electronic or printed prescription for a medication.

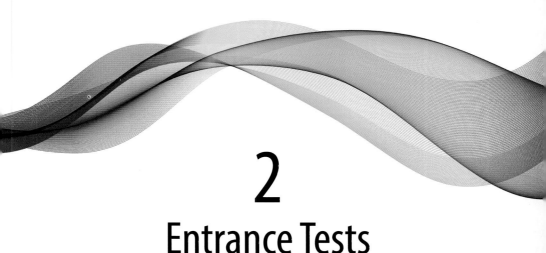

# 2
# Entrance Tests

Hilary Gaiser, OD, MSc / Jennifer Reilly, OD, MSc, FAAO / Benjamin Young, OD, FAAO

## 2.1 INTRODUCTION TO THE ENTRANCE TESTS

The entrance tests are the first procedures performed following the case history. The intentional selection of the procedures to be included in this sequence and the ongoing interpretation of the data gathered can make the difference in whether or not an efficient and accurate differential diagnosis is obtained at this point in the examination.

With the increasing pressures of healthcare economics, providers are adapting examination strategies that are primarily directed by symptomatology or positive test findings to maximize the efficiency of care and minimize the costs of delivery. The resulting decrease in the overall number of examination procedures performed on any given patient increases the importance of entrance test selection and their role of screening for visual disorders.

The entrance test sequence is usually composed of 6 to 12 procedures that have a low cost/benefit ratio, can be performed quickly, and do not depend on technologically sophisticated equipment. Typically, these tests have been used to elicit information that helps define the status of each of the primary problem areas: health, refraction, and functional vision. Frequently, entrance tests apply across categories and screen for problems in more than one area (**Table 2-1**).

| TABLE 2-1. Matrix Indicating the Primary and Secondary Areas of Diagnostic Significance for Each of the Entrance Tests | | | |
|---|---|---|---|
| | **Area of Diagnostic Significance** | | |
| **Entrance Tests** | **Refraction** | **Functional** | **Health** |
| Externals | | + | * |
| Visual acuity | * | + | * |
| Pinhole visual acuity` | * | + | * |
| Color vision | | + | * |
| Cover test | + | * | + |
| Stereopsis | + | * | |
| Near point of convergence | | * | |
| Hirschberg test | | * | + |
| Brückner test | | * | + |
| Extraocular muscle testing | | + | * |
| Pupils | | | * |
| Finger counting fields | | | * |

*, primary; +, secondary.

The entrance tests, considered a part of the minimum defined database, provide valuable information by screening for the presence of ocular anomalies in the absence of patient symptoms. Examples include neurological deficits as revealed by pupillary testing and visual field screenings, convergence insufficiency identified by near point of convergence (NPC) testing, or a muscle imbalance as noted by cover test. The information obtained from this testing also provides baseline diagnostic information for future comparison.

It is critical to emphasize that there is no one right set of entrance tests. Ask a number of eye care providers what they include in this sequence and you are likely to get a variety of answers. In fact, it is reasonable, and probably desirable, to expect that a given provider will have two or three lists that are age referenced. A test such as stereopsis serves a valuable role among children but may provide less useful information for the elderly. For the elderly, it may be far more useful to include an Amsler grid test to evaluate macular function as a part of the preliminary exam. The selection of tests for inclusion in the entrance tests must be based on a careful consideration of the cost of performing the test in terms of practitioner time and the return in terms of the utility of the information.

This chapter includes 15 procedures in addition to the introduction and summary. Three variations of visual acuity (VA) are included: the standard Snellen test, which is used in most primary care examinations; the logMAR VA, a method used widely in low vision and in clinical research; and the Massachusetts VA Test (Mass VAT), used for VA measurement or vision screenings in young children. Pinhole acuity is measured only in the event of decreased

VA. The Brückner test is included as an adjunct to the Hirschberg test and can be invaluable in screening infants and young children for strabismus, anisometropia, or media opacities.

There are tests included in other chapters that could be considered for inclusion as entrance tests. One of these, blood pressure measurement, is included as an entrance test with increasing frequency as optometrists assume responsibility for the detection of systemic diseases with related ocular manifestations. Other procedures to consider include the Amsler grid test, accommodative amplitude and facility testing, associated phoria, and the dominance sighting test.

Once the decision is made about what test to include for an individual patient, thought must be given to the arrangement of the tests to enhance efficiency. Factors that affect the sequencing include the equipment needed (many of the entrance tests use common equipment) and whether the test is done with or without the patient's correction. The flowchart in **Figure 2-1** illustrates an example sequence of entrance tests for a primary care examination on an adult patient.

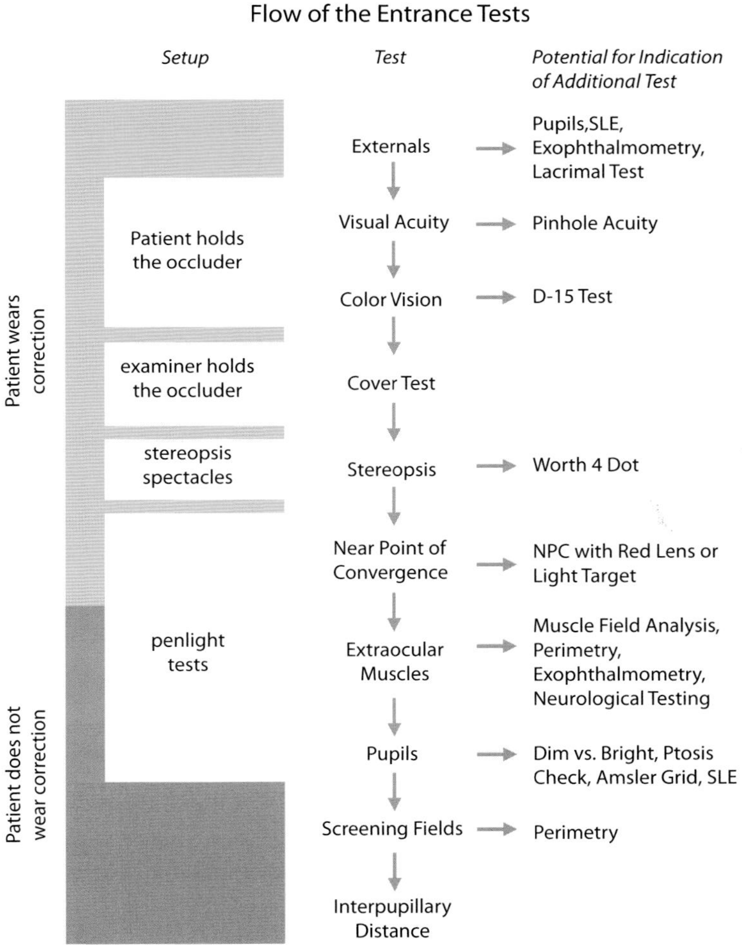

## Flow of the Entrance Tests

| Setup | Test | Potential for Indication of Additional Test |
|---|---|---|
| | Externals → | Pupils, SLE, Exophthalmometry, Lacrimal Test |
| Patient holds the occluder | Visual Acuity → | Pinhole Acuity |
| | Color Vision → | D-15 Test |
| examiner holds the occluder | Cover Test | |
| stereopsis spectacles | Stereopsis → | Worth 4 Dot |
| | Near Point of Convergence → | NPC with Red Lens or Light Target |
| penlight tests | Extraocular Muscles → | Muscle Field Analysis, Perimetry, Exophthalmometry, Neurological Testing |
| | Pupils → | Dim vs. Bright, Ptosis Check, Amsler Grid, SLE |
| | Screening Fields → | Perimetry |
| | Interpupillary Distance | |

*Patient wears correction* / *Patient does not wear correction*

**FIGURE 2-1** | Flowchart for the entrance tests. The main route or standard sequence of tests is shown in the center. Recommended side trips or secondary tests are represented to the right. Tests are grouped according to the need for correction and equipment on the left.

## 2.2 INFECTION CONTROL

### Purpose

Proper infection control practices are essential to preventing the transmission of infection and maintaining the health and safety of patients and healthcare personnel. In the eye care setting, it is important to be aware of communicable systemic diseases and infections of the eye in order to protect patients and healthcare providers. Please follow your local, regional, and national guidelines regarding infection control practices to ensure a safe environment for patient care. The recommended infection control practices listed below are adopted from the state of Massachusetts Department of Public Health and the Centers for Disease Control and Prevention (CDC).

### Indications

The CDC has defined several universal infection control measures called the *Standard Precautions*. Standard Precautions should be observed in all healthcare settings and for all patient encounters. The CDC has also outlined Transmission-Based Precautions which are applied in addition to Standard Precautions when a particular infectious agent is suspected to be present. These additional infection control measures are specific to the method of transmission of the suspected infectious agent. Examples of Transmission-Based Precautions include additional personal protective equipment (PPE), placement and isolation of patients, and additional measures of cleaning, disinfection, and sterilization beyond the routine methods outlined in the Standard Precautions below.

### Equipment

- Sink, hand soap, and alcohol-based hand sanitizer
- Disposable paper towels
- Isopropyl alcohol pads, swabs, or wipes
- Multi-purpose solution and hydrogen peroxide cleaning system for contact lenses
- Sterile saline solution
- Environmental Protection Agency (EPA) disinfectant wipes
- Latex-free examination gloves
- Protective eyewear
- Surgical masks or other medical grade masks
- Puncture resistant sharps container(s)
- Hazardous waste disposal bags and container
- Unit for sterilization (e.g., autoclave)

### Standard Precautions

1. *Hand hygiene:*

   a. Hands must be cleaned with soap and water or disinfected with hand sanitizer before and after patient contact. This is often considered the most important step in all of infection control.

   b. When using soap and water, hands should be vigorously rubbed together under running water for a minimum of 20 seconds. Hands should be thoroughly dried with disposable paper towels.

   c. Soap and water is the preferred method for hand hygiene when hands are visibly dirty, before eating, after using the restroom, or when handling contact lenses.

2. *Use of PPE:*

   a. PPE should be worn when healthcare personnel may come into contact with an infectious agent. All blood and bodily fluid should be treated as if they are infectious. Healthcare personnel should appropriately cover or bandage any broken skin.

   b. Examples of PPE include wearing a surgical mask, gloves, or eye protection. The specific PPE required for a patient encounter is often dictated by the method of transmission of the suspected pathogen, or by the potential for exposure, e.g., wearing eye protection if a bodily fluid splash is possible.

   c. Hand hygiene should be performed before donning (putting on) and after doffing (removing) PPE. PPE should be disposed of in a biohazard bin if suspected contact with an infectious agent, otherwise into a trash receptacle.

   d. PPE must be worn properly to be effective. Please consult CDC guidelines for recommended PPE in specific situations and for specific diseases.

3. *Respiratory hygiene:*

   a. Respiratory hygiene aims at preventing the spread of infection through the respiratory system including the nose and mouth.

   b. One measure of respiratory hygiene is cough etiquette which includes sneezing and/or coughing into your elbow, then performing hand hygiene (see #1 above).

   c. Respiratory hygiene may also include donning appropriate PPE such as a surgical mask or other medical grade mask to prevent disease transmission from one person to another.

4. *Sharps safety:*

   a. Sharps safety includes proper handling and disposal of sharp instruments including jeweler's forceps or needles. Sharps must be sterile to use in patient care.

   b. Sharps should always be disposed of or stored in a puncture resistant container immediately after use.

   c. If a needle must be recapped, the "single hand scoop" technique should be used where the provider uses one hand to scoop up the cap of the needle with the needle itself and using the same hand to secure the cap.

5. *Safe injection technique:*

   a. This technique applies the sharps safety measures listed above while also observing sterile or aseptic technique when performing an injection on a patient. The practitioner must don appropriate PPE.

   b. Injections should always be performed in a clean area with new sterile materials.

   c. Needles used for injection must be placed in a puncture resistant biohazard container immediately after use.

   *Note:* Injections often require additional certification or licensure for the eye care provider.

6. *Cleaning, disinfection, and sterilization of shared patient equipment:*

   a. Shared patient equipment is broken down into three categories: critical, semi-critical, and noncritical. Critical instrumentation penetrates soft tissue or bone, such as a scalpel, and must be sterilized after each use. Semi-critical instrumentation touches mucous membranes, such as a tonometer tip, and must be disinfected after each use. Non-critical instrumentation touches intact skin, such as an occluder or chin rest, and must be cleaned or disinfected after each use.

    b. Critical equipment should be soaked in the proper detergent, solution, or enzymatic cleaner immediately after use and prepared for sterilization. After sterilization, the instrumentation should be stored in sterile packaging for reuse.

    c. Semi-critical instrumentation should be cleaned according to manufacturer guidelines. This may include a dilute bleach solution or hydrogen peroxide soak followed by a rinse. If the equipment touches the ocular surface, it is imperative that any disinfecting solution is thoroughly rinsed before use to prevent chemical burns or ocular surface irritation.

    d. Noncritical instrumentation involved in patient contact, such as a phoropter, slip lamp, or fundus camera, must also be disinfected or cleaned before and after use at all patient contact points. Please refer manufacturer cleaning and disinfection recommendations for each piece of your particular equipment and instrumentation. Most touch points and high touch surfaces can be cleaned with 70% isopropyl alcohol or an EPA-registered disinfectant. Ensure to allow time for drying before use.

7. *Environmental cleaning:*

    a. The exam room and testing environment should be subject to routine cleaning including cleaning floors and surfaces.

    b. Disinfection of the space may be required if there is the potential for infectious material to remain in the exam room or area. It is important to clean high touch surfaces such as counters, chairs, keyboards, and light switches on a routine basis.

## Notes

- Failure to follow infection control guidelines can leave patients and healthcare providers at risk for acquiring or transmitting an infection.
- Infection control training should be routine in all healthcare settings and repeated at appropriate intervals.
- As always, using evidence-based procedures and protocols is paramount in healthcare and should apply to all patient encounters.
- Apply the aforementioned Standard Precautions and appropriate infection control protocols when performing all of the following procedures included within this text.

## 2.3 EXTERNAL OBSERVATION

### Purpose

The aim of this procedure is to identify gross abnormalities of the eye and adnexa.

### Equipment and Setup

- A penlight or transilluminator may facilitate observations, but no specific equipment is needed.
- There is no specific setup.

### Procedure

1. Observe the patient as they walk into the exam room and sit down in the exam chair. Specifically take note of:

    a. The patient's posture, including head tilts, gait, and carriage.

2. Look for anything odd or unusual about the patient and any asymmetries between one side of the body and the other, paying particular attention to the face and eyes, specifically:

    a. The patient's head, face, and accessory ocular structures.

    b. The patient's eyes: their placement in their head, the conjunctiva, cornea, iris, and lens.

3. Compare the patient's features to your knowledge of an expected normal appearance.

### Recording
- If in your professional judgment, the patient is normal in areas observed, record "no gross abnormalities or asymmetries."
- Record any pertinent negatives that may be relevant to the patient and their differential diagnosis:
  - E.g., (-)facial asymmetries, (-)skin lesions, (-)ptosis
- Describe any abnormalities or asymmetries you observe.

### Examples
- External observation (Ext): no gross abnormalities or asymmetries
- Ext: bilateral and symmetrical erythematous rash on right and left upper cheek
- Ext: Right-sided facial droop
- Ext: 1-cm globe displacement inferior OD

### Notes
- Some acceptable recording variations include "WNL" and "Normal," but specificity is encouraged for more thorough documentation.

## 2.4 VISUAL ACUITY: MINIMUM LEGIBLE

### Purpose
The aim of this procedure is to measure the clarity of vision or the ability of the visual system to resolve detail. A patient's VA depends on the accuracy of the retinal focus, the integrity of the eye's neural elements, and the interpretive faculty of the brain.

### Indications
VA should be done on all patients as the first procedure following the case history with very few exceptions. *Note:* It is important to understand that there are a number of ways by which a patient's visual function may be measured. The procedure described below, although the most common clinically, may not be applicable in certain circumstances (e.g., infants, low-vision patients, and illiterate patients).

### Equipment
- Computer-generated acuity chart, projector with VA slide, or wall-mounted acuity chart. Computer-generated charts allow the examiner to vary the letters, reducing the possibility of the patient memorizing lines of letters.
- Near point VA card
- Occluder
- Lamp
- Computer-generated or projector charts should be calibrated for the distance from the patient to the chart. In a 20-ft room, in order to subtend an angle of 5 minutes of arc, the 20/20 letter should have a height of 8.87 mm

### Setup
- The patient wears their habitual correction for the distance being tested. When the examiner wants to measure the patient's VA both with (cc) and without (sc) correction, the acuity should be measured without correction first to reduce the likelihood of memorization on charts that cannot randomize letters.
- The patient holds the occluder.
- An acuity chart, with lines from 20/50 to 20/15 exposed, is shown to the patient.

- Room illumination should maximize contrast on the VA chart used. (Higher illumination is needed for printed charts and dimmer illumination is needed for projected or computerized charts.)

## Procedure

1. Always observe the patient, not the chart. You can quickly glance at the chart to ensure that the patient is identifying the letter correctly but should be looking at the patient for the majority of the test.

2. Instruct the patient to cover their left eye and not to squint.

3. Instruct the patient to read the smallest line of letters that they can. If using a computer-generated chart or an acuity slide in a projected chart and the patient is unable to read 20/50, reposition the chart so the 20/60 line becomes the lowest line. Single lines of letters or single letters should only be used in special cases.

4. Encourage the patient to read the letters on the next smaller line, even if they have to guess. Stop the patient when more than half the letters on a line have been missed.

5. Have the patient cover their right eye and repeat steps 3 and 4.

6. Instruct the patient to uncover their right eye and repeat steps 3 and 4 with both eyes unoccluded. If the patient was able to read the largest letter with each eye and both eyes open, proceed to step 9. If the patient was unable to read the largest letter with either eye or both eyes, proceed to step 7.

7. Sometimes the patient will be unable to read even the largest letter on the chart. In this event, have the patient walk toward the chart until they can just make out the largest letter (usually a 20/400 E). Record the distance at which this occurs. *Note:* If using an exam room with a mirror system, remember to add the distance from the patient to the mirror to the distance of the mirror to the chart.

8. If the patient cannot see the largest letters at any distance, initiate the following testing, stopping at the level at which the patient can accurately respond.

   a. *Counting fingers* (CF): At a distance of approximately 1 ft (30.5 cm), expose a selected number of fingers in the center of the patient's vision. Ask the patient to tell you how many fingers you are holding up. Increase the distance from the patient until their responses are no longer accurate. Move back toward the patient until they can reliably report the number of fingers presented. Counting fingers at 2 ft is roughly equivalent to Snellen acuity of 20/2000.

   b. *Hand motion* (HM): Using your moving hand as the target, ask the patient if they can see the hand moving. Begin at approximately 1 ft and increase the distance until the patient reports they no longer detect the motion. Then move back toward the patient until they detect the motion once again.

   c. *Light projection* (LProj): Holding a penlight or transilluminator at a distance of approximately 20 inches from the patient, position the light in different areas of the patient's visual field. Each time ask the patient to point at the light and note the areas of the field in which the patient has vision.

   d. *Light perception* (LP): Direct a penlight or transilluminator at the patient and ask if they can see the light. If the patient cannot see the light, record no light perception (NLP).

9. Now test near VA. Repeat steps 1 through 6 at near using the following setup:

   a. Provide high illumination on the near point card. The light source should be either above or slightly behind the patient. Care should be taken that the light is not directed at the patient's eyes.

b. Instruct the patient to hold the card at the appropriate distance for which the card is calibrated, 16 in (40 cm) for a reduced Snellen Acuity Card.

## Notes

- The fraction 20/20 indicates that at distance of 20 feet (the numerator), the patient is able to see the letter size (denominator) that should normally be seen at that distance. 6/6 indicates the same as above except in meters.
- Many types of charts are available for measuring near VA including reduced Snellen charts, logMAR charts, tumbling E charts, near Lea symbols, cards with words or paragraphs, and samples of newsprint, playing cards, or musical staff notation (see **Figure 2-2**).
- Near VA can be recorded in Snellen notation, logMAR, N units (used by printers), decimal notation, or M units. Some near charts show several notations for the same line of letters or symbols.

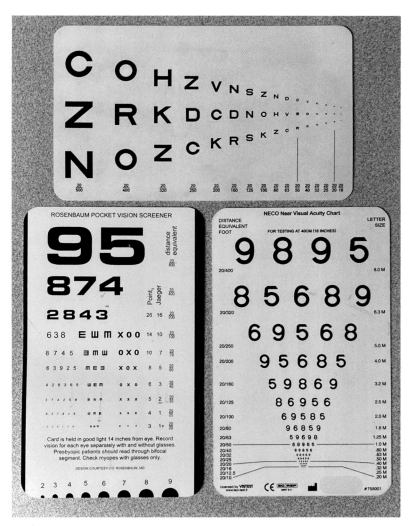

**FIGURE 2-2** | A variety of near point cards.

- M units are frequently used for assessing near VA in low-vision patients and increasingly used for primary care patients. (M units can also be used for distance acuity.) Cards with M units have a geometric progression of letter sizes between lines, which makes calculations easy to do. Near VA in M notation is written as a fraction with the numerator being the distance in meters and the denominator being the M letter size. For example, VA of 20/20 tested at 40 cm is recorded as 0.4/0.4M; 20/50 at 40 cm is recorded as 0.4/1.0M.
- Jaeger notation should be avoided since the difference between the sizes of letters on different lines is not consistent.

## Recording
- Write VAcc: cc means "with correction." If the VA is taken without correction, use sc instead of cc. If the patient's acuity is taken through contact lenses, use with contact lens (cCL).
- Record the patient's distance acuity first (DVA), followed by the near acuity (NVA) including the near distance in inches or centimeters.
- Record each eye separately and then both eyes together. Use the abbreviation of OD for the right eye, OS for the left eye, and OU for the two eyes together.
- For each eye, record the Snellen fraction or print size for smallest (lowest) line in which more than half the letters were correctly identified. (See the additional techniques described in this section if the patient could not see any of the letters at the 20-ft testing distance.)
- If the patient reads additional letters on the next line, follow the fraction or print size with a + (plus) sign and the number of letters read. If letters were missed, follow the fraction or print size with a "−" (minus) sign and the number of letters missed. When recording, "+" and "−" signs may be used simultaneously.
- Record the quality of the patient's response if it was abnormal, e.g., slow.
- When single lines or single letters are used, that should be recorded.
- If the patient had to walk toward the chart to discern the largest letter, record the distance at which they could first read the letter as the numerator and the letter size (usually 400) as the denominator.
- If the patient's distance vision is so poor that a Snellen acuity could not be obtained, measure using the sequence of techniques listed below and record the acuity that applies:
  - Counting fingers (CF) @_____ (distance)
  - Hand motion (HM) @_____ (distance)
  - Light projection (LProj). Record the areas of the visual field for which this was true.
  - Light perception (LP)
  - No light perception (NLP)

## Examples
- DVAcc    OD 20/40$^{+1}$      NVAcc    OD 20/30
         OS 20/25$^{-2}$             OS 20/30$^{-2/+2}$
         OU 20/25                 OU 20/25$^{-2}$ @ 40cm
- DVAsc    OD 20/25$^{-2}$      NVAcc    OD 20/30$^{+2}$ @ 16″
         OS 20/25$^{-2}$             OS 20/40 @ 16″ (read very slowly)
- DVAsc    OD 20/200, chart    NVAsc    OD 20/200
               20/100, line
               20/80, isolated letter
         OS 20/100              OS 20/200
         OU 20/100             OU 20/200 @40cm
- DVAcc    OD CF @ 4 ft
         OS LProj all quadrants

| VISUAL ACUITY at a glance | |
|---|---|
| 1. Distance VA setup | • Patient wears habitual correction<br>• Patient holds occluder<br>• Appropriate room illumination<br>• Project appropriate chart |
| 2. Test distance vision | • Test right eye at distance<br>• Test left eye at distance<br>• Test both eyes at distance |
| 3. If the patient cannot read the largest letter on chart, proceed through | • Finger counting<br>• Hand motion<br>• Light projection<br>• Light perception |
| 4. Near VA setup | • Patient holds occluder<br>• Place card at appropriate distance<br>• Illuminate card |
| 5. Test near vision | • Test right eye at near<br>• Test left eye at near<br>• Test both eyes at near |

## Expected Findings

- A VA of 20/20 (6/6) or better is considered normal.
- The difference between the two eyes should be no greater than one line.
- Any abnormality in VA must be addressed in the course of the examination and explained in the assessment and plan list. In the event of a failure on screening, the child must be referred for an eye examination by a licensed professional.

## 2.5 VISUAL ACUITY: MINIMUM LEGIBLE USING A LOGMAR CHART

### Purpose

The aim of this procedure is to measure the clarity of vision or the ability of the visual system to resolve detail. In a logMAR chart, the incremental size of letters and spacing of letters is determined according to the base 10 logarithm of the critical detail in minutes of arc of the letters. The critical detail in minutes of arc of the smallest recognizable letters is the patient's minimum angle of resolution (MAR).

### Indications

LogMAR charts should be used when a precise, quantitative assessment of VA is needed. VA in logMAR should be used in all research studies where VA is a dependent variable. Since logMAR acuity is often more sensitive than Snellen acuity, care should be taken when comparing measurements made with different types of charts.

### Equipment

- VA charts calibrated according to the logMAR system have several special properties that render them more precise and accurate than Snellen charts; See *Notes* below for a discussion of the rules for constructing a logMAR VA chart
- Occluder
- Back-lit cabinet or lamp to illuminate the chart (see **Figure 2-3**)
- Score sheet for the chart being used (see *Notes* below)

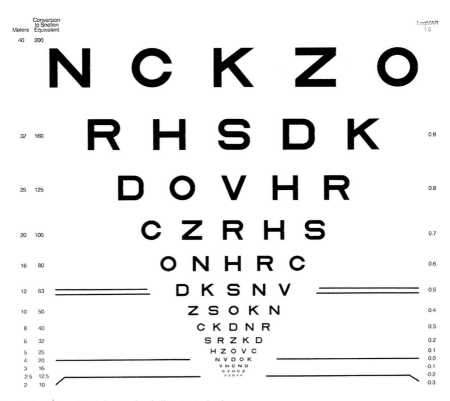

**FIGURE 2-3** | LogMAR chart in back illuminated cabinet.

## Setup

- The patient wears their habitual correction for the distance being tested. When the examiner wants to measure the patient's VA both with (cc) and without (sc) correction, the acuity should be measured without correction first to reduce the likelihood of memorization on charts that cannot randomize letters.
- The patient holds the occluder. The doctor holds the score sheet.
- A full logMAR acuity chart is shown at 4 meters. (Lines or individual letters are not isolated.)

## Procedure

1. Instruct the patient to cover their left eye and not to squint.
2. To the extent possible, observe the patient, not the chart. Because you must make marks on the score sheet as the patient reads the chart, it will be necessary to look at the score sheet some of the time. Nevertheless, it is necessary to ensure that the patient maintains occlusion of the non-tested eye and does not squint or in some other way modify their ability to read the chart.
3. Instruct the patient to read the letters on the chart (or identify the symbol in the case of charts using pictures), beginning at the top line. (See *Notes* below.)
4. On the score sheet, circle each letter correctly identified and put a line or "X" through each letter incorrectly identified. Adjacent to the letters, in the space provided, record the number of stimuli correctly identified on each line.

5. Encourage the patient to continue reading smaller and smaller letters, even if they have to guess.

6. Proceed until the patient incorrectly identifies at least four of the five letters on a line.

7. Instruct the patient to unocclude their left eye and occlude their right eye and repeat steps 2 through 6. *Optional*, repeat steps 2 through 6 with both eyes open. (See *Notes* below.)

8. When you have completed taking the VA on the patient's left eye, add up the number of letters or symbols correctly identified by each eye.

9. Apply the appropriate formula to calculate logMAR VA.

   *The formula:* In general, multiply the number of letters read correctly by 0.02 and subtract this product from 0.10 more than the logMAR of the first line read, as illustrated in the following examples:

   a. In the standard case in which the patient began reading at the top line of the chart (1.00 line), multiply the total number of letters read correctly by 0.02 and subtract this product from 1.10, or

   $$\text{LogMAR VA} = 1.10 - (0.02 \times \text{\# letters correctly read})$$

   b. If the patient began reading at the 0.80 line, the formula is

   $$\text{LogMAR VA} = 0.90 - (0.02 \times \text{\# letters correctly read})$$

   c. If they began reading at the 0.40 line, the formula is

   $$\text{LogMAR VA} = 0.50 - (0.02 \times \text{\# letters correctly read}).$$

   E.g., If the patient began reading at the top line and read 50 letters correctly, their log-MAR VA would be:

   $$\text{LogMAR VA} = 1.10 - (0.02 \times 50) = +0.10$$

10. If the patient cannot read any of the letters on the largest line, initiate the following testing sequence, stopping at the level at which the patient can respond accurately:

    a. *Counting fingers* (CF): At a distance of approximately 1 ft (30.5 cm), expose a selected number of fingers. Ask the patient to tell you how many fingers you are holding up. Increase the distance from the patient until their responses are no longer accurate. Move back toward the patient until they can reliably report the number of fingers presented.

    b. *Hand motion* (HM): Using a moving hand as the target, ask the patient if they can see the hand moving. Begin at approximately 1 ft and increase the distance until the patient reports that they can no longer detect the motion. Then move back toward the patient until they detect the motion once again.

    c. *Light projection* (LProj): Holding a penlight or transilluminator at a distance of approximately 20 in from the patient, position the light in different areas of the patient's visual field. Each time ask the patient to point at the light and note the areas of the field in which the patient has vision.

    d. *Light perception* (LP): Direct a penlight or transilluminator at the patient and ask if they can see the light.

11. Now test near VA. Repeat steps 1 through 9 at near using the following setup:

    a. Provide high illumination on a near point card calibrated according to the logMAR system. The light source should be either above or slightly behind the patient. Care should be taken so that the light is not directed at the patient's eyes.

    b. Instruct the patient to hold the card at the appropriate distance, usually 40 cm.

## Recording

- Write VAcc: cc, means "with correction." If the VA is taken without correction, use sc, instead of cc. If the patient's acuity is taken through contact lenses, record cCL.
- Record the patient's DVA, followed by the NVA including the near distance in inches or centimeters.
- Record each eye separately and then both eyes together. Use the abbreviation of OD for the right eye, OS for the left eye, and OU for the two eyes together.
- For each eye, record the result of the calculation of the formula (see step 9, above) as a decimal carried to the second decimal place. Because both + and − VAs are possible, always record the sign of the VA.
- If the patient could not correctly identify any of the letters on the VA chart, logMAR VA cannot be obtained. Proceed with the VA as described in step 10 above.
- If the patient's distance vision is so poor that a logMAR acuity could not be obtained, record the acuity that applies, as follows:
  - Counting fingers (CF) @_____ (distance)
  - Hand motion (HM) @_____ (distance)
  - Light projection (LProj). Record the areas of the visual field for which this was true.
  - Light perception (LP)
  - No light perception (NLP)

## Examples

- DVAcc    OD +0.26    NVAcc    OD +0.20
  OS  +0.14             OS +0.02 @ 40cm
- DVAsc    OD −0.02    NVAcc    OD  0.00
  OS  −0.12             OS +0.08 @ 40cm (read slowly)

## Expected Findings

- A logMAR VA of 0.00 (Snellen equivalent 20/20) or better is considered normal. Young, healthy adult patients can be expected to have a best-corrected logMAR VA of −0.10 to −0.20 (one to two lines better than 0.00) with a between-person standard deviation of approximately 0.10.
- LogMAR VA declines gradually as a function of age. Healthy seniors can be expected to have best-corrected VA of approximately 0.00 with a standard deviation of approximately 0.05.
- The difference between the two eyes should be no greater than 0.16 in a normal healthy patient.
- Like all measurements, logMAR VA is subject to variability or measurement error. In general, measurement error (standard deviation) of logMAR VA has been reported to be in the order of 0.08 to 0.10, which is equivalent to slightly less than one line on the chart. Therefore, interpreting these data very conservatively, consider that the patient's visual ability might have changed only if changes in their logMAR VA exceed 0.10.
- Any abnormality in VA must be addressed in the course of the examination and explained in the assessment and plan list. In the event of a failure on screening, the child must be referred for an eye examination by a licensed professional.

## Notes

- "LogMAR" is a system for calibrating the size increments of targets on a VA chart. Most such charts use block letters selected from the Roman alphabet. LogMAR charts are also available in Lea symbols. Theoretically, any type of stimulus can be used, provided it conforms to the rules of the system (see the following discussion and the section below,

Special Properties of LogMAR Charts). LogMAR charts obey the rule that spacing between stimuli is proportional to letter size. Therefore, logMAR charts are wide at the top, where the larger letters appear. As a result of the spacing requirement, it is very expensive to make a projected system calibrated according to logMAR, and most logMAR systems use printed charts. Both distance and near logMAR charts are commercially available. The most commonly encountered examples for distance VA measurement are black Roman letters on a white, translucent background designed to be viewed via back illumination. Most near charts are black stimuli printed on white plastic and are intended to be illuminated by an overhead lamp. The requirement for proportionality limits the practical maximum letter size on logMAR charts, because charts with stimuli with critical detail larger than logMAR 1.0 would be very large, difficult to make, and expensive.

- The score sheet (**Table 2-2**) contains the line-by-line identity of each letter or symbol on the chart and has a space to the right of each line to record the number of stimuli correctly identified on each line. It is useful to preprint the formula for calibrating VA at the bottom of the score sheet (see step 9, above).

**TABLE 2-2. Example of LogMAR Visual Acuity Recording Form**

| LogMAR | Snellen | | | | | | Number Correct |
|--------|---------|---|---|---|---|---|----------------|
| 1.00 | 200 | N | C | K | Z | O | _____ |
| 0.90 | 160 | R | H | S | D | K | _____ |
| 0.80 | 125 | D | O | V | H | R | _____ |
| 0.70 | 100 | C | Z | R | H | S | _____ |
| 0.60 | 80 | O | N | H | R | C | _____ |
| 0.50 | 63 | D | K | S | N | V | _____ |
| 0.40 | 50 | Z | S | O | K | N | _____ |
| 0.30 | 40 | C | K | D | N | R | _____ |
| 0.20 | 32 | S | R | Z | K | D | _____ |
| 0.10 | 25 | H | Z | O | V | C | _____ |
| 0.00 | 20 | N | V | D | O | K | _____ |
| −0.10 | 16 | V | H | C | N | O | _____ |
| −0.20 | 12.5 | S | V | H | C | Z | _____ |
| −0.30 | 10 | C | Z | D | V | K | _____ |
| | | | | | Total Number Correct | | _____ |

Line A = 0.1 more than LogMAR of start line.
Line B = 0.02 × number correct.
Subtract line B from line A = LogMAR Visual Acuity.

- To save time when taking acuity, it is permissible to start at a line lower than the top line; this requires a modification of the formula for calibrating VA described in detail in step 9. However, this is permissible only if the patient correctly identifies all five letters on the initial line read. If the patient fails to do so, then they must start reading the chart at a higher line with larger letters, such that they can correctly identify all five of the letters on the starting line. The only exception to this requirement is when the patient fails to read all of the letters on the top line of the chart. Because there is no larger line, they may begin on the top line (also, see step 10, above).

- It is desirable, but not necessary, to switch to a different logMAR chart when switching from the right eye to the left eye to minimize the effects of stimulus memorization.
- The formulas are to be applied literally. Thus, a patient can have a VA with a positive value, a VA with a negative value, or a VA of 0.00. A negative VA means that the critical detail, or MAR, is smaller than 1.0 minutes of arc, as is the case for any patient whose Snellen VA is better than 20/20.
- M units are frequently used for assessing VA in low-vision patients since M units are metric. VA measurements are done at 2 m or 1 m (20/20 at 1 m is designated as 1 M) and 40 cm or closer for near VA.

## Special Properties of LogMAR Charts

- The lines of letters on logMAR charts are in steps of equal difficulty of recognition rather than in steps proportional to their physical size. This is the rationale for adjusting letter sizes according to the logarithm of the critical detail of adjacent lines, which differs by exactly 0.10.
- Every 0.10 logMAR between the largest and the smallest targets is represented; no letter sizes are omitted. On most commercially available charts, the largest targets have a critical detail whose log is 1.0 (critical detail of 10 minarc, equivalent to 20/200 letters), and the smallest letters or symbols have a critical detail whose log is −0.30 (critical detail of 0.5 minarc, equivalent to 20/10).
- Letters are selected to be of a uniform difficulty of recognition.
- Each line contains the same number of letters or visual stimuli (usually five).
- In general, distance logMAR charts are calibrated for a 4 m viewing distance, and near logMAR charts are calibrated for a viewing distance of 40 cm.

## 2.6 VISUAL ACUITY: MINIMUM LEGIBLE USING THE MASSACHUSETTS VA TEST

### Purpose

The aim of this procedure is to screen or measure the clarity of vision of children who do not know the alphabet. Also, to screen for the presence of amblyopia and/or significant ametropia in 3- to 5-year-old children.

### Equipment

- Mass VAT
- Occluder or eye patch or occluder glasses
- Lamp

### Setup

- The patient wears their habitual correction for the distance being tested. When the examiner wants to measure the patient's VA both with (cc) and without (sc) correction, the acuity should be measured without correction first.
- The child holds the occluder, wears occluder glasses, or one eye is patched during testing (see **Figure 2-4**).
- The child also holds a square sheet containing large versions of the same four symbols tested to point as needed.
- Establish accurate communication between yourself and the child, as follows:
  - Standing 2 to 3 ft from the patient in normal room illumination, hold up one of the large cards with an isolated symbol.
  - Ask the child to name the picture they see, noting what word they use for each symbol. Note that there is no "right" or "wrong" name for a picture; for example, the child may call the square "square," or "box," or something else. The purpose of this step is to ensure

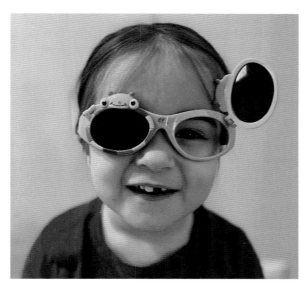

**FIGURE 2-4** │ Patient wearing occluder glasses to perform a vision screening.

that the child uses a different word for each of the four symbols and to identify the word the child will use when they correctly identify the symbol.

- If the child will not name the symbols they see, ask them to point to the symbol on the card they are holding that matches the symbol you are holding.
- Expose cards until you have gone through the full set of four symbols.
- Once the child is responding appropriately, proceed to screening or to VA measurement.
- As an alternative, use one of the cards marked "P" (for practice) in the upper corners instead of the small cards with isolated symbols.

## Procedure

*VA Measurement*

1. Have the patient cover their left eye and tell them not to squint.

2. To the extent possible, observe the patient, not the chart. Throughout the procedure, point to each symbol as you want the patient to identify it, making sure you unambiguously point to only one symbol at a time. As you point to each symbol, do not break the contour interaction bar with your finger or other pointer.

3. From a distance of 3 m (10 ft) with bright light illuminating the test card, show the child the +0.50 (equivalent to Snellen 10/32) card with "R" in the upper corners. If they correctly identify the first two symbols, flip to the +0.40 card for the right eye (this may require flipping more than one card).

4. If the child correctly identifies the first two symbols on that card, proceed to the next smaller card of symbols for the right eye. (The symbols are incremented in steps of 0.10 logMAR when viewed from 3 m) Continue showing incrementally smaller targets until the child misses one of the first two symbols on a line.

5. At that point go back to the card with the next larger set of symbols and ask the child to identify all of the symbols. If the child correctly identifies four or five of these symbols, go to the next smaller set of targets, and so on, until the child misidentifies more than one of the five symbols.

    a. The child's VA is the card with the smallest targets on which they accurately identify four or more symbols. If they miss one of the five targets, it is permissible to record a "−1" after the VA. Acuity can be recorded in Snellen equivalent, in logMAR, or in one of the other notations at the bottom of each card.

6. Instruct the child to cover their right eye and tell them not to squint.

7. To the extent possible, observe the patient, not the chart.

8. From a distance of 3 m with bright light illuminating the test card, show the child the +0.50 (equivalent to Snellen 10/32) card with "L" in the upper corners. The "L" indicates that this card is for testing the left eye. If they correctly identify the first two symbols, flip to the +0.40 card for the left eye (this may require flipping more than one card).

9. If the child correctly identifies the first two symbols on that card, proceed to the next smaller card of symbols for the left eye, and so on, until the child misses one of the first two symbols on a line.

10. At that point, go back to the next larger card of symbols for the left eye and ask the child to identify all of the symbols. If the child correctly identifies four or five of these symbols, go to the next smaller set of targets, and so on, until the child misidentifies more than one of the five symbols.

    a. The child's VA is the card with the smallest targets on which they accurately identify four or more symbols. If they miss one of the five targets, it is permissible to record a "−1" after the VA. Acuity can be recorded in Snellen equivalent, in logMAR, or in one of the other notations at the bottom of each card.

## Screening

1. Have the patient cover their left eye and tell them not to squint. If the patient is unable to hold the occluder, patch their left eye or use occluder glasses that cover their left eye. To the extent possible, observe the patient, not the chart.

2. From a distance of 3 or 4 ft show the child one of the flip charts marked with a "P" in the upper left or right corner. As you point to each symbol ask the child either to name it or to point to the one just like it on the square sheet containing large versions of the four symbols.

3. If the child correctly identifies all symbols, move back to a distance of 3.0 m (10 ft) and show them the card with "R" in the upper corner and the corresponding critical line for the age of the patient in the bottom corner (e.g., 20/50 for 3 and younger, 20/40 for 4- to 5-year-old, and 20/32 if 5 and older). Once again ask them to name the one you are pointing to or to point to the matching symbol on the square chart that they are holding. As you point to each symbol, do not break the contour interaction bar with your finger or other pointer.

4. Correctly identifying four or five of the symbols is a pass. Identifying two or more symbols incorrectly is a "fail."

5. Have the child cover their right eye to test their left eye and show them the card with "L" in the upper corner and the corresponding critical line for the age of the patient in the bottom corner (e.g., 20/50 for 3 and younger, 20/40 for 4- to 5-year-old, and 20/32 if 5 and older). Once again ask them to name the one you are pointing to or to point to the matching symbol on the square chart that they are holding.

6. Correctly identifying four or five of the symbols is a pass. Identifying two or more symbols incorrectly is a "fail."

## Recording

- Write VA; "cc," means with correction. If the VA is taken without correction, use sc instead of cc.

- Record each eye separately. Use the abbreviation of OD for the right eye, OS for the left eye.
- Record the child's distance acuity followed by the distance at which the acuity was measured (even if the standard distance of 3 m was used).
- If recording in logMAR notation, because both + and − VAs are possible, always record the sign of the VA.
- If the child could not correctly identify any of the letters on the card with the largest symbols (the practice card has 0.60 targets), the actual VA cannot be obtained with the Mass VAT. Record "worse than +0.60" or "worse than 20/80."

### Examples

For VA measurement:
- VAsc (MassVAT)    OD 10/32    at 3 m
    OS 10/8$^{-1}$
- VAsc (MassVAT)    OD 0.00    at 10 ft
    OS −0.10
- VAcc (MassVAT)    OD +0.20    at 10 ft
    OS +0.30

For screening:
- OD 5/5 pass, OS 4/5 pass, 10/32 at 10 ft
- OD 3/5 fail, OS 4/5 pass, 10/20 at 10 ft

### Notes

- This procedure is specific to our current state guidelines. Consult your local and regional guidelines for procedures used to screen vision in children.

## 2.7 PINHOLE VISUAL ACUITY

### Purpose

The aim of this procedure is to determine if a decrease in vision is due to uncorrected refractive error. Viewing the acuity chart through a pinhole will increase the patient's depth of focus and decrease the retinal blur. If the retina and visual pathway are free of abnormalities, the patient's acuity will improve.

### Indications

Pinhole acuities are taken when the VA is worse than 20/30 at distance through the habitual or induced correction.

### Equipment

- Computer-generated acuity chart, projector with VA slide, or wall mounted acuity chart
- Pinhole (PH) disc with 1.0- to 1.5-mm diameter pinhole(s)
- Occluder

### Setup

- The patient wears their habitual correction while looking at the distance VA chart.
- With the exception of the potential acuity pinhole, pinhole acuities are taken only at distance.

### Procedure

1. The patient is asked to occlude the eye not being tested. If both eyes are to be tested, test the right eye first.
2. Instruct the patient to position the PH disc until the chart is as clear as possible for the patient and then to read the smallest line of letters they can. (See **Figure 2-5**).

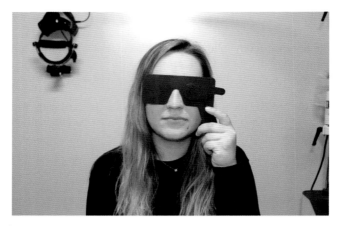

**FIGURE 2-5** | Patient using the pinhole occluder while viewing the distance VA chart.

3. Encourage the patient to read the next smallest line, even if they have to guess. Continue until the patient has missed more than half the letters on a line.

### Recording
- Write "PH" followed by the VA. This notation is usually recorded next to the distance VA through correction.
- "PHNI," or "PH: NI" may be used to indicate no improvement in VA with the pinhole.

### Examples
- DVAcc       OD  20/50$^{+2}$       PH: 20/30$^{+2}$
            OS  20/40               PH: 20/25
- DVAsc       OD  20/40$^{+1}$       PH: NI
            OS  20/100              PH: 20/50

### Expected Findings
- If the cause of the patient's decreased acuity is due to an uncorrected refractive error, VA is expected to improve through the pinhole.
- If the cause of decreased acuity is not optically based, no improvement, and possibly a decrease, will occur through the pinhole.
- A refraction should improve the acuity level of the patient at least to the level obtained through the pinhole.

## 2.8 COLOR VISION

### Purpose
The aim of this procedure is to screen for acquired or hereditary color vision defects. These clinical screening tests are particularly significant for the assessment of macular cone and optic nerve function.

### Equipment
- Occluder
- Overhead lamp
- Test book containing pseudoisochromatic plates (PIPs)
  - Common versions of PIPs include Ishihara or Hardy-Rand-Rittler (HRR) Edition 4

## Setup
- The patient wears their habitual correction for near.
- The patient holds the occluder.
- The examiner holds the test booklet 40 cm or 75 cm from the patient. *Note:* The original research to develop some tests used a 75 cm working distance, but many examiners in a clinical setting will perform the test at 40 cm for patient comfort and ease of use.
- The overhead lamp is on and pointed at the booklet.

## Procedure
1. Instruct the patient to occlude their left eye to test their right eye. It is essential to test color vision monocularly so that the two eyes can be compared to one another.
2. Observe the patient to make sure that only one eye can see the test plates.
3. Turn the pages one at a time at a rate of one every 3 seconds, asking the patient to identify the figure and the location of the figure on each page. *Note:* if available, give the patient the brush that comes with the test book to show the examiner where on the page they see the figures to prevent the patient from touching the plates.
4. Instruct the patient to occlude their right eye and repeat steps 2 and 3 to test the left eye.
5. If using HRR#4, use plates 5 through 10 for screening. Plates 5 and 6 test for blue-yellow defects and plates 7 through 10 test for red-green defects.
   a. If the patient misses plate 5 or 6, they have a blue-yellow defect and plate 21 through 24 should now be tested.
   b. If the patient misses any of the plates 7 through 10, they have a red-green color defect and plates 11 through 20 should now be tested.
   c. If the patient misses plates in both sections, 5–6 and 7–10, then all remaining plates (11–24) should be tested.

## Recording
- For each eye, write the number of correctly identified plates, a slash mark, and then the number of plates tested (i.e., a fraction) when a screening test is done. In the HRR #4 test, the first four plates are for demonstration and are not scored. Plates 5 through 10 are screening plates. Plates 11 through 24 are used to diagnose the type of defect and the extent of the defect. Use the recording sheet that comes with the HRR #4 test when plates 11 through 24 are used (see **Table 2-3**).
- Record the name of test used.

## Examples
- Color Vision (HRR #4): 6/6 OD, 6/6 OS
- Color Vision (HRR #4): 8/16 Strong Deutan OD, 9/16 Medium Deutan OS
- Color Vision (Ishihara): 6/6 OD, 6/6 OS

## Expected Findings
- Consult the manufacture guidelines for the specific PIP test booklet used for color vision testing. The instructions should be read to ascertain what is considered normal for the particular test. In some tests it is normal for the patient to make some mistakes.
- Approximately 8% of the general population will have congenital color vision anomalies; most of these patients are males as color vision is x-linked. In these patients, the color vision in each eye is usually the same and is most often a protan or deutan defect. These defects remain stable over time. In patients with acquired color vision anomalies due to ocular disease, the two eyes are often different from one another.

**TABLE 2-3.  HRR Recording Form**

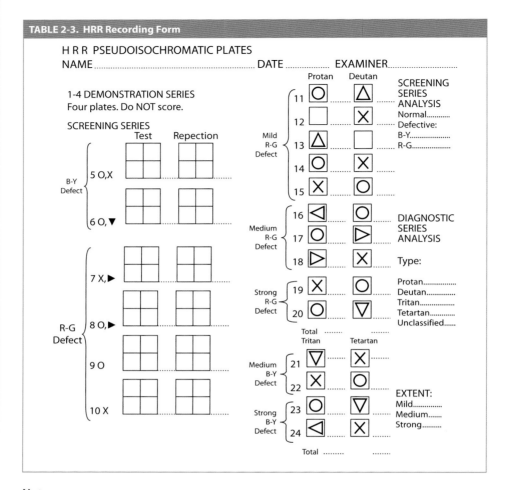

## Notes

- The HRR test, Edition 4, is recommended for screening since it has plates to screen for protan, deutan, tritan, and tetartan defects, making other color vision screening tests obsolete since they only screen for protan and deutan defects. The HRR test is available in both adult and pediatric versions.

## 2.9 COVER TEST

### Purpose

This is an objective test used for assessing the presence, type, and magnitude of ocular deviation (strabismus or heterophoria) under dissociated conditions. It is considered the gold standard to quantify the deviation when motor fusion is absent (strabismus) and to determine the demand (heterophoria) placed on the patient's fusional vergence system.

### Equipment

- VA chart
- Accommodative target (isolated letter 1-2 lines larger than optimal VA in worse seeing eye)
- Occluder (translucent or opaque)

- Overhead lamp
- Horizontal and vertical prism bars or loose prisms

## Setup

- The patient should wear their habitual correction (or alternative Rx) for the distance being tested.
- The room illumination can either be full or at minimum sufficient to allow the examiner to observe the eye movements of the patient.
- The examiner must be positioned to see the patient's eyes easily without interfering with the patient's view of the target.

## Procedure

*Unilateral Cover Test (Cover-Uncover)*

This is used to determine if the ocular deviation is a strabismus or heterophoria and the frequency, laterality, and direction of the strabismus if present.

1. Instruct the patient to look at the target, with both eyes open and to keep it clear.
2. Cover the patient's right eye (3 to 4 seconds) and observe the left eye for movement (refixation) as soon as the right eye is covered. No movement in the left eye (uncovered eye) indicates there is no strabismus of the left eye. Remove the occluder and allow 2 to 3 seconds for the two eyes to resume fixation. Repeat cover-uncover of the right eye 2 to 3 times.
3. Repeat the procedure now covering and uncovering the left eye. Repeat cover-uncover of the left eye 2 to 3 times.
   a. If the patient has a strabismus, determine the laterality and frequency of the deviation.
   - Same eye continually refixates → constant unilateral strabismus
   - Same eye intermittently refixates → intermittent unilateral strabismus
   - Each eye continually refixates → constant alternating strabismus
   - Each eye intermittently refixates → intermittent alternating strabismus
   b. Determine the direction of the deviation by observing the movement of the eye(s) when it refixates (uncovered eye).
   - Eye moves inward → exo (phoria/tropia) deviation
   - Eye moves outward → eso (phoria/tropia) deviation
   - Eye moves downward → hyper (phoria/tropia) deviation
   - Eye moves upward → hypo (phoria/tropia) deviation
   c. Determine the magnitude of the strabismus by either estimating or measuring with the alternating prism cover test as described below.

*Alternating Cover Test*

This determines the direction and magnitude of a strabismus or heterophoria if present but does not differentiate between strabismus or a heterophoria.

1. Instruct the patient to look at the target with both eyes open and to keep it clear. Cover the patient's right eye for 3 to 4 seconds and then quickly move the occluder from the right eye to the left while observing the just-uncovered eye for any movement.
2. Continue to move the occluder quickly between the two eyes while maintaining occlusion for a full 3 to 4 seconds on each eye alternatively. Note the direction of movement of the eyes to determine the direction of the deviation.
3. Determine the magnitude of the deviation by either estimating or measuring with the alternating prism cover test as described below.

### Alternating Prism Cover Test

This measures (neutralizes) the magnitude of the deviation of any strabismus or heterophoria. The magnitude of the deviation can be measured using either a prism bar or loose prisms. Both horizontal and vertical deviations can be measured, and the test can be done at both distance and near.

1. In the case of heterophoria, the prism can be held over either eye to measure the deviation while in strabismus the prism should be held over the deviating eye. (This is true for both vertical and horizontal deviations.)

2. Place the base (in reference to the patient's nose) of the measuring prism in the correct position depending on the orientation of the deviation (see **Figure 2-6**).
   - Exo → base in
   - Eso → base out
   - Hyper → base down
   - Hypo → base up

3. While performing the alternating cover test, slowly increase the magnitude of the prism until movement is no longer observed. The amount of prism needed to neutralize (no movement) the deviation represents the magnitude of the deviation. Once neutrality is achieved, the magnitude of the prism should be increased, until the movement is reversed.

4. The amount of prism needed to neutralize the deviation before reversal of movement should be recorded as the magnitude of the deviation.

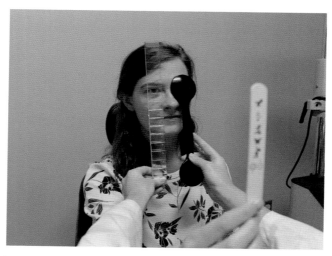

**FIGURE 2-6** │ The examiner neutralizes an ESO deviation with the near alternating prism cover test using base out prism. The patient holds the target.

### Measuring Cover Test in All Positions of Gaze

Determining comitancy in strabismus is important in the diagnosis of many visual conditions. Deviations are considered non-comitant if the deviation varies by more than 5Δ in any two positions of gaze. The alternate prism test is used to measure the deviation in all 9 positions of gaze; primary (straight ahead), inferior, superior, left, right, inferior left, superior left, superior right and inferior right (see **Figure 2-7**). In some instances, testing only in 5 positions of gaze; primary, inferior, superior, left and right is sufficient.

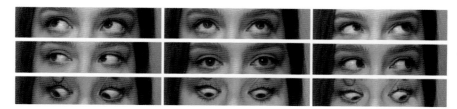

FIGURE 2-7 | The nine positions of gaze to be used when testing for comitancy.

## Recording

- Record the name of the test and at what distance the test is being performed. This can be abbreviated DCT and NCT for distance cover test and near cover test respectively. The near testing distance should include the distance in cm or inches e.g., NCT @ 40 cm or NCT @ 33 cm.
- Record the Rx through which the cover test was performed (habitual, subjective, add) Write "sc" for without correction and "cc" for with correction.
- Record the direction, laterality, frequency, and magnitude of the deviation as applicable. Only strabismus needs the laterality and frequency described as heterophorias are always constant and always affect each eye equally.
- Record the amount of prism needed to neutralize the deviation in prism diopters (pd or Δ). If the magnitude of the deviation was estimated (not measured) use a tilde (~) to denote this e.g., DCT cc (habitual) ~ 4 pd esophoria, NCT @ 40 cm cc (+1.00) 12pd R exotropia.
- The following abbreviations can be used:
  - EP – esophoria
  - XP—exophoria
  - ET—esotropia
  - XT—exotropia
  - Hyper or hypo for vertical deviations
  - ⊕—orthophoria (no deviation)
  - L—Left
  - R—Right
  - Alt—alternating
  - Int or (T)—intermittent
  - Con—constant
- Vertical deviations are designated based on the hyper eye. The terms *right hyper* or *left hyper* are used for heterophorias or alternating strabismus. The term *hypo* is used for downward-deviating unilateral strabismus.
- For intermittent strabismus an estimation of the percentage of time it is present should be recorded e.g., DCTcc (habitual) ~7 pd int. (50%) LXT.
- For alternating strabismus, the eye that is preferred for fixation and for what percentage of time should be recorded e.g., NCTcc @ 40 cm (habitual) ~7 pd alt. (80% R fixation) XT.
- If the patient has non-comitant strabismus the magnitude should be measured and recorded for each position of gaze. This can be recorded on a grid.

## Examples

- DCTsc ⊕, NCTsc @ 40cm 4 pd XP
- DCTcc (habitual) ~8 pd int. (50%) LXT
- NCTcc @ 40 cm (habitual) ~6 Δ alt. (80% R fixation) XT
- NCTcc @ 33 cm (+1.00) 10 pd constant LXT
- NCTsc @ 40 cm ~12 pd EP

## Expected Findings
- 1 $\Delta$ exophoria ($\mp$ 2 $\Delta$) at D; 3 $\Delta$ exophoria ($\mp$ 3 $\Delta$) at N.

## Notes
- Depending on the fusional vergence reserves of the patient, a large phoria may decompensate into strabismus. If no cover test abnormalities are noted in symptomatic patients, it is recommended to repeat the cover test procedure several times, at the end of the exam, or at a second visit scheduled for the end of the day.
- The heterophoria of the patient can be observed during unilateral cover test by looking at the eye that is underneath the occluder (translucent occluder or examiner peeking behind occulder). This is sometimes referred to as the latent deviation.
- Presbyopes may have a larger exophoria at near than the non-presbyopic population.

| COVER TEST at a glance | |
| --- | --- |
| **Technique** | **Purpose** |
| Unilateral Cover Test | Determines if strabismus is present and if present, the laterality and frequency |
| Alternating Cover Test | Determines if a heterophoria is present and the direction. A heterophoria is only present if there is no strabismus found on the unilateral cover test. |
| Alternating Prism Cover Test | Measures the magnitude of a deviation when present. |

## 2.10 STEREOPSIS

### Purpose
This is a subjective test used to measure the ability of the patient to fuse stereoscopic targets and to measure the magnitude of fine depth perception.

### Equipment
- Validated stereo-test and associated stereo glasses if needed
- Examples of validated stereo-tests include but are not limited to the following: Random Dot 3, Titmus, Random Dot E, Randot, and Preschool Assessment of Stereopsis with a Smile (PASS). See section "Considerations" for further details.

### Setup
- The patient wears the appropriate stereo glasses, if needed, for the chosen stereo-test. Stereo glasses are worn over habitual correction for distance or near depending on the distance at which the test is performed (see **Figure 2-8**).
- Consult the manufacturers guide for the distance at which the test should be performed as this may vary from test to test.
- The overhead lamp is directed toward the target so as not to create glare.

### Procedure
Always consult the manufacturer's instructions for directions regarding your specific stereo-test. The procedure presented here is for the Random Dot 3 test and can be applied to most near random dot test booklets.

### Adult Patient
1. It is very important to instruct the patient to not tilt or move their head once the test is set up. This can give cues that could lead to an artificially high measured value of stereopsis.

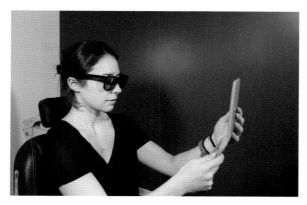

FIGURE 2-8 | A patient viewing the stereo booklet with stereo glasses on over habitual correction.

2. Direct the patient's attention to the smallest set of targets. Typically, this is a set of circles. Start with the first circle and ask the patient to identify in which position a smaller circle seems to be floating above the page (up, down, left, or right).

3. Continue testing each subsequent target until the patient gives an incorrect answer. If the patient gives an incorrect answer, retest the preceding target to ensure the patient was not guessing. If the patient misses this target, end the test and record the level of stereopsis associated with the last correct target. If they give a correct answer to the preceding target, record that preceding target as the endpoint.

4. If the patient is unable to correctly identify any of the smaller targets, have them try the medium targets, typically a medium-sized box with shapes and three levels of difficulty, and continue testing as described previously. If they are unable to identify the medium sized targets, have the patient try the largest targets, typically a large grid with four boxes and larger shapes, and continue testing as described previously.

## Pediatric Patient

1. The test should be performed in reverse order of the adult patient above, with the largest targets shown first and continuing with increasing levels of difficulty. *Note:* Specially designed pediatric tests can also be used.

## Recording

- Record the name of the test, the distance at which the test was done, and if the test was done with (cc) or without correction (sc). E.g., Random Dot 3 @ 40 cm cc.
- If the test was done with a new or modified refraction, record the refraction in place of cc or sc. For example, Titmus Fly (40 cm) with +1.00.
- Findings should be recorded in seconds of arc and can be abbreviated with the symbol (″) e.g., PASS 3 (40 cm) sc 100 arcsec or 100″.
- If the patient does not perceive any of the stereo targets, record "(no stereo)," e.g., Frisby (1 m) cc (no stereo).

## Examples

- Random Dot 3 @ 40 cm cc 20″
- Random Dot 3 @ 40 cm cc 20 seconds of arc
- Titmus Fly @ 40 cm cc 150″
- PASS 3 (40 cm) sc 100 arcsec
- Frisby (1 m) subjective (no stereo)

### Expected Findings (General)
- Adults: 20 seconds of arc with decreasing stereoacuity in elderly adults.
- Children (3 to 5): 168 (at 150 cm) to 126 (at 200 cm) seconds of arc (Random Dot E).
- *Note:* It is inappropriate to compare the results from different stereo tests as they cannot be used interchangeably. Additionally, the normative findings for the specific test used should be used if possible.

### Notes
- Stereopsis may be repeated with the subjective refraction findings particularly if there is a large change from the habitual Rx, and/or VA and alignment are improved.
- There are a number of stereo-tests on the market, including online versions, that may be performed at distance or near and, with or without stereo glasses (Polaroid or red-green) and versions for pediatric patients. In selecting a stereo-test, it is important to choose a test which has been clinically tested and validated. Random dot tests are preferred because they have few monocular cues, which can lead to an artificially high measurement of stereopsis.
- Vision screening stereo-tests are also in use and it is important to denote this in records as these tests may use only one threshold measure.

## 2.11 NEAR POINT OF CONVERGENCE (NPC)

### Purpose
This is a subjective and objective test used to determine the patient's absolute convergence ability. NPC is recommended as an entrance test for all comprehensive pediatric exams.

### Equipment
- Appropriate target (transilluminator, red lens, red-green glasses, or accommodative target).
- If an accommodative target is used, one should be selected with a line or isolated letter one to two lines above the patient's near VA in the worse seeing eye.
- An accommodative rule or standard ruler may be used to measure the break and recovery findings.

### Setup
- The patient wears their habitual near correction. The test can be repeated using the new manifest subjective findings if significant changes or improvement from the habitual VA of binocular status is noted.
- The overhead lamp is directed toward the target.
- An accommodative (or other target) is held by the examiner at 40 cm.

### Procedure
1. Instruct the patient to look at the accommodative target (or other target) and to follow the target as it moves closer to the patient while keeping the target clear and single.
2. Move the target toward the patient, observing the patient's eyes until the patient reports that the target appears double or until you see one eye lose fixation. Measure the distance from the spectacle plane at which the patient reports that the target doubles or at which you note that the patient loses bi-fixation. This is the break point.
3. Move the target away from the patient's eyes and measure the distance at which the patient's deviated eye regains fixation. The patient would report single vision at this distance if they reported diplopia in step 2. This is the recovery point.
4. The procedure can be repeated (steps 1 through 3) with other targets as needed. A transilluminator or penlight can be used as a non-accommodative target. Additionally, red-green glasses or a red lens over the right eye can be used with the light target.

5. Measurements should be obtained from the spectacle plane and not from the end of the patient's nose.

## Recording
- Red-green glasses can be abbreviated (RG), red lens (RL), accommodative target (acc.), and transilluminator (light).
- Record "diplopia" if the patient reported seeing two targets. Record "suppression" if the patient did not report seeing two targets but a break, or deviated eye, was observed. The eye that is observed to lose fixation is the eye that is suppressing.
- Record the name of the test, the target used, with or without correction, the break and re-covery values, and if suppression or diplopia occurred. It is highly recommended to record the eye that lost fixation as applicable. For example, NPC cc (acc.) 6 cm/10 cm suppression (OD out) or NPC sc (light) 4 cm/7 cm, diplopia, OS out.
- If the examiner was able to move the target to the bridge of the patient's nose without the patient's losing fixation, record TTN ("to the nose").
- If the patient breaks at a distance larger than the ruler used record greater than, e.g., >12 cm.

## Examples
- NPC cc (acc.) TTN
- NPC cc (acc.) 6 cm/10 cm suppression (OD out)
- NPC cc (RG) 6 cm/10 cm diplopia, OS out
- NPC sc (acc.) >12 cm diplopia (OD out)

## Expected Findings
- Accommodative Target: 5 cm break and 7 cm recovery.
- Light Target: 7 cm break and 10 cm recovery.
- Light Target with red-green glasses: 5 cm break and 7 cm recovery.
- Light Target with red lens: norms to be determined (TBD), expected to be similar to light with red-green glasses.

## Notes
- Patients who have symptoms consistent with convergence insufficiency should be retested with either the red lens or red-green glasses. It has been recommended (Schieman and Wick, 2013) to repeat NPC twice, first with an accommodative target and then with red-green glasses, as previous recommendations to repeat the NPC test 4-5 times have been shown to be of limited value clinically.
- It is important to bring the target forward to the bridge of the patient's nose and measure break/recovery from the spectacle plane and not the tip of the patient's nose as anatomical variations may create inconsistencies when expected findings are applied.

## 2.12 HIRSCHBERG TEST AND KRIMSKY TEST

### Purpose
These are objective tests used to determine the approximate positions of the visual axes of the two eyes under binocular conditions at near. These tests are used to identify the magnitude and type of strabismus when the gold standard cover test cannot be used, such as with children under the age of two.

### Equipment
- Penlight or transilluminator
- Prism bars if performing the Krimsky Test

## Setup
- These tests are performed without correction.

## Procedure
1. Direct the penlight toward the patient's eyes from a distance of 50 to 100 cm.
2. Instruct the patient to look at the light.
3. While the patient is looking at the light, observe the corneal light reflex in each eye individually by briefly covering each eye alternatively with either a hand or occluder. The corneal light reflex in each eye should be judged in relation to the center of the pupil. In most cases the corneal light reflex will fall slightly nasal to the center of the pupil (positive angle lambda).
4. Next, compare the locations of the corneal reflexes with both eyes open. The light source must be directly beneath the visual axis of the observer's fixating eye. If the reflexes are in the same relative position in each of the two eyes the patient does not have strabismus (see **Figure 2-9**). If the patient has strabismus the reflex will fall in the direction opposite to the strabismus (see **Figure 2-10**).

   a. Reflex centered nasally → exotropia

   b. Reflex centered temporally → esotropia

   c. Reflex centered superiorly → hypotropia

   d. Reflex centered inferiorly → hypertropia
5. There are two methods of determining the magnitude of the deviation. One is to estimate using the following equation: 1 mm of deviation = 22 prism diopters and the second is to utilize the Krimsky Test. The Krimsky Test is performed by placing prism over the fixating eye and increasing the amount of prism until the corneal reflex is in the same relative position in the deviating eye.

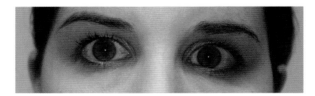

FIGURE 2-9 | The appearance of Hirschberg reflexes in a patient with no manifest deviation (ortho).

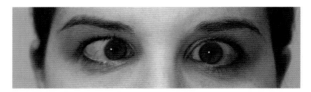

FIGURE 2-10 | The appearance of the Hirschberg reflexes in the patient with a right esotropia.

## Recording
- Record the name of the test used, e.g., Hirschberg.
- If there is no strabismus, record "symmetry" or "ortho."
- If there is a strabismus, record the eye that is deviated, the size of the deviation, and the direction of the deviation. For example, Hirschberg: ortho or Hirschberg: ~22 pd LXT;

Krimsky 25Δ LXT. *Note:* Hirschberg magnitude is estimated and should be recorded using a tilde (~), while Krismsky is measured and should be recorded using prism diopters (pd) or the delta (Δ) symbol.

### Examples
- Hirschberg ortho
- Hirschberg ~22 pd LXT; Krimsky 25Δ
- Hirschberg ~10 pd RET

### Notes
- Hirschberg and Krimsky should only be relied upon in cases where the examiner is unable to use cover test.
- Hirschberg reflexes can frequently be observed during other testing, e.g., Brückner and EOMs and can be used as supporting findings.

## 2.13 BRÜCKNER TEST

### Purpose
This is an objective test used to assess and screen for asymmetry of refractive error, media opacities, anomalies of the posterior pole, and strabismus in young preverbal children and other individuals who may not be able to participate in other testing.

### Equipment
- Direct ophthalmoscope

### Setup
- Performed without correction and without dilation
- Dim room illumination
- Ophthalmoscope with a large spot beam and +1.00 D lens (at 1 m distance)

### Procedure
1. Direct the ophthalmoscope toward the patient's eyes from an appropriate distance. It is recommended to use both a 1-m and 4-m distance as 1 m is more sensitive to the detection of strabismus, media opacities and other retinal abnormalities and 4 m is more sensitive for the detection of ametropia and anisometropia.
2. Instruct the patient to look directly at the light.
3. The examiner positions their eye directly behind the viewing window of the ophthalmoscope and dials in the lens that gives a clear view of the patient's pupils (e.g., for a distance of 1 m, this should be a +1.00 D lens.)
4. Compare the brightness of the glowing red reflexes in each of the two eyes to check for asymmetry (see **Figure 2-11**).
   a. If the two reflexes are equally bright see recording section.
   b. If the two reflexes are not equally bright, determine the anomalous eye:
      - Darker/dull reflex → patient may have anisometropia. The duller reflex is the affected eye.
      - Bright white reflex → patient may have strabismus or posterior pole abnormality, e.g., retinoblastoma. The brighter reflex indicates the non-fixating eye or eye with posterior pole abnormality.
      - Asymmetric shadowing/blockage of red reflex → patient may have a media opacity.

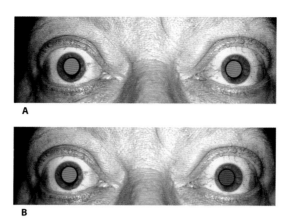

**FIGURE 2-11** | Appearance of the red fundus reflex in the Brückner test. (A) demonstrates equal reflexes or bifixation. (B) demonstrates reflex asymmetry which could indicate anisometropia greater in the left eye, or that that the patient is fixating with the left eye (right eye is deviated).

5. To determine the type of refractive error, observe the red reflex of both eyes and look for the presence of dark/white crescents.

   a. In hyperopes the white crescent will be in the upper portion of the pupil, the darker crescent lower in the pupil.

   b. In myopes the white crescent will be in the lower portion of the pupil and the darker crescent in the upper portion.

   c. In astigmatism the crescents may be slanted or twisted.

   The crescents of both eyes can be examined for asymmetry and magnitude. The larger the magnitude of refractive error the larger the white crescent will appear. In cases of high ametropia, myopes will have a dark fundal reflex while hyperopes will have a brighter fundal reflex. In both cases of high ametropia the crescents will be entirely absent.

## Recording
- If the reflexes are equal, Brückner can be recorded as Brückner OD = OS.
- If the reflexes are unequal, Brückner can be recorded qualitatively.
- If the reflexes are equal and significant crescents are observed the type of refractive error can be recorded.

## Examples
- Brückner: OD = OS
- Brückner: OD brighter than OS; R tropia
- Brückner: hyperopia OD > OS
- Brückner: cataract centrally OS
- Brückner: OD = OS; myopia OU

## Notes
- The Hirschberg reflexes can also be observed during the Brückner test and can aid in the determination of the non-fixating eye (see Procedure 2.12).
- Changes in the appearance of the reflex can also be created by the presence of anisocoria.
- The Brückner test is inaccurate in children under the age of 8 months.
- The Brückner test can be unreliable for small angle strabismus but can be used as an adjunct to determine the fixating eye in patients uncooperative with cover test.

- Differences in the pigmentation of the fundus between individuals cause variations in the brightness of the red reflex.

## 2.14 EXTRAOCULAR MOTILITIES (EOMS)

### Purpose
The aim of this procedure is to assess the patient's ability to perform conjugate eye movements.

### Equipment
- Transilluminator (or penlight)

### Setup
- The patient removes their spectacles.
- The examiner holds the transilluminator.

### Procedure
1. Perform the Hirschberg procedure as described in Procedure 2.12.
2. Give instructions to the patient:

   "Follow the light with your eyes without moving your head. Tell me if you ever see two lights instead of one or if you feel any pain or discomfort."
3. Start with the light on and pointed directly at the patient while holding the transilluminator 40-50 cm away. This is called the "primary position of gaze."
4. Move the light to the eight additional positions shown in **Figure 2-12**. *Note:* The order in which the positions are tested is not important. It is critical, however, to test gaze in all nine positions. In this step you are tracing the pattern of a large letter H bisected by a vertical line. It is important to maintain a sooth movement of the light across the patient's midpoint.

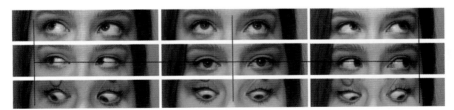

FIGURE 2-12 | Schematic diagram showing the positions of gaze for EOM testing seen from the perspective of the examiner looking at the patient. The double H pattern is marked with the black lines.

5. Throughout step 4, ensure the light is pointed at the patient's eyes. Look for changes in the relative positions of the corneal reflections, as in the Hirschberg test. *Note:* Do not move the light too far. At a test distance of 30 to 40 cm, a movement of the light 30 to 40 cm from the primary position will detect ocular deviations of about 40°. This is sufficient to uncover weak extraocular muscles.
6. Throughout the procedure, observe the following:

   a. the smoothness of movement;

   b. the accuracy of following the penlight; and

   c. the extent of movement.
7. If the patient reports diplopia in any position of gaze, perform Park's 3-step method for a paretic vertical muscle, or the red lens test to identify a paretic horizontal muscle (see Procedures 8.6 and 8.7, respectively).

## Recording

- If the patient follows the light smoothly to all positions of gaze with both eyes and never reports diplopia (double vision) or discomfort, write SAFE (or FESA). These letters stand for: S: Smooth, A: Accurate, F: Full, and E: Extensive.
- If the patient shows any problem, record only the letters that apply and describe the problem, for example, "jerky, unsteady, nystagmoid," "failure to follow into (give the location)," or "restricted, lagging, non-comitant."
- Identify the direction(s) of gaze that result in diplopia and/or discomfort.
- If only one eye is the abnormal one, be sure to identify it.
- If a muscle restriction is noted, estimate the percentage of restriction present.

## Examples

- EOMs: SAFE
- EOMs: diplopia in upper right gaze, 50% SR restriction OD, FESA OS
- EOMs: FESA, OD pain on left gaze
- EOMs: 70% LR restriction OS, SAFE OD

## Expected Findings

- SAFE or FESA
- No pain or diplopia
- At the extreme limits of a healthy patient's gaze, it is normal to observe a low-amplitude nystagmus, known as an *endpoint nystagmus.*

## Notes

- During step 4 above, instead of following a double-H pattern, you may instruct the patient to follow the light while you move it in the pattern of a large letter X. Extend the transilluminator from the patient's lower right gaze to their upper left gaze and then from the patient's lower left gaze to their upper right gaze. *Note*: You are still looking for under action or over action in one eye compared to the other as you move the transilluminator to these four secondary positions of gaze.

## 2.15 PUPILS

## Purpose

The aim of this procedure is to assess the afferent and efferent neurological pathways responsible for pupillary function.

## Equipment

- Penlight or transilluminator
- Pupillary distance (PD) ruler or pupillary gauge
- Overhead lamp
- Distance fixation target (e.g., 20/400 E)

## Setup

- The patient removes their glasses (if applicable).
- The examiner is ~25 cm away from patient out of the line of sight (i.e., off to one side, sitting or standing).
- The overhead lamp is as dim as possible but permits a clear view of both patient's pupils and irides.

## Procedure

1. Instruct the patient to look at the distance fixation target.

2. In dim illumination, compare the size, shape, and location of the pupil in each eye. If a difference in pupil size is observed (anisocoria), then measure the size of each pupil by placing the pupillary gauge next to the patient's pupil of the right eye. Repeat on the left eye. (**Figure 2-13**).

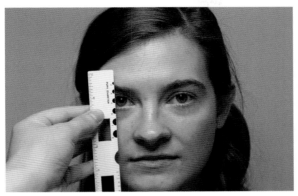

**FIGURE 2-13** | Measurement of pupil size with a pupillary gauge.

3. Move the overhead lamp so the light is shining on both eyes equally. Observe the size, shape, and location of the pupil in each eye. If a difference in pupil size is observed or was observed in step 2, measure each pupil by placing the pupillary gauge vertically next to the patient's pupil of the right eye. Repeat for the left eye.

4. *Direct pupil response*: Dim the overhead light or direct it away from the patient's eyes. Remind the patient to look at the distant target. Shine the transilluminator light into their right eye and observe the size and the speed of the pupillary constriction in this (ipsilateral) eye. Repeat one or two more times.

5. *Consensual pupil response*: Shine the transilluminator light into the right eye and observe the size and the speed of the pupillary constriction in the left (contralateral) eye. Repeat one or two more times.

6. Repeat steps 4 and 5 shining the transilluminator light into the left eye, again observing the direct and consensual responses of the appropriate pupils.

7. *Swinging flashlight test (afferent pupillary defect test)*: Move the transilluminator light between the eyes rapidly, leaving it on each eye for ~3 seconds. Observe the response (dilation or constriction) and the size of each pupil immediately when the light first arrives there and during the 3-second observation period. Be sure to shine an equal intensity of light into each eye on the same relative part of the retina and point the light slightly temporally to avoid spillover into the other eye. Repeat one or two more cycles.

8. If either or both pupils fail to respond directly or consensually, or if their responses are sluggish, test the near (accommodative) response of the pupil (see Procedure 8.4).

**Notes**
- If your patient is having trouble keeping their eyes open during pupil testing, you can modify the procedure by asking the patient to look slightly up during testing. This activates the levator palpebreae superioris muscle, which may diminish the blink reflex in some patients.

## Recording

- If all the pupillary responses are normal, record PERRL, (-)RAPD (Pupils Equal Round Reactive to Light, no Relative Afferent Pupillary Defect).
- Record only the letters that apply, omitting the others (e.g., if anisocoria is present, omit the E and record pupil sizes instead).
- If immediate dilation or pupillary escape is observed on the swinging flashlight test, record (+)RAPD (positive relative afferent pupillary defect) followed by the affected eye.

## Examples

- PERRL, (–)RAPD
- PERRL, (+)RAPD OS
- PRRL, (–)RAPD, OD > OS by 1 mm in dim and bright
- PRRL, (–)RAPD; dim: OD 5 mm OS 8 mm, bright: OD 4 mm OS 6 mm

## Expected Findings

- Pupil sizes should be equal between eyes in bright and dim light.
- Pupillary reaction should be the same during direct, consensual, and swinging flashlight test.
- Pupil size in bright illumination is expected to be 1.5–4.0 mm.
- Pupil size in dim illumination is expected to be 3–8.5 mm.

## 2.16 FINGER COUNTING VISUAL FIELDS

### Purpose

The aim of this procedure is to screen for previously unnoted visual field defects. This technique is generally effective only for substantial field loss.

### Equipment

- Overhead lamp
- Occluder

### Setup

- The patient removes their spectacles.
- The examiner faces the patient at eye level 60–80 cm from the patient.
- The space between the patient and the examiner should be brightly illuminated, but the light should not shine directly into either the patient's or the examiner's eyes.

### Procedure

1. Instruct the patient to cover their left eye with the occluder.
2. Close your right eye and keep your left eye open. Use an eyepatch if you are unable to close only one eye.
3. Instruct the patient to look at your open left eye while being aware of their side vision. Tell the patient that you will be holding up one, two, or four fingers in their side vision, and ask them to tell you how many fingers you are holding up. *Note:* Avoid holding up three fingers because this stimulus is too easily confused with two or four fingers.
4. Place your closed fist in the peripheral visual field. Your hand should be in the far periphery, but at a location where you will be able to distinguish the number of fingers exposed. Finger counting fields are actually a form of VA of the peripheral visual field, so the fingers should not be moved or wiggled. In finger counting fields, the patient's visual field is compared to the examiner's field, which is presumed to be full.

5. Expose one, two, or four fingers, taking care that they are brightly illuminated, that the darkened exam room (not your hand or arm) provides the background, that they are not pointing toward the patient, and that the fingers are in a plane midway between you and the patient (**Figure 2-14**).

6. Repeat step 5 in the appropriate eight locations in the field, on each side of the four visual field meridians. Be mindful not to expose fingers directly along or straddling the meridians.

7. When you have mapped the field for the right eye, have the patient occlude their right eye and repeat steps 4 through 6 on the patient's left eye. As the examiner, close your left eye or move the eye patch to cover your left eye and have the patient fixate on your open right eye.

8. Throughout the test, monitor the patient's fixation and keep reminding them to maintain fixation on your open eye.

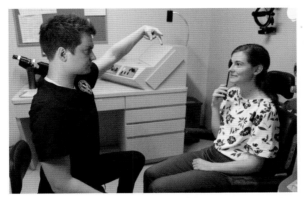

**FIGURE 2-14** | An example of finger counting visual fields. The examiner is exposing two fingers in the superior nasal field of the patient's left eye. Although it cannot be seen in the image, the examiner's left eye is closed.

### Recording
- If the patient accurately identifies your fingers in all eight meridians without looking directly at your hand, record Full or FTFC (Full To Finger Counting).
- Use FCF (Finger Counting Fields) to identify the procedure.
- If the field is abnormal, record "restricted" followed by the location of the restriction.

### Examples
- FCF: Full OD, Full OS
- FCF: FTFC OD, FTFC OS
- FCF: restricted temporally OD, restricted inferior-nasally OS

### Expected Findings
- Full visual field in the right and left eye

### Notes
- If the patient has a large refractive error preventing them from seeing the examiner's fingers, the patient may keep their spectacles on.

## 2.17 SUMMARY OF EXPECTED FINDINGS

Table 2-4 summarizes the expected findings of the core entrance tests.

| TABLE 2-4. Expected Findings for Entrance Tests | |
| --- | --- |
| **Procedure** | **Expected Findings** |
| **Visual Acuity** | 20/20 or better<br>No more than one line difference between eyes |
| **LogMAR VA** | 0.00 or better (a negative value)<br>No more than 0.16 difference between eyes |
| **Massachusetts VA Test** | Appropriate for child's age:<br>20/50 3 years old and younger<br>20/40 4–5 years old<br>20/32 5 years old and older |
| **Color Vision** | No errors or difference between eyes |
| **Cover Test** | 1Δ XP at distance (±2Δ)<br>3Δ XP at near (±3Δ) |
| **Stereopsis** | 20 seconds of arc |
| **Near Point of Convergence** | • Acc: 5/7 cm<br>• Light:7/10 cm<br>• R/G: 5/7 cm<br>• R/L: norms TBD expected to be similar to light with red/green glasses |
| **Hirschberg Test** | 0.5 mm nasal OD and OS |
| **Extraocular Motilities** | SAFE OD and OS |
| **Pupils** | PERRL, (–)RAPD |
| **Screening Visual Fields** | FTFC OD and OS |

FTFC, full to finger counting; PERRL, (–)RAPD, pupils equal round reactive to light, no relative afferent pupillary defect; SAFE, smooth, accurate, full, and extensive; VA, visual acuity

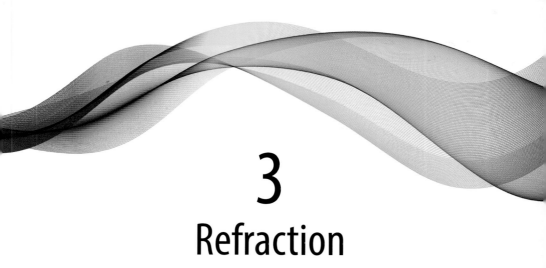

# 3

# Refraction

Hilary Gaiser, OD, MSc  /  Jennifer Reilly, OD, MSc, FAAO  /  Anita Gulmiri, OD, FAAO

## 3.1 INTRODUCTION TO REFRACTION

Refraction is as much an art form as it is a science. It is the basis of optimal vision and a proper and well thought out refraction must meet the patient's essential needs and visual function. Above all, refraction must be a well-considered process involving clinical decision-making skills and incorporating both the patient's subjective responses and the functional needs of the patient. All good refractions must first start with a careful history of both the patient's avocational and occupational visual requirements. Comfort is also a consideration and 20/20 clear acuity does not always translate to 20/20 happy and comfortable.

The procedures outlined here (**Figure 3-1**) are designed to guide the budding refractionist through the main steps and side roads of the subjective refraction procedure. It is not an exhaustive list of all the methods that can be used for refraction but rather designed to form a solid foundation for which other methods can be incorporated as the refractionist gains the relevant clinical experience. Clinical experience is perhaps the best teacher of refractive decision-making skills and it is highly recommended that the novice consults an experienced mentor to help guide their educational journey.

There are several main steps to consider when performing the subjective refraction procedure to determine the lenses that will allow the patient to achieve the most clear and comfortable vision with the easiest adaptation to glasses. These important steps are as follows: determination of the most appropriate starting point and method of refraction, the refraction procedure itself including an appropriate endpoint, confirmation or comparison of the refraction results as needed, and determination of the final spectacle prescription (SRx or Rx) of the patient.

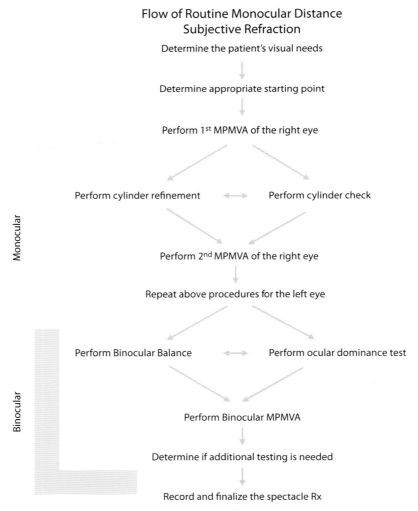

FIGURE 3-1. | Flowchart of routine distance subjective refraction.

Determination of the most appropriate starting point begins with an understanding of who the patient is sitting in your examination chair, their visual goals, and their current refractive status. Based on this information, the clinician makes an informed decision regarding the refractive starting point, e.g., retinoscopy, auto-refraction, or habitual Rx, and the most appropriate method of refraction, e.g., trial frame, phoropter, and/or use of cycloplegia.

The next part of the refractive process is the refinement of the starting point. This includes gathering the subjective responses of the patient in regard to changes in the power of lenses used during the refractive process, i.e., subjective refraction. Although the subjective responses of the patient are important, it is critical that the clinician understand the role of objective findings in the refraction process and when to use them in determining the most appropriate spectacle Rx for the patient. In some cases, the objective findings may be the best or only determinant for the final prescription, such as with small children.

Lastly, the end goal of the refractive process is to determine the final Rx for the patient. This may involve performing binocular balancing or demonstration of the final Rx in a trial frame. It cannot be stressed enough how a simple demonstration of the final Rx in a trial frame can build rapport and trust in your abilities with your patients. The trial frame can also be used to reassess the visual needs and goals of the patient which will aid in the discussion of the best method of correction, e.g., bifocal, progressive addition lenses, distance vision only, and the most appropriate lens options, e.g., polycarbonate lenses or anti-reflective coating. Promoting the idea of spectacles being an individualized tool to aid the patient with their visual and occupational needs is of benefit to all patients and their refractionists.

## 3.2 INTERPUPILLARY DISTANCE (PD)

### Purpose
The aim of this procedure is to determine the distance in millimeters between the entrance pupils of the two eyes for a given viewing distance. This is performed most often to fit spectacle lenses or set up and align a trial frame or phoropter.

### Equipment
- An easy-to-hold ruler marked in millimeters or a pupillometer

### Setup
- The examiner sits directly in front of the patient at eye level.
- The examiner's face should be located at the patient's customary near working distance (usually 40 cm).
- The near PD is typically measured before the distance PD when using a ruler.

### Procedure
*Near PD*

1. Close your right eye and instruct the patient to look at your open left eye. Align the zero-point of the ruler at the temporal edge of the patient's pupil margin of their right eye. Stabilize the ruler by resting two or three fingers on the patient's face and by lightly resting the ruler flat on the bridge of the patient's nose.

2. While the patient maintains fixation on your open left eye, measure from the temporal pupil margin of the patient's right eye to the nasal edge of the pupil margin of the patient's left eye. (**Figure 3-2**). This measurement is the near PD. For pupil irregularities, the temporal and nasal limbus can be used instead of the pupil margin.

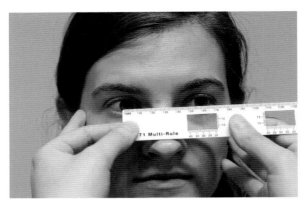

**FIGURE 3-2.**    Photo of the examiner measuring the near PD; the zero is aligned with the temporal pupil margin of the patient's right eye and the measurement is taken at the corresponding point, the nasal pupil margin, of the patient's left eye. The near PD is 57 mm as measured here.

*Distance PD*

1. While keeping the ruler in the same position as step 1 above, close your left eye and instruct the patient to look at your now open right eye. *Note:* The patient's eyes have moved, and the ruler is no longer aligned with the temporal pupil margin of their right eye; this is on purpose and the ruler should remain in place.

2. With the patient maintaining fixation on your open right eye, determine the measurement of the nasal pupil margin of the patient's left eye, or corresponding ocular landmarks as described in step 2 above. This is the distance PD. Again, the zero marker is no longer aligned with the patient's temporal pupil margin of their right eye, the examiner is only observing where the nasal pupil margin of the left eye aligns on the ruler.

3. Recheck the entire procedure by repeating steps 1 and 2 for near PD and distance PD.

   *Note:* By following steps 1 and 2, listed above, although the patient never looks at distance, you measure their distance PD, with each eye pointing straight ahead, as if the patient had been looking at distance (**Figure 3-3**).

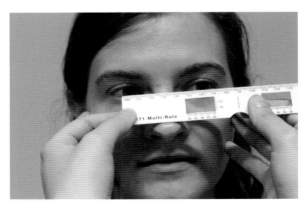

**FIGURE 3-3.**    Photo of the examiner measuring the distance PD; the zero *was* aligned with the temporal pupil margin of the patient's right eye when the patient was looking at the examiners left eye (near PD measurement); but now the patient is looking at the examiner's right eye and the examiner kept the ruler in place to record the measurement at the nasal pupil margin. The distance PD is 60mm as measured here.

## Pupillometer

Pupillary distance can also be measured with an instrument called a pupillometer, which is used like a pair of binoculars.

1. Use the dials to set the instrument to the desired distance to be measured, distance ($\infty$) or near (may have several options for the desired working distance in cm), and binocular or monocular PD.

2. Instruct the patient to rest their forehead on one end of the instrument with their nose in the groove and to look through the two eye pieces.

3. Instruct the patient to look at the target inside the instrument, often rings with a white or green dot in the center.

4. Look through the eyepiece at the opposite (examiner) end of the pupillometer and use the slides on the top or bottom of the instrument to align a vertical mire (hairline) with either the center of each of the patient's pupils or the corneal light reflex depending upon manufacturer guidelines for the specific pupillometer used.

5. Remove the instrument and record the binocular and/or monocular PD readings. The procedure can be repeated for other desired distances, e.g., intermediate, if multiple measurements are indicated.

## Recording

- Write the distance PD in millimeters, a slash, then the near PD in millimeters. *Note:* Although the near PD is measured before the distance PD with the ruler, the distance PD is recorded first, followed by the near PD (see Examples below). Recording may also omit the "mm" units due to standard unit use for the procedure.

- Sometimes the eyes are not centered with respect to the nose and separate monocular PDs are recorded for each eye relative to the center of the bridge of the patient's nose. Monocular PD's are also indicated for progressive additional lens (PAL) measurements.

## Examples

- PD 64/61
- PD 62/58 mm
- PD OD 30/28, OS 32/30

## Expected Findings

- The average measurement for adults is 63/60 mm.
- The near PD is typically 3–4 mm smaller than the distance PD.

## 3.3 LENSOMETRY

### Purpose

The aim of this procedure is to measure the back vertex refractive power, the cylinder axis, the optical center, and the prismatic power of prescription lenses and spectacles. *Note:* This procedure is also referred to as *focimetry* or *vertometry*.

### Indications

- To measure, or neutralize, a patient's habitual correction or an unknown lens.
- To verify a prescription before dispensing from an optical shop.

### Equipment

- Lensometer
- Eyeglasses or lenses to be measured

## Basic Components of a Lensometer

Since lensometers differ, the examiner should review the location of the components and the specific instructions provided by the manufacturer for the lensometer they are using. The following components are common to all lensometers and are important to the examiner in reading a lens prescription:

### External Parts

The external parts include (see **Figure 3-4**):

A. Adjustable eyepiece for focusing the instrument for the examiner's eye.

B. Lens holder and lens table to support the lens that is being measured.

C. Power wheel for reading the refractive power of the lens.

D. Axis wheel in 1° increments from 1° to 180° to read the axis of cylindrical lenses.

E. Marking device which includes an inkwell and pens for dotting the optical center of the lens.

### Internal Parts

The internal parts include (see **Figure 3-5**):

F. The reticle focuses and determines prism power. The reticle is focused by the eyepiece of the instrument.

G. The mires consists of two sets of lines perpendicular to one another for reading the power of the lens. These lines are focused by the power wheel. One set of lines corresponds to the sphere power of the lens and the other to the cylinder power.

To distinguish the sphere and cylinder lines for your particular lensometer, with no lenses in place, set the axis wheel to 180° and focus the mires. The vertically oriented mires are the "sphere lines" and the horizontally oriented mires are the "cylinder lines." At this time, it is also useful to see what the power wheel actually reads; the reading should be 0.00 D, but often a small offset may be detected. Findings should be adjusted for any offset observed at this time.

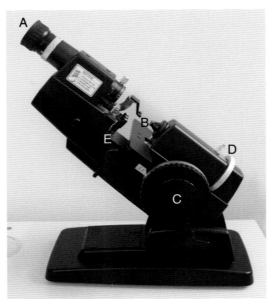

**FIGURE 3-4.** Example of external lensometer parts with corresponding labels: (A) eye piece, (B) lens holder and table, (C) power wheel, (D) axis wheel, and (E) inkwell with pens.

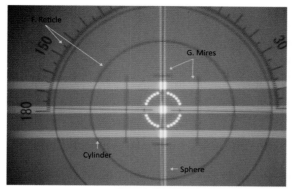

**FIGURE 3-5.** Example of internal lensometer parts with corresponding labels, (F) reticle (black lines), (G) mires (green lines).

## Setup

- With the power wheel set to zero, the examiner focuses the eyepiece by turning the eyepiece as far counterclockwise as possible, and then slowly turning it clockwise until the reticle first comes into sharp focus.
- Determine which part of the mires is used for determining the spherical power of the lens and which part is used for determining the cylindrical power of the lens. This varies depending on the manufacturer of the lensometer.
- If testing a pair of glasses, always check the right lens first (by convention).
- Place the lens or pair of glasses in the lensometer with the ocular surface of the patient's right lens away from you (temples pointed away from you). The lens is held in place by the lens holder and is held level on the lens table (see **Figure 3-6**).
- Center the lens by moving it so that the image of the lensometer mires is aligned in the center of the eyepiece reticle. *Note:* If the lens has been made with prism ground into it, it may be impossible to center the mires in the reticle, see Prism below.

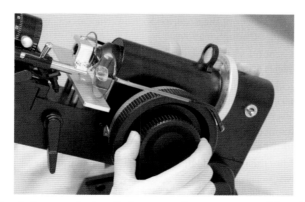

**FIGURE 3-6.** Spectacles properly placed in lensometer for measurement of the right lens.

## Procedure

*Single-Vision Lenses*

1. Once the lens is centered, rotate the power wheel to high plus (around +5.00 D to +8.00 D) and adjust the power wheel in the minus direction until the mires come into sharp focus. If the spherical and cylindrical lines of the mires come into focus at the same time,

the lens is spherical. Read the power of the lens from the power wheel and record. *Note:* If the mires are coming into better focus as you approach +5.00 D, but not yet sharp, you may have to increase the power wheel beyond +5.00 D to neutralize the lens.

2. If the spherical and cylindrical lines do not come into focus at the same time, the lens has a cylindrical component. To read the power of a spherocylindrical lens, start with enough plus power to blur the lensometer mires (around +5.00 D to +8.00 D), then rotate the power wheel toward less plus until the sphere lines come into focus. At the same time, orient the axis wheel of the lensometer so that the sphere lines are perfectly continuous. Read the power from the power wheel and record it as the spherical portion of the prescription. *Note:* If the cylinder lines come into focus first when moving the power wheel in the minus direction, the axis wheel should be rotated 90°. The sphere lines should then come into focus before the cylinder lines, which is necessary for measuring glasses in minus-cylinder form.

3. Focus the cylinder lines by continuing to rotate the power wheel toward more minus power. The difference between the power when the sphere lines are in focus and the cylinder lines are in focus is the amount of minus-cylinder power in the lens. Only the power wheel is moved to determine the cylinder power; the axis wheel was adjusted when the sphere lines were brought into focus and is not adjusted again. The axis of the cylinder is read directly from the lensometer's protractor.

4. *Optional:* before moving the glasses, dot the optical center (OC) of the lens with the lensometer's marking device.

5. Repeat steps 1 through 4 for the left lens.

6. If necessary, when both lenses have been measured and dotted, measure the distance between the optical centers of the lenses and compare it to the patient's PD. If the patient's PD and the PD of the spectacles are not the same, or if there is a vertical discrepancy in the heights of the optical centers of the two lenses, calculate the amount of induced prism using *Prentice's rule* (see step 4 under Prism).

7. The power of rigid and soft contact lenses can also be read in the lensometer. These procedures are described in Chapter 6.

### Multifocal Lenses

1. Read and record the power of the distance portion (the carrier) of each of the two lenses as described in steps 1 through 6 above.

2. Turn the glasses around so that the ocular surface faces you (temples are toward you). Ensure the spectacles are again placed flat and level on the stage.

3. Recheck one meridian in the carrier and compare the power in this meridian to the power in the *same meridian* through the near portion (the segment) of the lens (e.g., compare the spherical power to the spherical power or the cylindrical power to the cylindrical power). The difference between these powers is the add. It is often necessary to reset the axis orientation during this step.

4. Although the add in the right and left lenses is usually the same, the add should be determined separately for each lens.

5. Progressive addition lenses are read in the same manner as other multifocal lenses, but the examiner must use the guidelines of the manufacturer for locating the near portion of the lens.

### Prism

#### Prescribed Prism

1. If the lens has been made with prism ground into it, it may be impossible to center the target in the reticle. In this case, have the patient wear the glasses and dot the lens at the

location of the patient's line of sight for each eye. Position the lens in the lensometer so the dot is in the center of the reticle. Read the amount of prism using the prism scale in the lensometer. It is important to realize that the center of the mires will be displaced toward the BASE, not the apex, of the ground in prism.

*Note*: With high amounts of prism, it is difficult or impossible to locate the center of the target. In this case, handheld prisms are added to center the target and to determine the amount of prism in the lens.

2. Record the amount and direction of prism in the glasses for each lens separately.

### Induced Prism

1. Locate the center of the mires in the center of the eyepiece reticle.
2. Dot this location on the lens; this is the optical center of the lens.
3. Subsequently dot the location of the patient's line of sight on the lens (patient wears the spectacles to do so).
4. When the optical center of the lens and the location of the patient's line of sight do not coincide, compute the induced prism using Prentice's rule:

$$\Delta = DC/10$$

where D is the power of the lens in diopters and C is the linear distance between the patient's line of sight and the optical center of the lens in mm. Vertical and horizontal prisms are calculated separately.

*Note*: Calculate the prism induced by each lens separately. The prism induced by the spectacles is the net discrepancy between the prism induced by each of the two lenses.

## Recording

- Record the prescription (Rx) for each lens separately in standard Rx form.
- Record the amount and direction of the prescribed prism or induced prism in the glasses, if applicable.

## Examples

- OD: −2.75 sph
  OS: −2.25 − 1.00 × 010
- OD: +1.00 − 1.50 × 090, Add +2.00
  OS: +1.25 − 0.75 × 105, Add +2.00
- OD: −1.00 − 1.00 × 180, 2 Δ BI, Add +2.25
  OS: −1.25 − 0.75 × 170, 2 Δ BI, Add +2.25
- OD: +1.00 − 2.50 × 095, Add +1.00
  OS: +1.25 − 2.75 × 102, Add +1.50

## 3.4 INTRODUCTION TO THE MANUAL PHOROPTER

### Purpose

The phoropter is an instrument used to test individual lenses on each eye during the refraction procedure to determine an appropriate spectacle prescription (SRx or Rx) for the patient. In addition to lenses, there are a number of auxiliary lenses and other dials for various procedures.

### Setup

Prior to performing testing in the phoropter it must first be fit to the patient using a variety of knobs, levers, and levels. Failure to adequately fit the phoropter to the face of the patient can

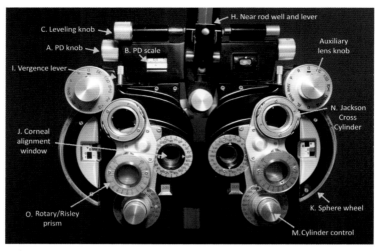

**FIGURE 3-7.** | Photo of a manual phoropter in common use today with labeled parts.

lead to inaccurate results and discomfort for the patient. The controls to fit the phoropter to the patient are as follows (see **Figure 3-7**):

**A.** PD knob: used to adjust the pupillary distance of the patient

**B.** PD scale: where the PD value is read

**C.** Leveling knob: used to level the phoropter before the patient's eyes

**D.** Vertex distance control: used to control the distance of the phoropter from the patient's face (not pictured above)

**E.** Pantoscopic tilt knob: used to adjust the angle of the plane of the phoropter before the patient's face (not pictured above)

**F.** Locking knob: used to lock the phoropter in place before the patient (not pictured above)

**G.** Rotation knob: used to adjust the phoropter around the vertical axis (not pictured above)

**H.** Near rod well and lever: used to place and lock the near rod in place for testing and raise and lower the near rod as needed

**I.** Vergence levers: used to adjust the PD from distance to near for near tests

**J.** Corneal alignment window: to ensure proper setup and vertex distance

*Auxiliary Lens Knob*

The auxiliary lens knob is used to change apertures and other lenses used during various procedures (see **Figure 3-8**). There is a secondary dial located on the rim of the auxiliary lens knob, which changes the spherical lenses by increments of 3 D, this is referred to as the strong sphere control. Please note that not all phoropters may have all of the described lenses. The remaining auxiliary lens options are described below:

**O:** the open position with a zero powered lens

**R:** retinoscopy lens; +1.50 lens used to compensate for working distance during retinoscopy

**P:** polarized lens; used for some binocular vision testing procedures; axis is typically 135° in the right eye and 45° in the left eye

**WMV/RMV:**  vertical Maddox rod for binocular vision testing; typically, white for the left eye and red for the right eye

**WMH/RMH:**  horizontal Maddox rod for binocular vision testing; typically, white for the left eye and red for the right eye

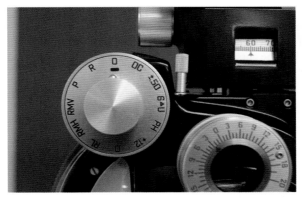

**FIGURE 3-8.** | Auxiliary lens knob.

**RL/GL:** red and green lenses for binocular vision testing

**O:** secondary open aperture for convenience

**+0.12 D:** spherical plus lens in 1/8th D step

**PH:** single pinhole aperture (see Procedure 2.7)

**10 BI/6 BU:** 10Δ base in left eye 6Δ base up right eye; dissociating prisms

**±0.50:** fixed Jackson Cross Cylinder (JCC); axis is preset for binocular vision tests

**OC:** occluding lens

*Lens Control Knobs*

The phoropter has two sets of lens controls, one for sphere (typically, +16.75 D to −19.00 D) and one for plano-cylindrical lenses (typically, 0.00 D to −6.00 D or 0.00 D to +6.00 D) depending on if the phoropter is in minus cylinder or plus cylinder. In general, plus power is typically indicated by black type on the dials while minus power is indicated by red type.

*Spherical Lens Control*

The large wheel **K** is commonly referred to as the *weak sphere dial* (increments of +/− 0.25 D) in contrast to the strong sphere dial (increments of 3.00 D) **L** (see **Figure 3-9**). The weak sphere dial is more commonly used during the refraction procedure to refine the spherical component of the patient's refraction.

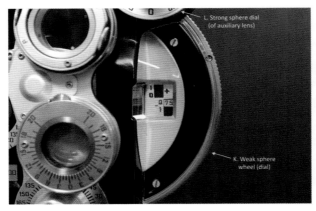

**FIGURE 3-9.** | Diagram of spherical lens controls.

### (Minus/Plus) Plano-cylinder Control

(Minus/plus) plano-cylindrical lenses (increments of 0.25 D) and axis control (increments of 5°) are located on dial **M** (see **Figure 3-7**). The cylindrical power is manipulated by using the center dial, while the outside sleeve of the dial is used to rotate the axis (see **Figure 3-10**).

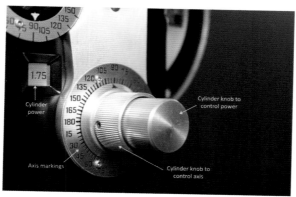

**FIGURE 3-10.**  Diagram of cylindrical lens controls.

### Additional Controls

In addition to adjustment/setup controls, auxiliary lenses, and sphere and cylinder dials, the phoropter contains other controls for additional testing. These are:

**N.** JCC: primarily used for refinement of the cylindrical component of the patient's Rx. The standard JCC is typically +/− 0.25 D and the red dots indicate the minus-cylinder axis and the white dots the plus-cylinder axis. The roll knob can be utilized for rapid flipping of the cross cylinders and is placed 45° away from the cylinder axes (see **Figure 3-11A**).

**O.** Rotary/Risley Prisms: primarily used for the introduction of prism during the refraction procedure and during binocular vision testing. Each rotary prism has a range of up to 20Δ and when paired give a total of 40Δ in any base direction. The scale is marked in increments of 1Δ and can be oriented to determine base up, base down, base in, or base out prism. With the zero positioned in the horizontal meridian (at 180°) the indicator arrow can be placed superiorly for BU prism and inferiorly for BD prism. When the zero is placed in the vertical meridian (at 90°) the indicator arrow can be placed medially for BI prism and laterally for BO prism (see **Figure 3-11B**).

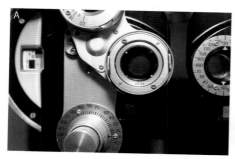
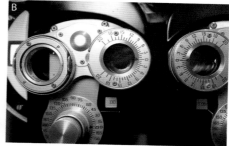

**FIGURE 3-11.**  Diagram of (A) JCC and (B) Risley prism.

## 3.5 STATIC RETINOSCOPY

### Purpose

This is an objective technique used to determine the refractive error of the patient at distance. This procedure is considered static as the patient's accommodation is not directly stimulated during the procedure. The results of retinoscopy may serve as a starting point for the subjective refraction procedure or as an objective determination of the glasses prescription if the patient is unable to respond to subjective testing. Optically, the far point of the patient is moved to the plane of the retinoscope using lenses, while the patient views a non-accommodative distance target.

### Equipment

- Retinoscope
- Phoropter, lens rack, or loose lenses
- Non-accommodative fixation target (e.g., 20/400 isolated Snellen letter)
- *Optional* red/green filter projected over the fixation target

### Setup

- Retinoscopy is performed binocularly, without glasses, behind a clean, well-fit phoropter with the proper distance PD of the patient dialed into the phoropter.
- The examiner positions themselves in front of the patient at their working distance (see **Table 3-1**) along the patient's visual axis without blocking the fixation target.
- The patient should be instructed to keep both eyes open during retinoscopy and to inform the practitioner if their head blocks the fixation target at any time. The phoropter may be rotated to allow the patient to see the target while the examiner maintains alignment along the patient's visual axis.
- During retinoscopy, the examiner keeps both eyes open and examines the patient's right eye with their right eye while holding the retinoscope in their right hand and vice versa for the left eye.
- Retinoscopy is most easily done in dim illumination.

| TABLE 3-1. Explanation of Retinoscopy Working Distance (WD) |
| --- |
| **Working Distance** |
| The "working distance" of the practitioner is the distance from the patient to the plane of the retinoscope. Since the far point of the patient is moved to the plane of the scope during the procedure while the patient is fixating on a distance target, the working distance must be compensated for in the final retinoscopy findings. |
| Common working distances are 20 in (50 cm) and 26 in (67 cm) representing −2.00 D and −1.50 D adjustments to the gross findings respectively. |
| "Gross results" refer to the power of the lens needed to neutralize the reflex without subtracting the working distance, while "net results" refer to the final findings compensating for the working distance. |
| Although 50 cm and 67 cm are common working distances (WD), alternatives dependent upon the practitioner's preference and stature are acceptable. This can be determined by measuring the distance of the patient to the plane of the retinoscope and converting to diopters: WD = 100/measurement in cm. |
| It is also acceptable to have two different working distances, e.g., longer distance for retinoscopy in the phoropter versus retinoscopy when using a retinoscopy rack (ret rack). |

## Procedure

*Retinoscopy in the Phoropter*

Initial Steps

1. With the patient seated behind the phoropter and at eye level with the examiner, quickly scope both eyes in succession with the streak oriented vertically making note of any differences in the brightness of the two reflexes. If the two reflexes are relatively equal, then the patient is not likely to have a large amount of anisometropia. The streak should then be rotated 360° in each eye while observing for any "breaks" or "scissoring" of the reflex. Breaks, differences in motion, or scissoring of the reflex indicate that the patient is likely to have astigmatism (**Figure 3-12**).

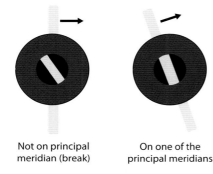

Not on principal
meridian (break)

On one of the
principal meridians

**FIGURE 3-12.** │ Diagram of the appearance of the retinoscopic reflex when using the break phenomenon to locate the principal meridians of an astigmatic eye.

Fogging

1. Appropriate fogging is critical to control the patient's accommodation, particularly in young adults and children. Inappropriate control of accommodation can lead to a more minus powered finding than what the patient actually has. Fogging can be accomplished with one of the techniques below.

   a. In a patient of unknown Rx or no Rx, fogging can be achieved by performing retinoscopy quickly on the left eye of the patient with the goal of a "rough" neutrality in a single meridian (typically 180°). The working distance is not removed at this stage leaving the patient fogged by the amount of the examiner's working distance. See **Table 3-2** for a description of neutrality.

**TABLE 3-2. Explanation of Neutrality of the Retinoscopy Reflex**

| Neutrality |
| --- |
| The desired endpoint for retinoscopy is "neutralization" of the reflex. When determining neutrality look for a bright, white, full reflex in the center of the pupil. |
| Larger pupils may have peripheral distortions making neutrality harder to determine. In these cases, focus on the center of the reflex of the pupil when determining neutrality. |
| A "range" of neutrality may be noted, i.e., more than one lens over which the reflex looks neutral. In these cases, the most plus lens can be selected. |
| Bracketing of the reflex is frequently used by experienced retinoscopists. In this technique, lenses are added until reversal of motion is noted. The most plus lens used before reversal can be used as the endpoint. |
| A dull, dim reflex (which indicates high refractive error) can be misinterpreted as a neutralized reflex. Look for a full, bright, reflex. If the motion of the reflex is hard to determine, use the "strong" power knob on the phoropter to add +/− 3.00 D of power to search for a better reflex. |

b. If the Rx of the patient is known, more plus power of 0.75 to 1.00 D can be added to the Rx of the left eye of the patient in order to fog the patient. Confirm that the patient is fogged by quickly measuring visual acuity (VA) OS (expect ~3–4 lines of decreased VA).

While appropriate fogging is crucial, too much fogging can stimulate tonic accommodation which can skew the retinoscopy results. This can be avoided by confirming that the patient can continue to see the 20/400 target.

*Note:* An alternative to the above fogging techniques is the "three-eyed-method." In this method, retinoscopy is performed thoroughly on the right eye, then the left eye, and then again on the right eye. This should ensure that the patient is fogged in the right eye while performing retinoscopy on the left eye and then the initial retinoscopy results of the right eye are rechecked while the left eye is fogged. A reminder that the working distance is only "removed" at the end of the retinoscopy procedure as this ensures the patient is fogged by the amount of the doctor's working distance.

### Neutralization

1. Once the left eye is fogged, begin scoping the reflex of the right eye. If a break, change in motion, or scissoring is observed, proceed to step 2. If no break, variation in motion between meridians, or scissoring is noted (lack of astigmatism), proceed to neutralize the reflex using the spherical lenses in the phoropter. Starting with the retinoscope in the sleeve down position (see **Figure 3-13**), observe the reflex for with or against motion. With motion appears as the light reflex within the pupil moving in the same direction as the retinoscope streak, while against motion appears as the light reflex within the pupil moving in the opposite direction of the retinoscope streak. If with motion is noted, plus power is added until the reflex is neutralized (full, bright, white, central reflex) while if against motion is noted, minus power is added until the reflex is neutralized. *Note:* The retinoscope can also be used in the sleeve up position. If the sleeve up position is used the motion and lenses needed to neutralize the reflex will be reversed, i.e., against motion will need plus power and with motion will need minus power. Some practitioners find it easier to determine neutrality while working in with motion.

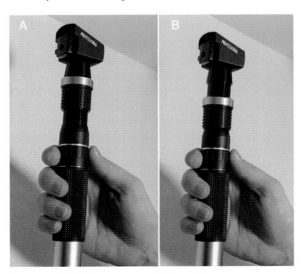

**FIGURE 3-13.** Retinoscope with (A) sleeve up and (B) sleeve down.

2. If a break, variation in motion between meridians, or scissoring of the reflex is noted when scoping an eye 360°, then the patient has astigmatism, and the two principal meridians will need to be identified and neutralized separately. These can be determined by looking for alignment of the retinoscopy reflex, i.e., the reflex within the pupil will move parallel to the movement of the streak on the patient's face or eye when the streak is aligned with one of the two principal meridians. *Note:* The orientation of the streak of the retinoscope is 90° away from the meridian being neutralized, e.g., when the streak of the retinoscope is vertical the horizontal meridian is being neutralized.

a. When performing retinoscopy in a minus cylinder phoropter, the most plus meridian (most with motion or least against motion) should be neutralized first with spherical lenses and then the more minus meridian (less with motion or more against motion) with the minus cylinder lenses. The orientation of the axis should be set in conjugate with the orientation of the most plus meridian. To determine the most plus meridian in the sleeve down position, look for the reflex that is closest to neutrality if against motion is noted in both principal meridians and the meridian that is furthest from neutrality if both principal meridians have with motion (see **Figure 3-14**). If there is opposing motion, i.e., against and with, the principal meridian noted to have with motion is the most plus meridian.

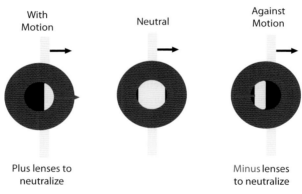

With Motion · Neutral · Against Motion

Plus lenses to neutralize · Minus lenses to neutralize

**FIGURE 3-14.**   Schematic demonstrating the range of motion of the retinoscopy reflex. *Note:* this assumes the sleeve down position.

b. If the most plus meridian has been appropriately neutralized, then when moving to neutralize the cylindrical component, against motion should be noted (sleeve down position). It may be difficult to determine the most plus meridian when first learning retinoscopy. If with motion is noted when moving to neutralize the cylindrical component then the meridians have been switched; rotate the axis 90° away from the original orientation, return to the sphere wheel and re-neutralize, then return to the cylinder. Against motion should now be noted and can be neutralized with minus cyl.

*Note:* A plus-plano cylinder phoropter is used in a manner consistent with the minus-plano cylinder phoropter with the exception that the most minus principal meridian is neutralized first, followed by the most plus principal meridian for the cylinder.

3. When neutrality is observed, recheck all meridians in both sleeve up and sleeve down position to confirm neutrality before moving to the left eye. The reflex should be neutral in both sleeve orientations. When moving to the left eye do not remove the dioptric amount of the working distance, as this will serve as the fogging lens for the right eye during left eye retinoscopy. Now perform retinoscopy (neutralize the reflex) as described above on the left eye.

4. To convert the gross retinoscopy results to net, algebraically add a minus lens equal to your working distance in diopters to the spherical lens that produced neutrality, e.g., add −2.00 D for a working distance of 20 in/50 cm and −1.50 D for a working distance of 26 in/67 cm. Make this adjustment in the phoropter before checking VA.

5. Measure the VA OD and OS through the net results.

*Retinoscopy with Retinoscopy Racks or Loose Lenses*
The procedure for retinoscopy in free space is essentially the same as that in a phoropter with the notable exception that the most plus meridian need not be neutralized first (see **Figure 3-15** for setup). An optical cross is recommended for beginners to record the gross and net findings before converting to prescription form (see **Figure 3-16**). *Note:* the working distance must be subtracted from both meridians when calculating the net retinoscopy in free space since the cylinder is not accounted for as it is in a minus-plano phoropter.

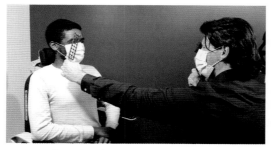

**FIGURE 3-15.** Retinoscopy performed with retinoscopy rack. The patient is viewing a non-accommodative target in the distance, past the examiner.

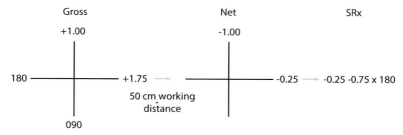

**FIGURE 3-16.** Optical cross example from retinoscopy rack or loose lens findings. In this example, the examiner found neutrality with +1.75 sph in the 180° meridian and +1.00 sph in the 90° meridian; accounting for a working distance of 50 cm (or −2.00 D sph), the net retinoscopy result in spectacle prescription format is −0.25 −0.75 ×180.

*Free Space Retinoscopy Tips*
- Fogging can be achieved with loose lenses over the patient's glasses in trial lens clips, or by using a trial frame. Additionally, when performing retinoscopy with a retinoscopy rack the examiner can start with lenses in the high plus range and "work down."
- Axis orientation can be gauged with the use of a protractor commonly found on many models of retinoscopy racks.
- Bracketing is often helpful for use in retinoscopy racks that have power increments larger than −0.25 D.

## Recording
- Record the net retinoscopy results and VA of each eye separately.

## Examples

- Retinoscopy:
  OD: $-2.00 - 1.00 \times 180$    20/30
  OS: $-1.50 - 0.75 \times 175$    20/20
- Retinoscopy:
  OD: +2.50sph                  20/15
  OS: +2.00 $-1.00 \times 090$    20/20[+2]

## 3.6 ROUTINE DISTANCE SUBJECTIVE REFRACTION WITH THE MANUAL PHOROPTER

### Purpose

This is a subjective technique used to determine the patient's refraction. After subjective refraction is complete, light rays from a stimulus should form a point image on the retina while accommodation is fully relaxed. Although subjective refraction is a critical component of the determination of a patient's refractive error, it may not be the final spectacle prescription. The examiner must rely on their clinical judgment when determining the final, written spectacle prescription.

### Equipment

- Phoropter
- VA chart: computer generated, projector, or printed chart

### Setup

- A clean phoropter with the appropriate distance PD of the patient should be placed in front of the patient, leveled, and adjusted to fit to the patient comfortably (see Procedure 3.4). The patient should be at a comfortable height so as not to lean over, slouch, or raise themselves to see through the eye pieces.
- A full VA chart should be displayed with the 20/15 line at the bottom.
- The starting point should be dialed into the phoropter; either the net retinoscopy results, previous/habitual Rx, or results from autorefraction.

### Procedure

The steps outlined below will instruct the examiner in the entire "main road" monocular distance subjective refraction. The refraction flowchart (**Figure 3-1**) serves as a guide for the various refraction procedures. As clinical experience is gained, modifications of this procedure may be warranted. For additions and modifications to the routine distance subjective refraction procedure, see Procedures 3.7 through 3.13.

1. **Starting Point**

   Before beginning the refraction procedure, a starting point must be determined. Generally, if the patient is functioning well, VA is good, and the patient has no complaints with their current eyeglass prescription, the previous or habitual Rx can be used as the starting point. If the patient is new and autorefraction or keratometry results are desired, autorefraction results may be an appropriate starting point. Either retinoscopy or autorefraction should be considered if vision is reduced or the patient has visual complaints. In all children and those unable to sit behind an autorefractor, retinoscopy should be used.

2. **Initial (First) Monocular Maximum Plus to Maximum Visual Acuity (MPMVA)**

   This step determines the maximum amount of spherical plus power the patient can accept to reach maximum VA. The full acuity chart is displayed.

a. The procedure is performed monocularly and with fogging. To fog the patient dial in 0.75 D to 1.00 D more plus power and confirm VA has been reduced ~ 3–4 lines from the entering VA. If visual acuity does not reduce 3–4 lines, more plus should be added until this is achieved.

b. Slowly but steadily increase the amount of minus power in 0.25 D steps, rechecking VA after each addition of minus power and encouraging the patient to read the next smaller line after each change of power, e.g., "what is the smallest line that you can read now." According to Egger's principle (see **Figure 3-17**), each 0.25 D more minus should allow the patient to read one line better and the patient should demonstrate improvement in VA. Having the chart look "better" to the patient is not sufficient justification to give them more minus.

| Egger's Chart | | |
|---|---|---|
| Distance Visual Acuity | Sph. Eq. Dioptric Blur | Simple WTR Astigmatism |
| 20/20 | 0.00 | 0.00 |
| 20/25 | 0.25 | 0.50 |
| 20/30 | 0.50 | 1.00 |
| 20/40 | 0.75 | 1.50 |
| 20/50 | 1.00 | 2.00 |
| 20/70 | 1.25 | 2.50 |
| 20/100 | 1.50 | 3.00 |
| 20/200 | 2.50 | 3.50 |

**FIGURE 3-17.** Egger's chart demonstrating expected improvement, or conversely reduction, in VA corresponding to dioptric power, blur, or defocus.

c. The endpoint of the initial MPMVA is when VA cannot be improved with any addition of more minus power. Note that VA may not always be 20/20 at this point in the refraction procedure.

d. In order to progress to the refinement of cylinder power and axis, it has been recommended to perform either the duochrome procedure, leaving the patient "one into the green" *or* by adding one additional increment of −0.25 D power to the initial MPMVA.

3. **Duochrome Procedure Prior to Cylinder Refinement**

This step provides a foundation for the refinement of cylinder found on your starting point (step 1).

a. Use the red-green filter over an isolated line of letters 1–2 lines above the patient's best corrected visual acuity (BCVA) from the initial MPMVA (see **Figure 3-18**). The procedure should be performed monocularly.

b. Instruct the patient to look from the green side to the red side and back to the green and let you know on which side the letters look sharper and clearer (not darker or brighter) or if they look equally clear.

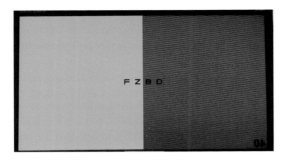

FIGURE 3-18. Duochrome target as seen by the patient.

c. If the letters on the red side are clearer or if the letters on both sides are equally clear, introduce an additional 0.25 D of minus-spherical power. If the letters on the green side are clearer, take away 0.25 D of minus (or add another 0.25 D of plus sphere).

d. The endpoint for the duochrome procedure prior to cylinder refinement is "one into the green," i.e., the minimum amount of minus power needed for the patient to report the green side of the chart has clearer letters.

*Note*: As this test relies on the optical principle of chromatic aberrations, it will still work for color anomalous patients. You may need to adjust your instruction to right and left side rather than green and red. Some patients are unresponsive to this test and seem to choose one side or the other, regardless of the lens powers in place. In this case, leave the patient over-minused by 0.25 D from the initial MPMVA (as this is another optional end point).

4. **Cylinder Refinement**

This step refines the cylinder found on the starting point according to the subjective responses of the patient and is performed after the initial MPMVA and duochrome test.

- It is generally recommended to refine the cylinder axis prior to the cylinder power if the cylinder power is > 0.50 D at the starting point. If only 0.50 D or 0.25 D of cylinder is found at the starting point, then power refinement can be performed prior to axis refinement. If the patient accepts more cylinder power when the power is refined first, then the axis may need to be refined before returning to a full power refinement.

**Cylinder Axis Refinement**

a. Isolate a line of letters 1–2 lines above the BCVA or use the circular dots target. Circular targets are preferred for the refinement of cylinder axis (see **Figure 3-19**).

b. Insert the JCC attachment over the right eye so that the thumb wheel of the JCC is in alignment with the axis of the cylinder found on the starting point. The JCC has two sets of dots located on the outside edge of the lens (red and white dots), which will straddle the thumb wheel and axis of the tentative correcting cylinder in the phoropter (see **Figure 3-20**).

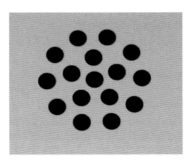

FIGURE 3-19. Circular dots target recommended for cylinder axis check.

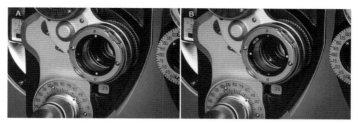

FIGURE 3-20.    Photograph of the JCC set for axis refinement, showing the JCC in its two positions or views (A and B) for tentative axis 45. Note that here the power dots straddle the axis.

c. Inform the patient that you will be showing them two views of the target and to let you know which view is clearer or if they are equal. The patient should be told that both views may be blurry, but they should select the view that is the least blurry.

d. Show the patient the two views (flip the thumb wheel) and associate each view with a number for the patient, e.g., one or two. Flipping the thumb wheel changes the orientation of the dots in relation to the axis found on the tentative starting point. Pause for 1–2 seconds to allow the patient to appreciate each view. This step may be repeated to allow the patient to compare choices.

e. Once the patient has made their selection, "chase the red" by moving the axis knob of the phoropter by 15° toward the direction of the red dots in the preferred orientation (view 1 or view 2) chosen by the patient. This will be either a clockwise or counter-clockwise direction.

f. Continue repeating steps d and e until the patient responds that both views are equal in clarity. Keep moving the axis by 15° until the preferred view switches direction (e.g., chase the red back in the direction from where you already came) and then bracket the axis change. The axis should be bracketed with the first selection being moved 15°, then 10°, 5°, and then 1°. If the patient does not respond that both views are equal in clarity but alternates between the clockwise and counterclockwise direction, select an axis in the middle of the range or the orientation that is closest to the axis in the pa-tient's habitual glasses.

g. Once the patient selects equality or the clinician selects a middle endpoint, move on to cylinder power refinement, or if power refinement has already been performed, proceed to step 5, second MPMVA.

*Note*: The greater the cylinder power, the greater the need for precision in the axis.

**Cylinder Power Refinement**

a. Insert the JCC so that one set of dots (either red or white) is aligned with the axis of the correcting cylinder set in the phoropter (see **Figure 3-21**).

b. Present two views to the patient by flipping the JCC lens using the thumb wheel and associate each view with a number for the patient, e.g., one or two. Flipping the thumb wheel changes the power of the cylinder, more or less power, in front of the patient. Ask the patient, "which view is clearer one or two or if they are equally blurry." The patient may need to be reminded that both views may be blurry but that they should select the view that is clearest of the two.

c. If the patient reports that the view with the RED dots (minus-cylinder axis) is "clearer," increase the power of the minus cylinder in the phoropter by −0.25 D. If the patient reports that the view with the WHITE dots (plus-cylinder axis) is "clearer," reduce the power of the minus cylinder in the phoropter by −0.25 D (more plus).

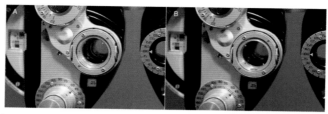

**FIGURE 3-21.** Photograph of the JCC set for power refinement, showing the JCC in its two positions or views (A and B) for power adjustment when the axis is set at 45. Note that here the power dots align with the axis.

d. Throughout the JCC power refinement, it is important to maintain the spherical equivalent of the refraction. To do this, increase or decrease the spherical power by 0.25 D in the opposite direction for each change of 0.50 D of cylinder power, e.g., the patient accepts −0.50 D more cylinder power, add +0.25 D spherical power to the refraction.

e. The endpoint of the cylinder power refinement is when both views are equally clear to the patient or the patient alternates between adding and removing cylinder power. If the patient alternates between power either select the power that is closest to the patient's habitual Rx or select the lesser powered option.

*Note:* It is recommended that if the cylinder power refinement changes by more than 0.75 D that the cylinder axis refinement be rechecked. Recall that the higher the magnitude of cylinder the more necessary it is to have the cylinder axis be refined in smaller increments.

**Cylinder Check**

A cylinder check is considered if no cylinder was found at the starting point (otherwise, continue to step 5).

a. If no cylinder was found during determination of the starting point, VA is 20/20 or better, and the patient is happy with their vision, cylinder check does not need to be performed.

b. If VA is reduced or the patient is unhappy with their vision and no cylinder was found during determination of the starting point, a cylinder check using either the clock chart or Polasky method may be used (see Procedures 3.8 and 3.9). An alternative cylinder check method recommended if VA is relatively good but lingering cylinder is suspected has been described by Bennet and Rabbetts. In this method, the JCC is placed in the phoropter at *axis* 90/180° without any additional cylinder power dialed in. The patient is then asked which view is preferred, e.g., *red dot* (power) at 45° or 135°. The procedure is repeated with the axis at 45/135°. Cylinder power of either −0.25 or −0.50 is then introduced between the axes in which cyl power was previously chosen, e.g., if 45° and 180° were selected choose axis 23° and cylinder refinement is performed as described previously. If the patient reports that both views look the same at 45/135° and 90/180° then it can be concluded that the patient does not need cylindrical correction.

5. **Second Monocular MPMVA**

This step is used to determine the maximum plus-spherical power which provides the patient with their maximum VA after cylinder refinement.

a. The patient should first be fogged by approximately 0.75 D to 1.00 D more plus spherical power. The VA should be confirmed to be around 20/40 to 20/50. If the VA is not adequately reduced with 1.00 D, more plus power should be increased until the VA is at an appropriate level and over-minusing during the preceding steps should be suspected.

b. After adequately fogging the patient the magnitude of plus power should be reduced slowly using 0.25 D minus at a time. Remember that the patient should obtain approximately one additional line of VA for each 0.25 D of minus sphere added (or each 0.25 D of plus sphere removed). Recall that simply looking "better" is not sufficient justification for giving the patient more minus or less plus.

c. The endpoint of the second MPMVA can be reached by any of the following endpoints.

### The Duochrome Endpoint

a. The duochrome procedure is performed as in step 3, with the exception that the endpoint for the second MPMVA is red-green balance *instead of* "one into the green;" i.e., both sides red and green look equally clear. Recall that when performing the test that if the red side is clearer more minus power is added and if the green side is clearer more plus power is added.

b. VA should be rechecked after the red-green filter is removed and before proceeding to the binocular balance step.

*Note:* Not all patients are responsive to the duochrome test and some will appear to have a preference for one side or the other regardless of the lens power in place. In this instance another endpoint is preferred.

### The Smaller/Darker Endpoint

a. Once the patient's VA is no longer improving with additional minus power during the second MPMVA introduce one more increment of −0.25 D power and ask the patient if this change makes the letters clearer, the same, or just smaller and darker. If the change makes the letters smaller, darker, or the same do not give the additional 0.25 D of minus power. If the patient reports that the letters are subjectively clearer it is recommended they demonstrate some improvement in VA, e.g., read more letters on the next line or read the current line more "smoothly" before giving any additional minus power.

### The 20/20 endpoint

a. Generally, if the patient has clear 20/20 vision or better, Egger's chart is followed throughout the refraction procedure (one line improvement for every one increment of 0.25 more minus power), and the refraction does not change significantly from the patient's habitual Rx, an endpoint of 20/20 VA can be used as the endpoint for the second MPMVA before transitioning to the binocular balance step.

After completing the initial MPMVA, cylinder refinement, and second MPMVA of the right eye, steps 2 through 5 should be repeated with the left eye before proceeding to binocular balance.

6. **Binocular Balance**

The primary purpose of binocular balance is to balance the accommodative stimulus between the two eyes while also relaxing accommodation binocularly. As the procedure requires the patient to compare a prism dissociated target of the same VA level for each eye, it should only be performed in patients who have relatively the same BCVA in both eyes after the second MPMVA. Additionally, if the patient is an absolute presbyope and no longer has accommodative ability, binocular balance can also be skipped.

a. The procedure is performed with both eyes open and with each eye fogged by approximately 0.75 D to 1.00 D more plus power. The patient's VA should be confirmed to be around 3–4 lines worse than BCVA before the addition of fogging lenses. If the VA is not sufficiently reduced, more plus power should be introduced until the patient's VA is confirmed to be 3–4 lines worse binocularly.

b. Once the VA is confirmed to be 3–4 lines worse than the VA found after the second MP-MVA, an isolated line of letters *one line above the fogged VA* should be used as a target.

c. Using the Risley Prism, introduce 3Δ base up prism over the right eye and 3Δ base down prism over the left eye (see **Figure 3-22**). It is recommended to either occlude the patient or have the patient close their eyes to minimize any discomfort while introducing the prism.

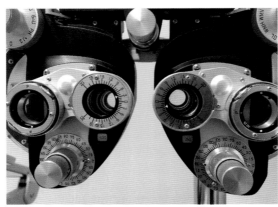

**FIGURE 3-22.** Photograph of the phoropter's Risley (rotary) prisms set to 3Δ base up over the right eye and 3Δ base down over the left eye for performing binocular balance. With the prisms set in this way, the right eye will see the lower image, except in the rare case of a left hyper deviation greater than or equal to 6Δ.

d. With both eyes open, confirm that the patient sees two lines of letters, one on top of the other. If the patient is having difficulty locating the images the examiner can alternate occlusion between the two eyes to help the patient find the images. Inform the patient that it is okay if the images are each a little blurry, but they should be able to make out or read the letters on each line.

e. Instruct the patient to look back and forth between the two lines of letters and tell you "which line is clearer, the top or the bottom." The examiner should add 0.25 D plus power to the eye which sees the clearer line, e.g., top line is clearer take away 0.25 D minus from the eye with the base down prism (left eye in this example).

f. The procedure should be repeated until the patient reports equal blur between the two lines or the patient alternates between the two lines. If it is not possible to achieve equality between the two lines, perform an ocular dominance check and leave the dominant eye with the clearer vision (see Procedure 3.10).

g. Once equality is reached or the more dominant eye is left clearer, remove the Risley prisms.

7. **Binocular MPMVA**

a. Once binocular balance if completed, bring the patient out of the fog binocularly until the binocular MPMVA is achieved. Remember that the patient should improve ~1 line of letters for every 0.25 D more minus power that is introduced. Any of the second MPMVA endpoints can be used as the binocular MPMVA endpoint.

*Note:* If binocular balance was skipped, fog each eye until the VA is 3–4 lines worse than BCVA and then proceed with step **a** above.

b. After the binocular MPMVA has been achieved, measure VA OD, OS, and OU and record the results of the refraction with VA.

## Recording

- Record the sphere power, cylinder power, and cylinder axis in the phoropter for each eye.
- Measure and record the VA for the right eye, the left eye, and for both eyes together.
- Any qualitative assessment during the procedure may also be recorded, e.g., "fluctuating vision OS."

*Note:* The final glasses prescription for a patient may differ from the final subjective refraction results found in the phoropter. It is important that the results of the subjective refraction, along with any subsequent modifications be recorded in the patient's chart.

## Examples

- Monocular distance subjective refraction:
  OD + 0.25 − 1.00 × 165    20/15
  OS − 0.50 − 0.75 × 010    20/15

| SUBJECTIVE REFRACTION FLOW at a glance | |
|---|---|
| **Technique** | **Procedure and Purpose** |
| **Starting Point** | Can use habitual Rx, retinoscopy, or autorefraction results; refined during the subjective refraction procedure. |
| **Initial MPMVA** | Finds the initial working sphere by fogging to 20/40–20/50 VA by adding more minus power. |
| **Preparation for Cylinder Refinement** | Use either the duochrome test "one into the green" *or* leave the patient with 0.25 D more minus from the initial MPMVA. |
| **Cylinder Refinement** | Perform either power or axis refinement first as applicable. If VA is reduced and cylinder was not found on the starting point, perform a cylinder check. |
| **Second MPMVA** | Determines the sphere power after cylinder refinement in preparation for binocular balance. |
| **Binocular Balance** | Balances the accommodative demand between the two eyes. The patient is fogged and shown two images created by introduction of Risley prism. |
| **Binocular MPMVA** | Slowly brings the patient out of the fog after the binocular balance is performed to complete the subjective refraction procedure. |

### Side Trips from the Routine Distance Subjective Refraction

The following procedures (3.7 through 3.14) are auxiliary tests often used as needed in addition to the distance monocular subjective refraction.

## 3.7 USE OF THE TRIAL FRAME TO MODIFY A PRESCRIPTION

### Purpose

The aim of this procedure is to demonstrate a new prescription to the patient and to modify the subjective refraction findings for maximum patient comfort.

### Equipment

- Trial lens set
- Trial frame (TF)
- Distance VA chart
- Near VA chart
- Reading material—e.g., book, music sheet, phone, tablet or computer screen

## Setup

- Place the trial frame on the patient. Adjust the trial frame so that it sits comfortably on the patient's face and the patient's eyes are centered relative to the lens wells of the frame. See the Trial Frame Refraction section in this chapter (Procedure 3.11) for labeled parts.
  *Note:* If the patient has a previous pair of glasses and the change is spherical, the trial lenses can be held directly over the patient's current glasses to demonstrate the change in prescription.

## Procedure

1. Instruct the patient to look at the distance acuity chart if the new prescription is for distance or at the near point card if the new prescription is for near. Alternatively, the patient may look at another distance target rather than at the distance acuity chart or at reading material rather than at the near acuity chart.
2. Ask the patient if things look clear and if they feel comfortable looking through the new prescription.
3. If the patient reports that things are not clear or are not comfortable through the new prescription, adjust the prescription in one of the following ways until the patient reports clear and comfortable vision:
   a. Increase the minus sphere in 0.25 D steps.
   b. Increase the plus sphere in 0.25 D steps.
   c. Move the axis of the cylinder toward the axis in the patient's previous prescription or toward 90° or 180° (see **Figure 3-23**).

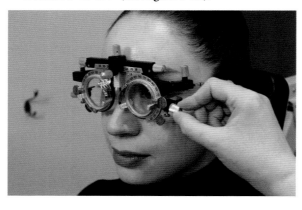

**FIGURE 3-23.**   The clinician adjusts the axis of a proposed prescription in the trial frame.

   d. Decrease the cylinder power in 0.25 D steps, making concurrent changes in the sphere to maintain the spherical equivalent of the prescription.
4. For prescriptions that are for near only, instruct the patient to move the reading material in toward themselves until it blurs and out away from themselves until it blurs to ensure that there is an adequate range for the patient's needs.
5. For prescriptions that are for near only, instruct the patient to look through the prescription at distance and explain that it is normal for distance objects to look blurry through a near prescription.

## Recording

- Record all of the prescriptions that were tested. If VA was measured in addition to assessing comfort, record the VA as well.
- Record the patient's response to each of the trial framed prescriptions.

## Examples

- TF:

  OD: −4.75 sph       20/20

  OS: −3.50 − 0.50 × 175    20/20

- TF for near:
  - OD: +1.00 − 0.50 × 010

    OS: +1.00 − 0.50 × 165
  - OD: +1.00 sph

    OS: +1.00 sph
  - OD: +0.50 sph

    OS: +0.50 sph

  Patient was 20/20 with each; most comfortable with +1.00 sph OU. Range adequate for patient's near needs.

- TF +0.25 OU and +0.50 OU over patient's current near glasses; patient prefers +0.50 OU.

- TF +2.00 OU for near; patient reports clear, comfortable vision for reading, but blurry at the computer screen. TF +1.50 OU and +1.25 OU for computer; patient most comfortable with +1.25 OU at the computer.

## 3.8 CLOCK CHART (SUNBURST DIAL)

### Purpose

This is an alternative, subjective method to determine the axis and power of the cylindrical component of the refractive error prior to refinement by the subjective refraction technique. The clock chart is sometimes referred to a cylinder check versus cylinder refinement procedure as it is utilized to determine the tentative cylindrical correction for cylinder refinement when 20/20 VA cannot be achieved with spherical lenses or when the starting point is suspected to be inaccurate.

### Equipment

- Phoropter (or loose lenses and trial frame)
- VA chart with clock chart or sunburst dial

### Procedure

1. The procedure is performed monocularly, with 2–3 lines of fog, and without any cylinder in the phoropter. The patient is then shown the clock chart (see **Figure 3-24**).

2. The patient is asked to identify the darkest set of lines on the clock chart according to their position on the face of a clock, e.g., 1 o'clock. If none of the lines are darker, i.e., all are equally blurry, the clock test did not detect any uncorrected astigmatism, the test is terminated and the monocular subjective refraction procedure is resumed.

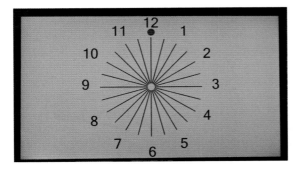

**FIGURE 3-24.** | Image of a typical clock chart, or sunburst dial target.

3. If one set of lines is determined to be darker or bolder, the smaller clock hour is multiplied by 30 and the resulting number is the axis of the tentative cylinder, which is then dialed into the phoropter; e.g., 2 o'clock (also equivalent of 8 o'clock) = 60° (2 × 30).

4. If two sets of lines (e.g., 1 o'clock and 2 o'clock) appear equally dark, select an axis value midway between the two calculated axes, e.g., 45°.

5. Once the axis is determined, a tentative cylinder power of 0.50 D can be placed in the phoropter and the cylinder refinement step of the monocular subjective refraction can be performed.

## Recording

Results of the clock chart test may be included as qualitative support of subjective refraction findings but are not required as they are considered an 'auxiliary step' in the procedure.

## 3.9 JACKSON CROSS CYLINDER (JCC) CHECK TEST FOR UNCORRECTED ASTIGMATISM

### Purpose

This is an alternative, subjective method to determine the axis and power of the cylindrical component of the refractive error prior to refinement by the subjective refraction technique. This procedure is referred to a cylinder check as it is utilized to determine the tentative cylindrical correction prior to cylinder refinement when 20/20 VA cannot be achieved with spherical lenses or when the starting point is suspected to be inaccurate, i.e., "checking for uncorrected cylinder."

### Equipment

Phoropter

VA chart: computer generated, projector, or printed chart

### Setup

The phoropter contains the sphere from the end of the initial MPMVA (see setup in Procedure 3.6). This check is performed monocularly.

### Procedure

1. After performing the initial MPMVA of the monocular subjective refraction procedure, dial −0.50 D of cylinder into the phoropter while maintaining the spherical equivalent.

2. With the axis of the cylinder first set to 180° ask the patient "which view is clearer, one or two" while alternatively showing the patient the white and red dots in alignment with the correcting cylindrical axis, i.e., cylinder power refinement procedure (see Procedure 3.6, step 4).

3. If the patient prefers the red dots in alignment with the correcting cylinder axis at 180°, the patient subjectively prefers cylindrical correction at that axis and the cylinder refinement procedure should be continued. If the patient prefers the white dots the patient has "kicked out the cyl" and does not want cylindrical correction at that axis and the other axes; 90°, 45°, and 135° should be tested in succession. Perform cylinder refinement if cylinder is accepted in any meridian.

4. If the patient prefers the white dots at all orientations, e.g., 180°, 90°, 45°, and 135°, then the patient does not have uncorrected astigmatism and the monocular subjective refraction procedure can be continued. When removing the cylinder be sure to again maintain the spherical equivalent.

## Recording
- Results of the JCC cylinder check are not typically recorded as they are considered an 'auxiliary step' in the distance monocular subjective refraction procedure.

## 3.10 OCULAR DOMINANCE TESTING

### Purpose
The aim of this procedure is to identify the patient's sighting-dominant eye. A variety of methods exist for the determination of the patient's dominant eye and there are two primary classifications, motor and sensory testing. Tests with a motor component require the patient to hold or otherwise utilize their hands as part of the procedure while sensory testing requires only the subjective responses of the patient. Sensory tests of ocular dominance are typically preferred as it is thought that tests that involve a motor component may skew the results in the direction of the patient's preferred hand dominance.

### Indications
Ocular dominance testing may be performed when a balance between the two eyes is not able to be achieved with the binocular balance procedure or when determining an appropriate monovision correction for a patient.

### Equipment
- The equipment and setup are determined by the procedure used below.

### Procedure
*Motor Tests of Ocular Dominance*

Triangle with Hands: Miles Test
1. The patient forms a triangular "window" with their hands held at an arms distance away and is instructed to fixate on a distance target. The patient is then instructed to alternatively close their eyes and note for which eye the target is still within the triangular "window"; e.g., if the patient reports the target is more centered in the triangular window with the right eye open then the patient is right eye dominant.

   *Note:* It is possible for patients to have equal eye dominance. In this case the target will appear to move equally when the eyes are alternatively closed.
2. An alternative method can be used in which the patient is asked to fixate on the examiner's dominant eye while at a distance of 10 feet. The examiner then notes which eye the patient is using to fixate the examiner's eye through the triangular window.

Hole in Card: Crider Test
1. The patient is asked to hold a piece of cardboard (20 ×12.8 cm) with a 3-cm diameter hole cut into the middle of the cardboard with both hands and asked to look at the examiner's open right eye while at a distance of 4 m.
2. The examiner then determines which eye the patient is using to view the target. This is the dominant eye.

*Sensory Tests of Ocular Dominance*

Blur Test
1. The patient is asked to fixate on a line of letters equal to one line above the best corrected VA of the worse seeing eye at a distance of 4 m.
2. The examiner holds a +1.00 D spherical trial lens alternatively in front of each eye for two seconds and asks the patient during which view (right or left eye with lens), is blurrier. The procedure can be repeated a few times before the patient makes their final selection.
3. The eye that sees blurrier throughout the procedure is the dominant eye.

Other Sensory Tests of Ocular Dominance

Other computerized methods exist for the determination of sensory ocular dominance; the discussion of which is outside the scope of this publication.

### Recording

- The dominant eye should be recorded as applicable, e.g., "OD dominant."

## 3.11 TRIAL FRAME REFRACTION

### Purpose

The aim of this procedure is to determine the refractive state of the eye when a phoropter is unavailable, contraindicated, or does not provide the best means to perform the procedure. The trial frame is also used to confirm and modify phoropter-based refraction results (see Procedure 3.7).

### Indications

This method of refraction is particularly useful for patients with low vision, high refractive error (including aphakes), accommodative instability, deafness, or ambulatory restrictions.

*Note*: The technique described here is a modification of a phoropter-based refraction. It is critical to point out that sub-steps of the procedure may be applied or eliminated depending upon the patient and the refractive error. The sub-step sequence may also be modified to enhance the efficiency of the trial frame refraction. Prior to reading this section, the examiner should be thoroughly familiar with routine distance subjective refraction with the phoropter.

### Equipment

- VA chart: computer generated, projector, or printed chart
- Trial frame
- Retinoscope and retinoscopy rack *(depending on starting point, see below)*
- Trial lens set
- Handheld JCC: handheld JCCs come in a variety of powers (±0.25 D, ±0.50 D, ±1.00 D). The power used will depend on the patient's acuity level. For patients with acuity of 20/25 or better in the eye(s) being tested, a ±0.25 D JCC is recommended. For patients with acuity poorer than 20/30, higher powered JCCs are needed.

### Setup

- Have the patient remove any corrective lenses.
- The *starting point* for the procedure can be the patient's habitual correction in the trial frame or the retinoscopy results found with retinoscopy racks or loose lenses (see Procedure 3.5).
  *Note:* If the starting point is the habitual correction or retinoscopy with loose lenses, the trial frame can be placed on the patient's face at the start of the procedure. If performing retinoscopy with retinoscopy racks, the trial frame can be fit once retinoscopy is complete.
- Place the trial frame on the patient. Be certain to adjust the trial frame so that it sits comfortably on the patient's face and the patient's eyes are centered relative to the lens wells of the frame. This is critical, especially for patients with high refractive error, as it will affect the final refraction result. This requires adjustment of the following (see **Figure 3-25**):
  - the temple length to minimize vertex distance; standard vertex distance is 10–13 mm;
  - the frame height via the nose pad adjustment;
  - the pantoscopic tilt and leveling of the frame; and
  - the PD.

A photograph of the trial frame on the patient is shown in **Figure 3-26**.

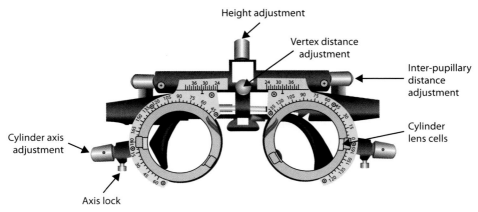

FIGURE 3-25.   Schematic diagram of a typical trial frame with the adjustment mechanisms labeled.

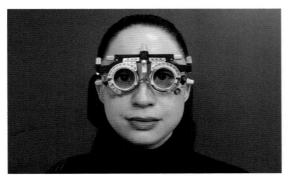

FIGURE 3-26.   Patient wearing a trial frame. The patient's eyes should be centered in the lens apertures and the temples adjusted to provide a snug fit.

## Procedure

*Monocular Subjective Refraction*

1. Insert your refraction starting point into the lens wells of both eyes in the trial frame. This will serve as the midpoint lens throughout the procedure.

   *Note:* Spherical lens powers are inserted into the most posterior lens well (closest to the patient's eye), and cylindrical powers are inserted into the anterior lens wells.

2. Occlude the patient's left eye with either the black or frosted occluding lenses within the trial frame set. Frosted occluders should be especially considered for pediatric patients, patients with esotropia, and patients with nystagmus.

3. Display the full acuity chart and perform the initial MPMVA on the right eye leaving the patient overminused by 0.25 D or "one into the green" in order to perform the cylinder check or refinement. This may be done by using handheld bracketing lenses (several in one hand, e.g., +0.25, +0.50, +0.75), or a lens rack. Modify the sphere in the trial frame to reflect the results of the MPMVA.

4. Isolate a single line of letters 1–2 lines above BCVA and perform the JCC test (cylinder refinement) using a handheld JCC. To increase manual control, a long handled JCC is recommended. If the cylinder power at the start of the JCC test is > 0.50 D, check the axis first (4.a below), if the cylinder power is < or = 0.50 D, check the power first (4.b below). If no cylinder is present, a cylinder check can be performed (4.c below). The JCC power

used will be based on the patient's acuity; typically, this can be determined using the "just noticeable difference (JND)" rule (see **Table 3-3**).

a. Refine the cylinder axis by flipping the JCC in front of the trial frame with the axes of the cross cylinders 45° away from the correcting cylinder axis. This is generally the case when the handle of the JCC is aligned with the correcting cylinder axis. Rotate the lens cell of the trial frame to change the cylinder axis in response to the results of the JCC axis test. Moving the cylinder axis toward the red lines on the JCC.

b. Refine the cylinder power using the JCC by aligning the axes of the JCC with the correcting cylinder axis. Adjust the power of the cylinder in the trial frame while maintaining the spherical equivalent. Unnecessary lens changes may be avoided by changing the cylinder power in the trial frame by an amount equal to twice the power of the JCC. For example, if a ±0.25 D JCC is being used, and the patient prefers minus, add −0.50 D to the correcting cylinder. If on the next comparison the patient prefers minus you will have saved a step. Similarly, if the patient prefers plus, you can extrapolate that the endpoint is 0.25 D less minus-cylinder power than the amount in the well.

c. A cylinder check can be performed if there was no cylinder found at the starting point. If the patient's acuity is 20/30 or better, a 0.50 D minus-cylinder lens can be used to perform the check, and higher powers can be used for poorer acuity; the same power JCC should be used to perform the check. Insert the minus cylinder lens into the anterior lens well with the axis at 180° and perform a power check (4.b above). If the cylinder is rejected, perform a power check at 45, 90, and 135°. If the cylinder power is rejected (patient prefers white dots), in all meridians, the cylinder can be removed, and the examiner can move on to step 5. If the patient accepts the cylinder in any meridian (patient prefers the red dots), the examiner can then perform a power and axis refinement as listed in 4.a and 4.b above.

| TABLE 3-3. Handheld JCC Selection Using the Just Noticeable Difference Rule | |
| --- | --- |
| **VA Range** | **Recommended JCC Power** |
| 20/20 to 20/50 | +/− 0.25 D |
| 20/60 to 20/100 | +/− 0.50 D |
| 20/120 and worse | +/− 1.00 D |

5. Displaying the full acuity chart, perform the second MPMVA using loose lenses or a lens rack and make the final adjustment to the spherical component of the patient's correction.

6. Record your monocular subjective results and the VA.

7. Unocclude the left eye and occlude the right eye and repeat steps 3 through 6 for the left eye.

*Binocular Balance*

Perform this step only if each eye achieved the same VA following the monocular subjective refraction. As with a phoropter-based refraction, the binocular balance may be done via prism dissociation using the loose prisms included in the trial lens set, or the modified Humphriss method which is described here.

1. Make sure neither eye is occluded and both eyes can see the VA chart. Fog one eye by +1.00 D.

2. Direct the patient's attention to a single line of letters, 1–2 lines above the patient's best VA and show them +0.25 D then −0.25 D sphere over the non-fogged eye allowing them to compare the views.

3. If the patient reports that the views are the same or the +0.25 D view is better, add +0.25 D to that eye. Repeat step 2 until the minus lens is preferred, then proceed to step 4.

4. If the patient prefers the −0.25 D view, stop the procedure and repeat on the fellow eye, e.g., remove the fog from the first eye and fog the other eye. Repeat steps 2 and 3 on the other eye.

*Binocular MPMVA*

1. Display the full acuity chart and perform a binocular MPMVA using loose lenses in each hand.

2. Measure and record the VA for the right eye, the left eye, and both eyes.

## Recording

- Record the technique used.
- Record the final correction for the right eye and the left eye.
- Record the VA for the right eye, the left eye, and both eyes.

## Example

Trial Frame Refraction:

OD    −3.00 −0.50 × 135    20/20⁻¹
OS    −2.75 −0.50 × 045    20/20

## Notes

Recommendations for performing efficient trial frame refractions:

- Avoid stacking or changing the lenses in the wells of the trial frame. This may be accomplished by holding lenses in front of the trial frame, rather than placing lenses in the lens wells. To avoid stacking, the midpoint should be adjusted according to patient responses, so the least number of lenses remain in the trial frame at a given time.
- Learn to insert and remove lenses smoothly to promote patient comfort (see **Figure 3-27**).
- Use the right hand to present plus lenses and the left hand to present minus lenses. This allows the examiner to be efficient when reacting to patient responses.
- If the patient has reduced VA, be sure to use lens increments and JCC powers that allow the patient to make comparative judgments. For example, if a patient can only see 20/40 try using a ±0.50 D JCC instead of a ±0.25 D JCC (see **Table 3-3**).

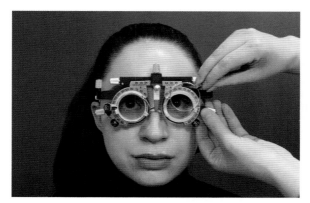

**FIGURE 3-27.** The insertion and removal of lenses in the trial frame should be done with care. The sphere is placed in the lens cell behind the facade of the frame and the cylinder in the cell before the facade. The examiner is adjusting the cylinder lens in this photo.

## 3.12 CYCLOPLEGIC REFRACTION

### Purpose

This is an alternative method to measure a patient's refractive error without an accommodative response. Cycloplegic drops that temporarily paralyze the ciliary body are used to eliminate the accommodative response. Cycloplegic refractions are particularly useful in pediatric eye exams, cases of latent hyperopia, strabismus linked to potential accommodative disorders, suspected accommodative spasm, or any visual symptoms/VA that do not match the objective assessment of the patient's refractive error. Any use of drugs, including eyedrops, requires the examiner to have an awareness of the contraindications and side effects of the selected drug. *Note:* If performing this procedure on a child, parental/guardian consent must be obtained for the use of diagnostic drugs.

### Equipment

- Retinoscope
- Phoropter, loose lenses and trial frame, or retinoscopy rack
- VA chart: computer generated, projector, or printed chart
- Topical anesthetic (optional)
- Cycloplegic agent: agents that may be used include cyclopentolate 1.0%, cyclopentolate 0.5% (particularly with infants), atropine 0.5% or 1.0%, homatropine 2% or 5%, or scopolamine 0.25%
  *Note:* Cyclopentolate 1.0% is recommended for routine cycloplegic refractions on patients above the age of 2 years. Atropine 0.5% or 1.0% has previously been recommended as the preferred agent when absolute cycloplegia is preferred, e.g., preschool accommodative esotropia. However due to concerns regarding the safety of atropine, alternative cycloplegic regimens have been recommended (Guo 2022), e.g., 1 drop 1% tropicamide, 1 drop 2.5% phenylephrine, 2 drops 1% cyclopentolate in pediatric patients. In adults, 2 drops Tropicamide 1% may be an effective agent for partial paralyzation of accommodation. Variations based on clinician's judgment exist.

### Procedure

In adults and some older children cycloplegic refraction is typically performed after non-cycloplegic retinoscopy and refraction. In children, non-cycloplegic retinoscopy should still be performed prior to cycloplegic retinoscopy and refraction. All typical precautions: VA, appropriate entrance testing, assessment of the anterior segment and anterior chamber angle of both eyes, assessment of intraocular pressure, review of medications, allergies, and pregnancy/breastfeeding should be performed prior to any mydriatic drop instillation. One drop of topical anesthetic, e.g., proparacaine 0.5% may be instilled prior to cycloplegic drops.

1. In general, two drops each separated by 5 minutes of 1.0% cyclopentolate are instilled in each eye; alternative cycloplegic regimens may be recommended.

2. On average, full cycloplegia is achieved after 30 minutes and the patient's accommodation should be checked prior to performing retinoscopy and refraction. Accommodation can be checked by either the push-up amplitude of accommodation or with screening by retinoscopy.

3. After determining that the patient is under full cycloplegia, perform retinoscopy and/or monocular subjective refraction as clinically indicated (see Procedures 3.5, 3.6, and 3.11 respectively).

## Recording

- When using pharmacological agents, the agent, concentration, number of drops, and time administered should always be recorded.
- Record the results of cycloplegic retinoscopy, refraction, and the resulting VA in the right eye, left eye, and both eyes when applicable.

## Example

- 2 gtts cyclopentolate 1% OD/OS @ 1:00 pm
  Cycloplegic Retinoscopy:
  OD +4.00 −1.00 × 180     20/30
  OS +4.50 −0.75 × 170     $20/25^{-2}$
  Cycloplegic Refraction:
  OD +3.50 −1.00 × 180     20/20
  OS +4.00 −0.75 × 170     20/20

## Expected Findings

- Typically, a more plus powered refraction and retinoscopy findings will be predicted under cycloplegia, particularly in cases where an accommodative spasm, latent hyperopia, or an accommodative esotropia is suspected. Additionally, due to the high accommodative ability found in many pediatric patients, the refractive error found during non-cycloplegic retinoscopy and refraction is typically inaccurate.

## 3.13 DELAYED SUBJECTIVE REFRACTION

### Purpose

This is a non-cycloplegic refractive technique used to maximize the acceptance of more plus power during the refraction process by more fully relaxing the patient's accommodation. This technique is particularly useful for patients with suspected latent hyperopia or an accommodative spasm and are unable to undergo cycloplegia.

### Equipment

- A phoropter and near point rod with near point card
- VA chart: computer generated, projector, or printed chart

### Procedure

Delayed subjective refraction is performed after the routine monocular subjective refraction and negative relative accommodation/positive relative accommodation (NRA/PRA) (see Procedure 4.10).

1. An isolated line of letters equal to the patient's best-corrected distance acuity should be used as a target.
2. Delayed subjective refraction is performed at distance with the results of the NRA procedure at near left in the phoropter. The patient should report that the target is blurry.
3. Minus power is added in 0.25 D increments until the target at distance is clear. Once the target is clear, display the full VA chart. Power should be changed slowly, and the patient should be encouraged to read down as far as the VA chart as possible after each change in 0.25 D.
4. The endpoint can be confirmed by the use of the duochrome test (see Procedure 3.6).

### Recording

- Record the name of the test and the results as a separate section from the routine monocular subjective refraction. Include the VA results OD, OS, and OU.

## Examples
- Delayed subjective refraction:

  OD   +1.25 − 0.25 × 010   20/20

  OS   +1.50 − 0.75 × 175   20/20

  OU                                  20/15

## Expected Findings
- The results of the delayed subjective refraction are typically more plus than the routine monocular subjective refraction particularly in cases of latent hyperopia and accommodative excess.

## 3.14 DETERMINING THE ADD FOR A PRESBYOPE

### Purpose
The aim of this procedure is to determine the near prescription (add) for the presbyopic patient. An add is the additional plus power needed for the presbyopic patient to see a near target and compensates for the decreasing accommodative ability. It is the difference between the distance and the near correction.

### Equipment
- Phoropter with near point rod and card
- Trial frame, loose lenses, and near card (optional)

### Setup
- The procedure is completed after the distance subjective refraction with the results of the distance refraction left in the phoropter.
- The PD is adjusted from distance to near and the near rod and near card are put into place and set at a distance of 40 cm.
- The near card should be fully illuminated.

### Procedure
1. **Tentative Add**

   A tentative add must first be selected and is used as the starting point for the near refraction. The tentative add can be determined by any of the following methods, although age is typically used due to ease of use.

   *Age*

   As accommodation decreases by a function of age the tentative add can be selected based on the patient's age. **Table 3-4** can be used as a guide when determining the tentative add based on the patient's age.

| TABLE 3-4. Tentative Add as a Function of the Patient's Age and Refractive Status | | | |
|---|---|---|---|
| Age | Myopia/Emmetropia | Low Hyperopia | High Hyperopia |
| 33–37 | pl | pl | +0.75 |
| 38–43 | pl | +0.75 | +1.25 |
| 44–49 | +0.75 | +1.25 | +1.75 |
| 50–56 | +1.25 | +1.75 | +2.25 |
| 57–62 | +1.75 | +2.25 | +2.50 |
| 63 and over | +2.25 | +2.50 | +2.50 |

*Fused Cross Cylinder (FCC)*

The endpoint of the FCC test (see Procedure 4.9) can be used as a tentative add. In presbyopic patients some plus may need to be added in order for the cross target to be seen when beginning the test.

*Half the Amp in Reserve Rule*

The difference between the dioptric equivalent of the patients preferred near working distance and half the patient's amplitude of accommodation can be used as the tentative add, e.g., a patient with a near standard working distance of 40 cm (2.50 D demand) and 4 D of total accommodative ability (can use 2 D comfortably) would need a tentative add of 0.50 D.

*Entering VA and Habitual Rx*

For each line of reduced near VA below 20/20, an additional +0.25 D is added to the patient's entering net near Rx. The examiner should be mindful of the initial net near Rx as any changes in the distance Rx will need to be taken into account when determining the calculation of the tentative add.

2. **Add Refinement**

   a. Once the tentative add has been determined and dialed into the phoropter, the NRA/PRA procedure should be performed (see Procedure 4.10).

   b. The results of the NRA/PRA procedure should be balanced in order to refine the add. To do this, the results of the NRA/PRA procedure should be added algebraically, e.g., +2.00/−1.00 → +1.00, and the sum divided by 2 e.g., +1.00/2 → +0.50, which is then added to the tentative add. *Note:* It is important to maintain the sign when adding the NRA/PRA results.

   c. The balanced add may be the endpoint if the patient's preferred working distance is the standard working distance of 40 cm. If the patient reads at a nonstandard working distance the balanced add may need to be further modified to meet the needs of the patient.

   *Note:* A good case history is critical to the success of a near add. The visual needs of the patient including vocation and avocation must be ascertained prior to writing the final near Rx. Patients may need multiple near prescriptions in order to meet their visual goals. Additionally, a patient's stature may play a role in any modifications of the near Rx. Taller individuals have a tendency to hold reading material further away while the converse is true with shorter individuals. It is highly recommended to show the patient the proposed Rx in a trial frame for any first time presbyopic refraction, large changes in near correction, and for specialized occupational or hobby related corrections.

   d. Trial frame modifications can be determined by having the patient wear the proposed near Rx in the trial frame and having the patient look at the preferred reading material, e.g., book, phone, or computer at their preferred reading distance. Plus power can be increased/decreased in 0.25 D increments depending on the needs of the patient. An increase in working distance from 40 cm would necessitate a decrease in plus power and a decrease in working distance would require an increase in plus power.

   e. The final modified near Rx and VA OD/OS/OU should be recorded in the patient's chart. Additionally, the range of clear near vision should be recorded if performed (see below).

3. **Range of Clear Near Vision**

   The range of clear near vision can be determined either in free space (trial frame and loose lenses) or in the phoropter. The recommended target is typically a line of letters 1–2 lines larger than BCVA but may be other appropriate near material for the patient's needs.

a. In free space the patient can be asked to bring the target material closer until blur is noted and then away from them until blur is noted. The distance in cm or inches is recorded in the patient's chart.

b. In the phoropter, the examiner can bring the target toward and away from the patient until near and distance blur are reported. This can easily be done with the near card on the near rod.

Note: The add can be modified in 0.25 D steps to shift the range closer or further from the patient as their individual working distance requires.

## Recording

- Write the word "add" followed by the dioptric power of the final add (not the net near Rx). This is typically next to or under the results for the distance subjective monocular refraction. If the add differs between eyes, although rare, be sure to specify for each eye as needed.
- Record the near VA for each eye through the final add.
- Record the range of clear near vision if performed.

## Examples

- Subjective refraction:
  OD  $+2.50 - 1.00 \times 090$    20/20
  OS  $+2.50 - 1.00 \times 090$    20/20
  Add  +1.00                         20/20 OD and OS; 20/15 OU
  Range of clear vision 22–54 cm

| DETERMINING THE ADD FOR THE PRESBYOPE at a glance | |
| --- | --- |
| **Purpose** | **Technique** |
| Select a tentative add (see step 1) | • Age and refractive status<br>• FCC<br>• Half the amp in reserve<br>• Rx + near VA |
| Refine the add | • Balance the NRA/PRA |
| Finalize the add | • Trial frame<br>• Measure the VA and range<br>• Adjust the near Rx as needed |

## 3.15 WRITING A SPECTACLE PRESCRIPTION

### Purpose

The aim of this procedure is to write a clear and comprehensive prescription for glasses that will be recognized, understood, honored, and filled by any optician or optical lab. An updated copy of a patient's glasses Rx is required by US law to be given to all patients after their examination regardless if the prescription has not changed from their habitual Rx.

### Equipment

- Computer for electronically generated or printed prescription, or prescription pad
- The prescription should contain the following provider or practice information:
  - Provider name and credentials
  - Practice name, address of practice and phone/fax number of practice
  - Provider license number

## Procedure

There are several key elements of the spectacle prescription which must be included. These are as follows:

1. The patient's full name and date of birth
2. The eye, right (OD) *and* left (OS), and the corresponding glasses Rx, including sphere, cylinder, and axis
3. Date of exam and expiration date of the prescription
4. Signature of prescribing doctor either electronically or in ink

Some additional elements may be required depending on the patient and recommendations by the prescribing doctor for the patient:

1. An "add" as required for near vision.
2. Type of glasses recommended to the patient, e.g., near vision only, distance vision only, bifocals, or progressives
3. Lens options recommended to the patient, e.g., transitions, high-index, polycarbonate. *Note:* In some US states polycarbonate lenses are required for all pediatric patients or monocular patients
4. Pupillary distance
5. Prism (magnitude and direction of base) as needed

## Examples

An example of an eyeglass prescription is seen in **Figure 3-28**.

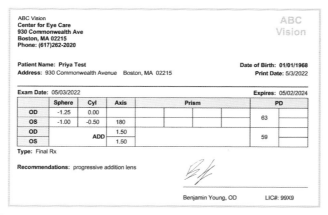

**FIGURE 3-28.** | Example of a glasses prescription electronically generated and printed.

## Notes

- A copy of every prescription should be maintained on file in the patient's chart.

## 3.16 KERATOMETRY

### Purpose

The aim of this procedure is to assess the curvature, power, and toricity of the central cornea. Keratometry may also be used to assess the integrity of the corneal/tear surface.

### Equipment

- Keratometer

## Basic Components of the Keratometer

Since keratometers differ, the examiner should review the specific instructions provided by the manufacturer for the keratometer they are using. The following components are common to all keratometers:

- Adjustable eyepiece for focusing the instrument for the examiner's eye
- Adjustable chin rest and forehead rest to support the patient's head comfortably during testing
- A knob to raise and lower the instrument to align it with the patient's eye
- Two power wheels to measure the corneal power in each of the two principal meridians
- An axis scale to indicate the location of the two principal meridians; the barrel of the instrument can be rotated to align the keratometer appropriately
- Target (known as *mires*) which is projected onto and reflected from the patient's cornea
- Focus control knob or joystick to focus the mires on the patient's cornea

## Setup

- Disinfect the chin rest and forehead rest of the keratometer by wiping it with alcohol and drying it with a tissue.
- The patient removes their glasses or contact lenses.
- Focus the eyepiece of the keratometer in the following manner:
  - Turn on the instrument's power.
  - Set the adjustable eyepiece as far counterclockwise as possible.
  - Place a white paper in front of the instrument objective to retroilluminate the reticle.
  - Turn the eyepiece clockwise until the reticle is first seen in sharp focus.
  - Adjust the height of the patient's chair and the instrument to a comfortable position for both the patient and the examiner.
  - Unlock the instrument controls. This is necessary on some keratometers.
  - Instruct the patient to place their chin in the chin rest and their forehead against the headrest.
  - Raise or lower the chin rest until the patient's outer canthus is aligned with the hash mark on the upright support of the instrument or with the pointer on the side of the instrument.

## Procedure

1. From outside the instrument, roughly align the barrel with the patient's right eye by raising or lowering the instrument and/or by moving it to the left or right until a reflection of the mires is seen on the patient's cornea (see **Figure 3-29**).
2. Instruct the patient to look at the reflection of their own eye in the center of the keratometer barrel.
3. Look into the keratometer and refine the alignment of the image of the mires (three circles) on the patient's cornea.
4. Focus the mires and adjust the instrument so that the reticle is centered in the lower right-hand circle.
5. Lock the instrument in place. This is necessary on some but not all types of keratometers.
6. Adjust the horizontal and the vertical power wheels until the mires are in close apposition.
7. To locate the two principal meridians of the patient's cornea, rotate the telescope until the two horizontal spurs on the mires are perfectly continuous with one another (see **Figure 3-30**).

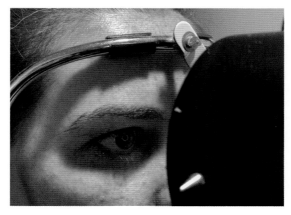

**FIGURE 3-29.** Alignment of the keratometer with the patient's right eye. The reflection of the mires is visible on the patient's cornea.

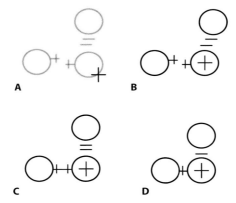

**FIGURE 3-30.** The appearance of the keratometric mires on the patient's cornea from inside the instrument. (A) The appearance of the blurry mires when the telescope has first been aligned with the patient's cornea. (B) The appearance of the mires when they have been focused and the reticle has been placed in the lower right-hand circle. (C) The appearance of the mires when the two principal meridians have been properly located. (D) The appearance of the mires when the horizontal and vertical power wheels have been properly adjusted.

8. Adjust the horizontal power wheel until the horizontal mires are coincident.

9. Adjust the vertical power wheel until the vertical mires are coincident.

   *Note:* If the corneal astigmatism is irregular, the two principal meridians will not be 90° apart. In this case, after the power reading for the horizontal meridian is made, the examiner must readjust the barrel of the instrument to align the vertical components of the mires before adjusting the power wheel.

10. Throughout the procedure, adjust the focus and recenter the reticle as needed.

11. Observe the integrity of the cornea by observing the condition of the mires.

12. Roughly align the telescope with the patient's left eye as described in step 1.

13. Repeat steps 2 through 11 on the patient's left eye.

## Extending the Range

Sometimes the power of a meridian falls outside the power range of the keratometer. In such cases, extend the range of the keratometer in the following manner:

- Tape or hold a +1.25 sph or a +2.25 sph (for corneal powers above the range of the keratometer), or −1.00 sph (for corneal powers below the range of the keratometer) lens over the opening of the keratometer barrel and perform the measurements, as described in steps 1 through 11. To calculate the actual power of the meridian, multiply the keratometer reading by the *correction factor* that corresponds to the extender lens used, as shown in **Table 3-5**.

| TABLE 3-5. Keratometry Correction Table for Extended Lens | | | |
|---|---|---|---|
| | Extender Lens Used | | |
| | +1.25 | +2.25 | −1.00 |
| Correction factor* | 1.166 | 1.3126 | 0.8576 |

*Actual correction factors vary with the specific brand of keratometer. However, the above multipliers are close to those of keratometers in common use and their use will probably not result in significant errors.

## Recording

- Record for each eye separately.
- Record the power and the meridian for the horizontal meridian first (the primary meridian).
- Write a slash mark after the primary meridian and record the power and meridian for the vertical meridian (the secondary meridian). *Note:* For keratometry, we record the power and the meridian along which it was found; we do *not* record the axis of power.
- Calculate and record the amount of corneal astigmatism in diopters.
- Record the type of astigmatism:
  - WTR or WR—with the rule (more corneal power in the vertical meridian)
  - ATR or AR—against the rule (more corneal power in the horizontal meridian)
  - OBL or Obl.—oblique (major meridians within ±15° of 45° and 135°)
  - Irregular—the two principal meridians are not 90° apart
- Record the conditions of the mires: mires clear and regular (MCAR) or mires irregular and distorted.

## Examples

- OD 42.50 at 180/43.50 at 090; 1.00 D WTR, MCAR
  OS 47.37 at 180/41.37 at 090; 6.00 ATR, mires distorted
- OD 41.75 at 180/43.75 at 070; 2.00 D irregular astig, mires distorted
  OS 43.12 at 135/41.87 at 045; 1.25 Obl., MCAR

If only the secondary meridian is recorded, the position of the primary meridian is assumed to be 90° away.

- OD 42.00/43.00 at 090; 1.00 D WR, MCAR
  OS 42.00/42.00 at 090; sphere, MCAR

If both meridians have exactly the same power, it is permissible to record that power a single time followed by the abbreviation "sph" rather than to record each meridian's power separately (e.g., 42.12 sph).

## Expected Findings

- Average K readings are 43.00 D to 44.00 D. Unless the cornea has been surgically altered, keratometry readings lower than 40.00 D or above 48.00 D are highly unusual and should be rechecked.
- The two principal meridians are expected to be 90° apart.

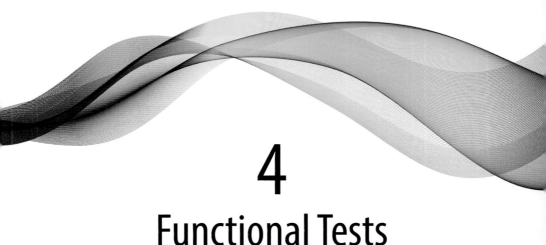

# 4
# Functional Tests

Hilary Gaiser, OD, MSc / Jennifer Reilly, OD, MSc, FAAO

## 4.1 INTRODUCTION TO THE FUNCTIONAL TESTS

To maintain clear, comfortable, binocular vision for all visual tasks, a patient needs a number of well-functioning visual skills. The patient must be able to align and maintain alignment of their two eyes in addition to having sufficient accommodation to sustain focus comfortably.

Additionally, the patient's accommodative system must be accurate and efficient. Due to the interconnection of the accommodative and vergence systems, both systems must function well and interact appropriately. To evaluate the patient's visual informational processing and binocular function status, tests of the accommodative and vergence system are performed. This chapter outlines a number of commonly used, basic functional tests that can be performed during a primary care, comprehensive eye exam. **Table 4-1** provides the expected findings for commonly performed entrance and functional tests.

| TABLE 4-1. Expected Findings for Functional Tests | |
| --- | --- |
| **Procedure** | **Expected Findings** |
| Cover Test | Distance: 1Δ exo (±2Δ)<br>Near: 3Δ exo (±3Δ) |
| Near Point of Convergence | Acc: 5/7 cm<br>Light: 7/10 cm<br>R/G: 5/7 cm<br>R/L: TBD expected to be similar to R/G |
| Stereopsis | Adults: ~ 20″ (seconds of arc)<br>Children 3 to 5 (Random Dot E): 168″ (150 cm) to 126″ (200 cm) |
| Amplitude of Accommodation | Hofstetter's Formulas:<br>Minimum = 15–0.25 × (age)<br>Average = 18.5–0.30 × (age)<br>Maximum = 25–0.40 × (age) |
| Distance Lateral von Graefe<br>Near Lateral von Graefe | Distance: 1Δ exo (±2Δ)<br>Near: 3Δ exo (±3 Δ) |
| Distance Vertical von Graefe<br>Near Vertical von Graefe | Distance: ortho<br>Near: ortho |
| Distance Horizontal Vergences (Smooth)<br>Near Horizontal Vergences (Smooth) | Distance: BI x/7/4 (±3/2); BO 9/19/10 (±4/8/4)<br>Near: BI 13/21/13 (±4/4/5); BO 17/21/12 (±5/6/7) |
| Distance Vertical Vergences (Smooth)<br>Near Vertical Vergences (Smooth) | Distance: 3–4 Δ/1.5–2 Δ<br>Near: 3–4 Δ/1.5–2 Δ |
| Fused Cross Cylinder | +0.50 D (±0.50 D in non-presbyopes) |
| Negative Relative Accommodation/<br>Positive Relative Accommodation | +2.00 D (±0.50)/ −2.37 D (±1.00) |
| Gradient AC/A Ratio | >2/1 and < 6/1 |
| Accommodative Facility | **Monocular**<br>Children 8–12 years: 7 cpm<br>Adults 13–30: 11 cpm<br>**Binocular**<br>Children 8–12 years: 5 cpm<br>Adults 13–30: 10 cpm |
| Monocular Estimated Method Retinoscopy | +0.25 D to +0.50 D  (+/− 0.25) lag |
| Associated Phoria | Ortho at distance and near |
| Maddox Rod | Distance: 1Δ exo (±2Δ)<br>Near: 3Δ exo (±3 Δ) |
| Modified Thorington | Distance: 1Δ exo (±2Δ)<br>Near: 3Δ exo (±3Δ) |
| 4Δ Base Out Test | No suppression |
| Pursuits and Saccades | See Tables 4-13 and 4-14 |

This chapter is non-exhaustive and for a more in-depth evaluation of the binocular vision status of the patient, the reader is encouraged to consult references focused on a more comprehensive binocular workup. The techniques outlined in this section allow the examiner to screen a patient's accommodative and vergence systems and determine if the patient may have a functional problem that warrants further investigation. The decision of which series of tests to use during a preliminary examination are based on the patient's age, symptoms, the results of the functional entrance tests, and the examiner's professional judgment. **Table 4-2** summarizes the purpose of each functional test.

**TABLE 4-2. Summary of Functional Tests.**

| Purpose | Set-Up | Test | Objective/ Subjective | Distance/Near |
|---|---|---|---|---|
| Accommodative accuracy | Free-Space | MEM | Objective | Near |
| | Phoropter | FCC | Subjective | Near |
| Accommodative ability | Free-Space | Amps | Subjective | Near |
| | Phoropter | NRA/PRA | Subjective | Near |
| Accommodative facility | Free-Space | BAF and MAF | Subjective | Near |
| Convergence and divergence ability | Free-Space | Lateral and Vertical Vergences with Prism Bars | Subjective and Objective | Distance and Near |
| | Phoropter | Lateral and Vertical Vergences with Risley Prism | Subjective | Distance and Near |
| | Phoropter | NRA/PRA | Subjective | Near |
| Absolute convergence ability | Free-Space | NPC | Subjective and Objective | Near |
| Strabismus vs. heterophoria | Free-Space | Cover Test | Objective | Distance and Near |
| Ocular deviation | Phoropter | Associated Phoria | Subjective | Distance and Near |
| | Phoropter and Free-Space | Maddox Rod | Subjective | Distance and Near |
| | Free-Space | Modified Thorington | Subjective | Distance and Near |
| Presence of microtropia | Free-Space | 4Δ BO Test | Objective | Near |
| Stereopsis | Free-Space | Stereopsis | Subjective | Near |
| Fusional ability | Free-Space | W4D | Subjective | Distance and Near |
| Ocular motility | Free-Space | Pursuits & Saccades | Objective | Near |

4Δ BO, four prism diopter base out; BAF, binocular accommodative facility; FCC, fused cross cylinder; MAF, monocular accommodative facility; MEM, monocular estimated method; NPC, near point of convergence; NRA, negative relative accommodation; PRA, positive relative accommodation; W4D, worth four dot

## 4.2 DISTANCE LATERAL AND VERTICAL DEVIATIONS BY VON GRAEFE (VG) TECHNIQUE

### Purpose

This is a subjective assessment of the horizontal and vertical oculomotor deviation of the patient at distance in the absence of fusion. This test may also be referred to as "von Graefe phorias."

## Equipment

- Phoropter
- Distance acuity chart

## Setup

- The distance correction that you are considering prescribing and distance pupillary distance are dialed into the phoropter. *Note:* It may be appropriate to perform testing with the habitual Rx, subjective refraction findings, or modified Rx.
- The appropriate target for distance is an isolated letter, 1-2 lines larger than the patient's best-corrected visual acuity in the poorer seeing eye.
- Insert the Risley prisms before both eyes and adjust the right eye prism to 12Δ base in (BI) and the left eye prism to 6Δ base up (BU) (**see Figure 4-1**). It is recommended to have the patient close their eyes while the prisms are being adjusted.

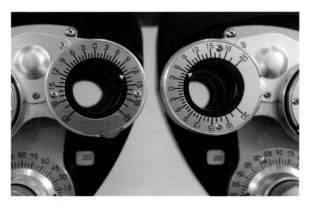

**FIGURE 4-1.** Proper setup of von Graefe phorias in the phoropter with Risley prisms set at 12 BI OD and 6 BU OS.

## Procedure

*Distance Lateral von Graefe*

1. Ask the patient how many targets they see and where they are in relation to each other. The patient should see two targets: one up and to the right, one down and to the left (**see Figure 4-2**). If they do not see the targets in the correct orientation refer to the troubleshooting section at the end of these procedures.

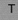

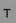

**FIGURE 4-2.** The von Graefe targets as viewed from the patient's perspective.

2. Instruct the patient to look at the lower target, and to keep it clear. Tell the patient to continue looking at the lower target while also paying attention to the upper target which you will be moving until the targets are aligned. Ask them to tell you when the two targets are lined up vertically, "like buttons on a shirt."
3. While the patient is looking at the targets, reduce the amount of BI prism (measuring prism) at a rate of about 2Δ per second until the patient reports vertical alignment of the

two targets. Make note of the amount of prism and direction of the base when the patient reports that the two targets are aligned.

4. Continue moving the prism in the same direction (overshoot) by approximately 10Δ and then reverse the direction of movement until the patient reports the two targets are vertically aligned again. Instruct the patient that you will be overshooting the target and they should inform you when the targets are re-aligned. Note the amount of prism and the direction of the base of the prism when the patient reports that the two targets are aligned again.

5. The results from lateral von Graefe testing are the average of the two values from steps 3 and 4, provided that they are within 3Δ of each other. If the two values are not within 3Δ of one another, repeat the measurement, emphasizing the instructions to the patient.

*Distance Vertical von Graefe*

Initial setup is the same for vertical as for lateral von Graefe. However, in this procedure, the disassociating and measuring prism are reversed and the instruction set is different.

1. Ask the patient how many targets they see and where they are in relation to each other. The patient should see two targets: one up and to the right, one down and to the left (**see Figure 4-2**). If the patient does not see the targets in the correct orientation refer to the troubleshooting section at the end of these procedures.

2. Instruct the patient to look at the upper target and to keep it clear. Tell the patient to continue looking at the upper target while also paying attention to the lower target which you will be moving until the targets are aligned. Ask them to tell you when the two targets are lined up horizontally, "like headlights on a car."

3. While the patient is looking at the targets, reduce the amount of BU prism (measuring prism) at a rate of about 2Δ per second until the patient reports horizontal alignment of the two targets. Make note of the amount of prism and direction of the base when the patient reports that the two targets are aligned.

4. Continue moving the prism in the same direction (overshoot) by approximately 5Δ and then reverse the direction of movement until the patient reports the two targets are aligned horizontally again. Instruct the patient that you will be overshooting the target and they should inform you when the targets are re-aligned. Note the amount of prism and the direction of the base of the prism when the patient reports that the two targets are aligned again.

5. The results from vertical von Graefe testing are the average of the two values from steps 3 and 4, provided that they are within 2Δ of each other. If the two values are not within 2Δ of one another, repeat the measurement, emphasizing the instructions to the patient.

*Troubleshooting*

- If the patient sees only one target, first check to ensure that both eyes are unoccluded. If the patient continues to see only one target, alternately occlude each eye to help the patient locate each of the images in space. *Note:* It is also possible that the patient may be suppressing.

- If the patient sees two targets but the orientation is reversed, one up and to the left and one down and to the right, increase the amount of BI prism on the right eye until the targets are in the correct orientation. *Note:* This typically occurs when the patient's deviation is larger than 12Δ exo.

- If the patient reports that the two targets become one during testing, then they are fusing, and you should end the test. You can record the magnitude and direction of prism at which fusion occurred.

### Recording
- Record the magnitude and direction of the deviation in prism diopters.
- Record if the test was performed with or without correction and the prescription through which the test was done, e.g., habitual, modified, or subjective.
- Results for von Graefe can be abbreviated as DLVG and DVVG for distance lateral von Graefe and distance vertical von Graefe, respectively.
- For vertical deviations, always record the eye with the hyper deviation.

### Examples
- DLVG cc (subjective): ortho
- DLVG sc: 2Δ exo
- DLVG cc (modified subjective): 4Δ eso
- DVVG sc: 2Δ right hyper
- DVVG cc (habitual): 1Δ left hyper

### Expected Findings
- DLVG: 1Δ XP (±2Δ)
- DVVG: Ortho (no deviation)

### Notes
- The Risley prisms used during the von Graefe procedure serve as both dissociating and measuring prisms during the test. In the lateral test, the 12Δ BI prism serves as the measuring prism while the 6Δ BU prism serves as a dissociating prism. The relationship is reversed for vertical von Graefe.
- Literature suggests that the von Graefe technique is the least repeatable of the oculomotor deviation methods available, and results for von Graefe have been found to be more exo than results obtained from other methods. However, the test can increase efficiency when many other tests are being performed in the phoropter. It is possible to perform von Graefe in free space with the use of a trial frame and changing the prism in 1Δ steps.
- When using von Graefe for gradient AC/A ratio, results tend to be higher than other methods.
- The results from von Graefe testing cannot be used interchangeably with other methods of oculomotor deviation. Practitioners should use the same measurement method when comparing previous patient results.

## 4.3 NEAR LATERAL AND VERTICAL DEVIATIONS BY VON GRAEFE (VG) TECHNIQUE

### Purpose
This is a subjective assessment of the horizontal and vertical oculomotor deviation of the patient at near in the absence of fusion.

### Equipment
- Phoropter
- Near acuity chart with accommodative block target and near rod

### Setup
- The near correction that you are considering prescribing and near pupillary distance is dialed into the phoropter. *Note:* It may be appropriate to perform testing with the habitual Rx, subjective refraction findings, or a modified Rx.

- The near rod should be in place and the accommodative block should be used as the near target for patients correctable to 20/20 (**see Figure 4-3**). An isolated letter or line, 1–2 lines larger than the patient's best-corrected visual acuity in the poorer seeing eye should be used for patients who are not 20/20. The card should be well illuminated.

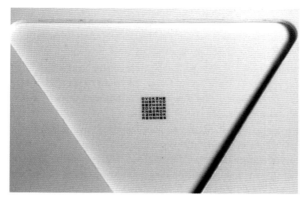

**FIGURE 4-3.** | Accommodative block target on near point card.

- Insert the Risley prisms before both eyes and adjust the right eye prism to 12Δ BI and the left eye prism to 6Δ BU. It is recommended to have the patient close their eyes while the prisms are being adjusted.

## Procedure

### Near Lateral von Graefe

1. Ask the patient how many targets they see and where they are in relation to each other. The patient should see two targets: one up and to the right, one down and to the left. If they do not see the targets in the correct orientation refer to the troubleshooting section at the end of Procedure 4.2.

2. Instruct the patient to look at the lower target, and to keep it clear. Tell the patient to continue looking at the lower target while also paying attention to the upper target, which you will be moving until the targets are aligned. Ask them to tell you when the two targets are lined up vertically, "like buttons on a shirt."

3. While the patient is looking at the targets, reduce the amount of BI prism (measuring prism) at a rate of about 2Δ per second until the patient reports vertical alignment of the two targets. Make note of the amount of prism and direction of the base when the patient reports that the two targets are aligned.

4. Continue moving the prism in the same direction (overshoot) by approximately 10Δ and then reverse the direction of movement until the patient reports the two targets are vertically aligned again. Instruct the patient that you will be overshooting the target and they should inform you when the targets are re-aligned. Note the amount of prism and the direction of the base of the prism when the patient reports that the two targets are aligned again.

5. The results from lateral von Graefe testing are the average of the two values from steps 3 and 4, provided that they are within 3Δ of each other. If the two values are not within 3Δ of one another, repeat the measurement, emphasizing the instructions to the patient.

### Near Vertical von Graefe

Initial setup is the same for vertical as for lateral von Graefe. However, in this procedure, the disassociating and measuring prism are reversed and the instruction set is different.

1. Ask the patient how many targets they see and where they are in relation to each other. The patient should see two targets: one up and to the right, one down and to the left. If the patient does not see the targets in the correct orientation refer to the troubleshooting section of Procedure 4-2.

2. Instruct the patient to look at the upper target and to keep it clear. Tell the patient to continue looking at the upper target while also paying attention to the lower target which you will be moving until the targets are aligned. Ask them to tell you when the two targets are lined up horizontally, "like headlights on a car."

3. While the patient is looking at the targets, reduce the amount of BU prism (measuring prism) at a rate of about 2Δ per second until the patient reports horizontal alignment of the two targets. Make note of the amount of prism and direction of the base when the patient reports that the two targets are aligned.

4. Continue moving the prism in the same direction (overshoot) by approximately 5Δ and then reverse the direction of movement until the patient reports the two targets are aligned horizontally again. Instruct the patient that you will be overshooting the target and they should inform you when the targets are re-aligned. Note the amount of prism and the direction of the base of the prism when the patient reports that the two targets are aligned again.

5. The results from vertical von Graefe testing are the average of the two values from steps 3 and 4, provided that they are within 2Δ of each other. If the two values are not within 2Δ of one another, repeat the measurement, emphasizing the instructions to the patient.

## Recording
- Record the magnitude and direction of the deviation in prism diopters.
- Record if the test was performed with or without correction and the prescription through which the test was done, e.g., habitual, modified, or subjective.
- Results for von Graefe can be abbreviated as NLVG and NVVG for near lateral von Graefe and near vertical von Graefe.
- For vertical deviations, always record the eye with the hyper deviation.

## Examples
- NLVG cc (subjective): ortho
- NLVG sc: 2Δ exo
- NLVG cc: (modified subjective): 4Δ eso
- NVVG sc: 2Δ right hyper
- NVVG cc (habitual): 1Δ left hyper

## Expected Findings
- NLVG: 3Δ XP (±3Δ); 8Δ XP (±3Δ) for presbyopes.
- NVVG: Ortho (no deviation).

## Notes
- See Procedure 4.2 for notes.

## 4.4 DISTANCE HORIZONTAL STEP AND SMOOTH VERGENCES

### Purpose
The aim of this procedure is to measure the patient's absolute ability to perform horizontal fusional vergence movements at distance. Vergences are simultaneous movements of both eyes in opposite directions to maintain single binocular vision. Vergence (supply)

allows the patient to compensate for a heterophoria (demand). Failure to have enough vergence ability to compensate for a heterophoria can lead to strabismus (decompensated phoria). Step vergence testing is both objective and subjective, while smooth vergences are subjective only.

### Horizontal Vergences

When testing negative fusional vergence (NFV) or divergence with BI prism, and positive fusional vergence (PFV) or convergence with base out (BO) prism, you are looking for three findings: blur, break, and recovery (see below). There is some variation in the literature on recommended order of vergence testing. Generally, BI should be performed prior to BO in order to avoid prism adaptation and stimulation of accommodation, which can affect findings. In cases of symptomatic patients with known *heterophoria*, it has been recommended to measure the compensating vergence first, e.g., BI for esophoria, to ensure the critical vergence range is assessed first.

*Note:* It has also been recommended by Rowe (2010) to perform vergences in the order of BO, BU, BI, then base down (BD) (see vertical vergence testing) in cases of unknown or normal deviation.

- **Blur:** May or may not occur during horizontal vergence testing. Since accommodation and vergence are linked, accommodation can add to the vergence supply. Blur represents the point when the accommodation supply has been exhausted and the target appears blurry and stays blurry for the patient.
- **Break:** The break represents the point at which the patient has used all fusional vergence reserves and can no longer compensate for the prism-induced retinal disparity, i.e., sees double.
- **Recovery:** The recovery represents the point at which the prism-induced retinal disparity has been reduced to the point that the patient can regain the use of the fusional vergence system and compensate for any retinal disparity, i.e., sees single again.

### Equipment

- Horizontal prism bars (step vergences) or phoropter (smooth vergences)
- A distance acuity chart that can isolate single letters
- Trial frame if measuring step vergences with something other than the habitual Rx

### Setup

- The patient should be wearing their habitual distance correction. *Note:* It may be appropriate to measure vergences with the most recent subjective refraction or a modified glasses Rx. In this case, a trial frame can be used, or the alternative Rx can be dialed into the phoropter. In both cases, the distance pupillary distance should be used.
- The target is an isolated letter or line of letters one to two lines above the patient's best-corrected visual acuity in the poorer seeing eye.
- *For testing with prism bars,* the prism is held with the base in the appropriate orientation; BI prism is oriented with the base towards the patient's nose and for BO the prism is oriented with the base towards the patient's ear. In both cases, testing should be performed starting with the lowest prism power first. Prism bars should be held to avoid tilt, which can induce vertical prism at high magnitudes (**Figure 4-4**).
- *For testing in the phoropter,* Risley prisms are put in place with the zero set at 90° in both eyes (**Figure 4-5**). It is recommended that the patient close their eyes while prisms are manipulated to minimize discomfort. For BI prism testing, the arrows of the Risley prism will be moved towards the patient's nose while for BO testing, the arrows of the Risley prism will be moved towards the patient's ears.

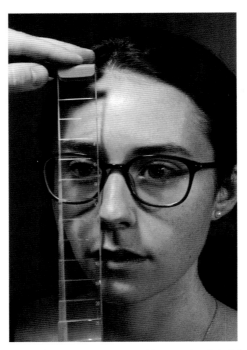

**FIGURE 4-4.** Distance horizontal step vergences setup. The examiner is holding the horizontal prism bar in front of the right eye oriented with the BO, while the patient is viewing the distant target.

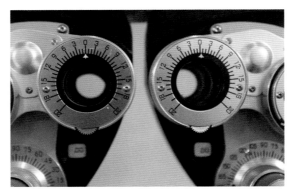

**FIGURE 4-5.** Horizontal smooth vergences setup in the phoropter with the Risley prism 0 set at 90° in front of both eyes.

## Procedure

### Step Vergences (Prism Bars)

Step vergence testing is performed in free space with the use of prism bars. This procedure is called *step* as most prism bars increase in magnitude in greater than 1Δ increments. This test is considered both objective and subjective as the practitioner can observe the patient's eyes for loss of fixation, which indicates a break, and a return to fixation, which indicates recovery. This method is recommended for all pediatric patients. See "*for testing with prism bars*" in setup above.

1. With both eyes unoccluded, the patient should see one image of the isolated letter or line of letters. Instruct the patient to look at the target and to try to keep it single and clear. Ask the patient to report if/when the target becomes blurry, splits into two, and comes back into one. This represents the blur, break, and recovery points, respectively. The patient should also be instructed to report if the target moves to the left or right at any time. If the patient reports that the target is moving, stop the test, and see "Notes" section below.

2. In horizontal step vergence testing the prism bars can be held over either the right or left eye. Since the eyes are innervated equally, the results of vergence testing in the right eye will be the same as the left. The prism should be held with the lowest amount of prism power first and slowly increased until the patient reports blur, break, and recovery.

3. Slowly increase the amount of prism while noting the amount of prism in front of the patient's eyes when blur and break occur, recall that blur may not occur in every patient. Ensure that the patient is looking through the full prism and not through the break marker between steps in prism power.

4. To determine recovery, overshoot the break point slightly by adding a little more prism in the same direction then reduce the prism until the patient reports that the target is single again. You may need to remind the patient to tell you when the target becomes single again.

5. Repeat the above steps on the same eye with the prism base in the opposite direction.

### Smooth Vergences (Phoropter)

Smooth vergences are performed in the phoropter with the addition of the Risley prisms. They are called *smooth* as the increments on the Risley prisms are in $1\Delta$ steps and the increase in prism can be performed "smoothly." Smooth vergences are considered a subjective test as the practitioner is not able to view the patient's eyes and the patient's responses must be relied upon. See "*for testing in the phoropter*" in setup above.

1. With both eyes unoccluded, the patient should see one image of the isolated letter or line of letters. Instruct the patient to look at the target and to try to keep it single and clear. Ask the patient to report if/when the target becomes blurry, splits into two, and comes back into one. This represents the blur, break, and recovery points, respectively. The patient should also be instructed to report if the target moves to the left or right at any time. If the patient reports that the target is moving, stop the test, and see "Notes" below.

2. In horizontal smooth vergence testing, unlike step vergences, the Risley prisms will be manipulated in both eyes simultaneously. The prism should be oriented with the zero positioned vertically and with the arrow of the Risley prism directed to the zero marker.

3. Slowly increase the amount of prism in both eyes simultaneously at the rate of about $2\Delta$ per second. BI is measured with the Risley arrows moved toward the nose in both eyes and BO with the Risley arrows moved toward the ears in both eyes. Note the total amount of prism, in both eyes, for blur, break, and recovery to occur, e.g., $3\Delta$ BO OD and $4\Delta$ BO OS equals $7\Delta$ BO.

4. To determine recovery, overshoot the break point slightly by adding a little more prism (4 to $5\Delta$ in each eye) in the same direction then reduce the prism until the patient reports that the target is single again. You may need to remind the patient to tell you when the target becomes single again.

5. Repeat the above steps with the prism in the opposite direction. Record your findings as indicated below.

## Recording
- Record the name of the test, e.g., step or smooth vergences, the distance, if the test was performed with or without correction, and with what correction, e.g., habitual, modified, subjective, or sc (no correction).
- Record the orientation of the prisms and the results of blur, break, and recovery separated by slashes, e.g., 4/10/8. If no blur point is observed, record an "x," e.g., x/10/8.
- If recovery values are in the direction opposite to what you expect (testing BO but had to go into BI for recovery), record as a negative value, e.g., 4/10/−2.

## Examples
- Dist. Step Vergences (subjective): BI x/10/4, BO 12/18/8
- Dist. Smooth Vergences (sc): BI suppression OD, BO: 6/14/10
- Dist. Smooth Vergences (modified; +2.25 OU): BI x/7/4, BO 10/18/−4

## Expected Findings
- The norms in **Table 4-3** represent population-based averages which vary as a result of testing distance, method of testing, age, and target size.
- It is expected to find no blur point for BI vergence testing at distance as blur represents relaxation of accommodation. Finding blur for BI testing at distance can indicate that the patient is over-minused or has latent/under-corrected hyperopia.

**TABLE 4-3. Expected Findings for Distance Smooth and Step Horizontal Vergences**

| Smooth Vergence Testing | | | |
|---|---|---|---|
| Distance BO | Blur | 9 | ∓4 |
| | Break | 19 | ∓8 |
| | Recovery | 10 | ∓4 |
| Distance BI | Blur | No blur | n/a |
| | Break | 7 | ∓3 |
| | Recovery | 4 | ∓2 |
| **Step Vergence Testing** | | | |
| Distance BO | Blur | Unknown | Unknown |
| | Break | 11 | ∓7 |
| | Recovery | 7 | ∓2 |
| Distance BI | Blur | No blur | n/a |
| | Break | 7 | ∓3 |
| | Recovery | 4 | ∓2 |

BI, base in; BO, base out

## Notes
- In order to compensate for the retinal disparity created by the use of prism, the eyes make simultaneous movements in opposite directions to maintain the images on the fovea.
- If the target moves during testing, the patient is suppressing an eye. The target will move in the direction of the apex of the prism over the eye that is not suppressing, e.g., during BI testing the target moves to the left when the right eye is being suppressed.
- It is not recommended to interchange the results of step vergence and smooth vergence testing. The same method should be used on the same patient in subsequent exams.

## 4.5 DISTANCE VERTICAL STEP AND SMOOTH VERGENCES

### Purpose

This test is a subjective and objective measurement of the patient's absolute ability to perform vertical fusional vergence movements at distance. Vergences are simultaneous movements of both eyes in opposite directions, to maintain single binocular vision. Vergence (supply) allows the patient to compensate for a heterophoria (demand). Failure to have enough vergence ability to compensate for a heterophoria can lead to a decompensated phoria (strabismus). Step vergence testing is both objective and subjective, while smooth vergences are subjective only.

### Vertical Vergences

When testing supra/hypervergence (BD) and infra/hypovergence (BU) you are looking for two findings, break and recovery. This is in contrast to horizontal vergences for which three findings, blur, break, and recovery, are expected. Blur is not expected as accommodation is not engaged during vertical fusional movements. Either BD or BU testing can be performed first.

- **Break**: The break represents the point at which the patient has used all fusional vergence reserves and can no longer compensate for the prism-induced retinal disparity, i.e., sees double.
- **Recovery**: The recovery represents the point at which the prism-induced retinal disparity has been reduced to the point that the patient can regain the use of the fusional vergence system and compensate for any retinal disparity, i.e., sees single again.

### Equipment

- Vertical prism bars (step vergences) or phoropter (smooth vergences)
- A distance acuity chart that can isolate single lines or letters
- Trial frame if measuring step vergences with something other than the habitual Rx

### Setup

- The patient should be wearing their habitual distance correction. *Note:* It may be appropriate to measure vergences with the most recent subjective refraction or a modified glasses Rx. In this case, a trial frame can be used, or the alternative Rx can be dialed into the phoropter. In both cases the distance pupillary distance should be used.
- The target is an isolated letter or line of letters one to two lines above the patient's best-corrected visual acuity in the poorer seeing eye.
- *For testing with prism bars,* the prism is held with the base in the appropriate orientation; BU prism is oriented with the base toward the patient's forehead and for BD the prism is oriented with the base toward the patient's chin (**see Figure 4-6**). In both cases, testing should be performed starting with the lowest prism power first.
- *For testing in the phoropter,* Risley prisms are set with the zero set horizontally (aligned with 180°) in both eyes (**Figure 4-7**). It is recommended that the patient close their eyes while prisms are manipulated to minimize discomfort. For BU prism testing, the arrows of the Risley prism will be moved toward the patient's forehead while for BD testing, the arrows of the Risley prism will be moved toward the patient's chin. *Note:* The second prism is placed before the contralateral eye (at zero) to equalize the quality of the image presented to the two eyes.

### Procedure

*Step Vergences (Prism Bars)*

Step vergence testing is performed in free space with the use of prism bars. This procedure is called *step*, as most prism bars increase in magnitude in greater than 1Δ increments. This test is considered both objective and subjective as the practitioner can observe the patient's eyes for loss of fixation, which indicates a break, and a return to fixation, which indicates

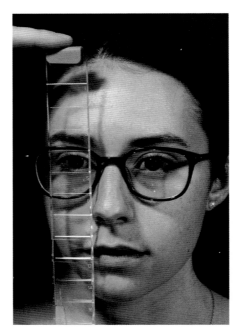

**FIGURE 4-6.** | Distance vertical step vergences setup. The examiner is holding the vertical prism bar in front of the right eye oriented with the BD, while the patient is viewing the distant target.

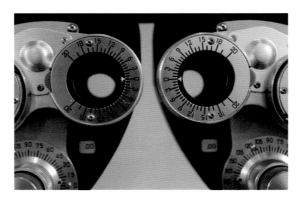

**FIGURE 4-7.** | Vertical smooth vergences setup in the phoropter with the Risley prism 0 set at 180° in front of both eyes.

recovery. This method is recommended for all pediatric patients. See *"for testing with prism bars"* in setup above.

1. With both eyes unoccluded, the patient should see one image of the isolated letter or line of letters. Instruct the patient to look at the target and to try to keep it clear and single. Ask the patient to report if/when the target splits into two and when it comes back into one. This represents the break and recovery points, respectively. The patient should also be instructed to report if the target moves up or down at any time. If the patient reports that the target is moving, stop the test, and see "Notes" section below.

2. In vertical step vergence testing it is recommended that the prism bars be held over the right eye for consistency although either eye can be chosen as both eyes are innervated

equally. BD OD results should equal BU OS results and vice versa. The prism should be held with the lowest amount of prism power first and slowly increased until the patient reports break and recovery.

3. Slowly increase the amount of prism while noting the amount of prism in front of the patient's eyes when break and recovery occur. Ensure that the patient is looking through the full prism and not through the break marker between steps in prism power.

4. To determine recovery, overshoot the break point slightly (2 to 3Δ) by adding a little more prism in the same direction, then reduce the prism until the patient reports that the target is single again. You may need to remind the patient to tell you when the target becomes single again.

5. Repeat steps 1–4 with the prism base in the opposite direction, but over the same eye. Record your findings as indicated below.

*Smooth Vergences (Phoropter)*

Smooth vergences are performed in the phoropter with the addition of the Risley prisms. They are called *smooth* as the increments on the Risley prisms are in 1Δ steps and the increase in prism can be performed "smoothly." Smooth vergences are considered a subjective test as the practitioner is not able to view the patient's eyes and the patient's responses must be relied upon. See "*for testing in the phoropter*" in setup above.

1. With both eyes unoccluded, the patient should see one image of the isolated letter or line of letters. Instruct the patient to look at the target and to try to keep it clear and single. Ask the patient to report if/when the target splits into two and when it comes back into one. This represents the break and recovery points, respectively. The patient should also be instructed to report if the target moves up or down at any time. If the patient reports that the target is moving, stop the test, and see Notes below.

2. In vertical smooth vergences, unlike horizontal smooth vergence testing, the Risley prisms only need to be manipulated in one eye. The prism should be oriented with the zero positioned horizontally and with the arrow of the Risley prism directed to the zero marker. It is recommended to use the measuring prism on the right eye for consistency. Recall that both eyes are innervated equally, and the BD OD results should equal BU OS results and vice versa. Either BD or BU can be performed first.

3. Slowly increase the amount of prism in the right eye at the rate of about 1Δ per second. BD findings are measured with the Risley arrows moved toward the patient's chin and BU with the Risley arrows moved toward the patient's forehead. Note the amount of prism needed for break and recovery.

4. To determine recovery, overshoot the break point slightly (2 to 3Δ) by adding a little more prism in the same direction, then reduce the prism until the patient reports that the target is single again. You may need to remind the patient to tell you when the target becomes single again.

5. Repeat steps 1–4 with the prism base in the opposite direction, but over the same eye. Record your findings as indicated below.

## Recording

- Record the name of the test, e.g., step or smooth vergences, the distance, with what correction, e.g., habitual, modified, subjective, or sc (no correction), and over which eye the prism was introduced.
- Record the orientation of the prisms and the results of break and recovery separated by slashes, e.g., 4/3.
- If recovery values are in the direction opposite to what you expect (testing BD but had to go into BU for recovery), record as a negative value, e.g., 4/−2.

### Examples
- Dist. Step Vergences (subjective): OD BU 4/2, OD BD 2/1
- Dist. Smooth Vergences (sc): OD BU suppression OD, OD BD 3/1
- Dist. Smooth Vergences (modified; +2.25 OU): OD BU 2/0, OD BD 4/2

### Expected Findings
- Break: $3\Delta$ to $4\Delta$
- Recovery: $1.5\Delta$ to $2\Delta$

### Notes
- If the target moves during testing the patient is suppressing the eye without the prism. If the patient does not note a change in the target when large amounts of vertical prism are introduced, consider suppression of the eye with the prism.
- It is not recommended to interchange the results of step vergence and smooth vergence testing. The same method should be used on the same patient in subsequent exams.

## 4.6 NEAR HORIZONTAL STEP AND SMOOTH VERGENCES

### Purpose
The aim of this procedure is to measure the patient's absolute ability to perform horizontal fusional vergence movements at near. Vergences are simultaneous movements of both eyes in opposite directions to maintain single binocular vision. The following description presumes the reader has read the procedure for horizontal vergences at distance, some information stated earlier is omitted here (see Procedure 4.4).

### Equipment
- Horizontal prism bars (step vergences) or phoropter (smooth vergences)
- A near acuity chart for step vergences
- A near rod with accommodative block target for smooth vergences
- Trial frame if measuring step vergences with something other than the habitual Rx

### Setup
- The patient should be wearing their habitual near correction. *Note:* It may be appropriate to measure vergences with the most recent subjective refraction or a modified glasses Rx. In this case, a trial frame can be used, or the alternative Rx can be dialed into the phoropter. In both cases the near pupillary distance should be used.
- The target is an isolated letter or line of letters one to two lines above the patient's best-corrected visual acuity in the poorer seeing eye. The accommodative block is recommended when testing in the phoropter if the patient is 20/20 OD and OS. The target should be well illuminated.
- The near card is placed at 40 cm/16 in. For near step testing, the patient can help the examiner by holding the near card at 40 cm/16 in.

### Procedure
*Step Vergences (Prism Bars)*
1. With both eyes unoccluded, the patient should see one image of the isolated letter or line of letters. Instruct the patient to look at the target and to try to keep it single and clear. Ask the patient to report if/when the target becomes blurry, splits into two, and comes back into one. This represents the blur, break, and recovery points, respectively. The patient should also be instructed to report if the target moves to the left or right at any time. If the patient reports that the target is moving, stop the test, and see "Notes" section of Procedure 4-4.

2. In horizontal step vergence testing, the prism bars can be held over either the right or left eye. Since the eyes are innervated equally, the results of vergence testing in the right eye will be the same as the left. The prism should be held with the lowest amount of prism power first and slowly increased until the patient reports blur, break, and recovery.

3. Slowly increase the amount of prism while noting the amount of prism in front of the patient's eyes when blur and break occur, recall that blur may not occur in every patient. Ensure that the patient is looking through the full prism and not through the break marker between steps in prism power.

4. To determine recovery, overshoot the break point slightly by adding a little more prism in the same direction, then reduce the prism until the patient reports that the target is single again. You may need to remind the patient to tell you when the target becomes single again.

5. Repeat the above steps on the same eye with the prism base in the opposite direction. Record your findings as indicated below.

*Smooth Vergences (Phoropter)*

1. With both eyes unoccluded the patient should see one image of the accommodative block target on the near rod. Instruct the patient to look at the target and to try to keep it clear and single. Ask the patient to report if/when the target becomes blurry, splits into two, and comes back into one. This represents the blur, break, and recovery points, respectively. The patient should also be instructed to report if the target moves to the left or right at any time. If the patient reports that the target is moving, stop the test, and see "Notes" section of Procedure 4-4.

2. In horizontal smooth vergence testing, unlike step vergences, the Risley prisms will be manipulated in both eyes simultaneously. The prism should be oriented with the zero positioned vertically and with the arrow of the Risley prism directed to the zero marker.

3. Slowly increase the amount of prism in both eyes simultaneously at the rate of about $2\Delta$ per second. BI is measured with the Risley arrows moved toward the nose in both eyes and BO with the Risley arrows moved toward the ears in both eyes. Note the total amount of prism, in both eyes, for blur, break, and recovery to occur, e.g., $3\Delta$ BO OD and $4\Delta$ BO OS equals $7\Delta$ BO.

4. To determine recovery, overshoot the break point slightly by adding a little more prism in the same direction, about $10\Delta$, then reduce the prism until the patient reports that the target is single again. You may need to remind the patient to tell you when the target becomes single again.

5. Repeat the above steps with the prism in the opposite direction. Record your findings as indicated below.

## Recording

- Recording is the same as distance horizontal vergence testing, with only the change in testing distance (see Procedure 4.4).

## Examples

- Near Step Vergences (subjective): BI 6/10/4, BO 12/18/8
- Near Smooth Vergences (sc): BI suppression OD, BO 14/16/12
- Near Smooth Vergences (modified; +2.25 OU): BI 4/7/4, BO 10/18/−2

## Expected Findings

- The norms listed in **Table 4-4** represent population-based averages which vary as a result of testing distance, method of testing, age, and target size. For near step testing there are variations in the norms between children and adults. Additionally, it has been recommended based on the current literature that the population-based vergence ranges measured with the step vergence method in children should not be used as one single criterion for diagnosis.

**TABLE 4-4. Expected Findings for Near Smooth and Step Horizontal Vergences**

| Smooth Vergence Testing | | | |
|---|---|---|---|
| Near BO | Blur | 17 | $\mp5$ |
| | Break | 21 | $\mp6$ |
| | Recovery | 12 | $\mp7$ |
| Near BI | Blur | 13 | $\mp4$ |
| | Break | 21 | $\mp4$ |
| | Recovery | 13 | $\mp5$ |
| **Step Vergence Testing** | | | |
| *Children 7–12* | | | |
| Near BO | Blur | Unknown | Unknown |
| | Break | 23 | $\mp8$ |
| | Recovery | 16 | $\mp6$ |
| Near BI | Blur | Unknown | Unknown |
| | Break | 12 | $\mp5$ |
| | Recovery | 7 | $\mp4$ |
| *Adults* | | | |
| Near BO | Blur | Variable | Variable |
| | Break | 19 | $\mp9$ |
| | Recovery | 14 | $\mp7$ |
| Near BI | Blur | Variable | Variable |
| | Break | 13 | $\mp6$ |
| | Recovery | 10 | $\mp5$ |

## 4.7 NEAR VERTICAL STEP AND SMOOTH VERGENCES

### Purpose
The aim of this procedure is to measure the patient's absolute ability to perform vertical fusional vergence movements at near. Vergences are simultaneous movements of both eyes in opposite directions to maintain single binocular vision. The following description presumes the reader has read the procedure for vertical vergences at distance, some information stated earlier is omitted here (see Procedure 4.5).

### Equipment
- Vertical prism bars (step vergences) or phoropter (smooth vergences)
- A near acuity chart for step vergences
- A near rod with accommodative block target for smooth vergences
- Trial frame if measuring step vergences with something other than the habitual Rx

### Setup
- The patient should be wearing their habitual near correction. *Note:* It may be appropriate to measure vergences with the most recent subjective refraction or a modified glasses Rx. In this case, a trial frame can be used, or the alternative Rx can be dialed into the phoropter. In both cases the near pupillary distance should be used.
- The target is an isolated letter or line of letters one to two lines above the patient's best-corrected visual acuity in the poorer seeing eye. The accommodative block is recommended

when testing in the phoropter if the patient is 20/20 OD and OS. The target should be well illuminated.

- The near card is placed at 40 cm/16 in. For near step testing, the patient can help the examiner by holding the near card at 40 cm/16 in.

## Procedure

*Step Vergences (Prism Bars)*

1. With both eyes unoccluded, the patient should see one image of the isolated letter or line of letters. Instruct the patient to look at the target and to try to keep it clear and single. Ask the patient to report if/when the target splits into two and when it comes back into one. This represents the break and recovery points, respectively. The patient should also be instructed to report if the target moves up or down at any time. If the patient reports that the target is moving, stop the test, and see section "Notes" of Procedure 4.5.

2. In vertical step vergence testing it is recommended that the prism bars be held over the right eye for consistency although either eye can be chosen as both eyes are innervated equally. BD OD results should equal BU OS results and vice versa. The prism should be held with the lowest amount of prism power first and slowly increased until the patient reports break and recovery.

3. Slowly increase the amount of prism while noting the amount of prism in front of the patient's eyes when break and recovery occur. Ensure that the patient is looking through the full prism and not through the break marker between steps in prism power.

4. To determine recovery, overshoot the break point slightly (2–3Δ) by adding a little more prism in the same direction then reduce the prism until the patient reports that the target is single again. You may need to remind the patient to tell you when the target becomes single again.

5. Repeat the above steps on the same eye with the prism base in the opposite direction. Record your findings as indicated below.

*Smooth Vergences (Phoropter)*

1. With both eyes unoccluded, the patient should see one image of the accommodative block target. Instruct the patient to look at the target and to try to keep it clear and single. Ask the patient to report if/when the target splits into two and when it comes back into one. This represents the break and recovery points, respectively. The patient should also be instructed to report if the target moves up or down at any time. If the patient reports that the target is moving, stop the test, and see section "Notes" of Procedure 4.5.

2. In vertical smooth vergences, unlike horizontal smooth vergence testing, the Risley prisms only need to be manipulated in one eye. The prism should be oriented with the zero positioned horizontally and with the arrow of the Risley prism directed to the zero marker. It is recommended to use the measuring prism on the right eye for consistency. Recall that both eyes are innervated equally, and the BD OD results should equal BU OS results and vice versa.

3. Slowly increase the amount of prism in the right eye at the rate of about 1Δ per second. BD findings are measured with the Risley arrows moved toward the patient's chin and BU with the Risley arrows moved toward the patient's forehead. Note the amount of prism needed for break and recovery.

4. To determine recovery, overshoot the break point slightly (2 to 3Δ) by adding a little more prism in the same direction then reduce the prism until the patient reports that the target is single again. You may need to remind the patient to tell you when the target becomes single again.

5. Repeat the above steps on the right eye with the prism base in the opposite direction and record your findings as indicated below.

### Recording
- Recording is the same as distance vertical vergence testing, with only the change in testing distance.

### Recording Examples
- Near Step Vergences (subjective): OD BU 4/2, OD BD 2/1
- Near Smooth Vergences (sc): OD BU suppression OD, OD BD 3/1
- Near Smooth Vergences (modified; +2.25 OU): OD BU 2/0, OD BD 4/2

### Expected Findings
- Break: 3Δ to 4Δ
- Recovery: 1.5Δ to 2Δ

## 4.8 AMPLITUDE OF ACCOMMODATION (AMPS)

### Purpose
This test is a subjective measurement, in diopters, of the patient's absolute ability to accommodate to a near stimulus.

### Equipment
- Near point visual acuity card or fixation stick with appropriate targets
- Tape measure or ruler
- Occluder

### Setup
- The patient is tested wearing their habitual distance correction and/or with the correction you would like to determine the patient's ability to accommodate, e.g., an updated manifest refraction.
- Either the patient or the examiner may hold the near point card.
- The near point card should be well illuminated.
- For children, a near fixation stick with Lea Symbols may be used.

### Procedure
1. Instruct the patient to occlude their left eye.
2. Direct the patient's attention to a row of letters one or two lines larger than their habitual near VA.
3. Instruct the patient to keep the letters clear. Children can be asked to call out the letters or pictures to ensure clarity.
4. Slowly move the target closer to the patient and ask the patient to report when the letters first become and stay blurry, known as the *first sustained blur*. The patient should just be able to read the letters (slowly). If the patient cannot read the letters the target should be moved further away so as not to overestimate the amps.
5. Measure the distance from the target to the patient's spectacle plane in centimeters, this is the near point of accommodation.
6. Convert the near point of accommodation to diopters by dividing 100 by the distance measured in cm. This is the patient's absolute amplitude of accommodation in diopters.
7. Occlude the right eye and repeat the procedure for the left eye.

## Recording
- Record the amplitude of accommodation in diopters (round off to the nearest half diopter).
- Separately record the results for the right and left eye.

## Examples
- Amps OD 7 D and OS 8 D
- Amps OD 10.5 D and OS 11 D

## Expected Findings
- The amplitude of accommodation decreases as a function of age. Hofstetter's Formulas are frequently used clinically to determine the expected amplitude of accommodation based on age.
  - Minimum expected amplitude = $15 - 0.25 \times$ (age)
  - Average expected amplitude = $18.5 - 0.30 \times$ (age)
  - Maximum expected amplitude = $25 - 0.40 \times$ (age)
- Donder's Table is also used to determine if amps match expected norms (**see Table 4-5**).

| **TABLE 4-5. Donder's Table for Age-Referenced Amplitude of Accommodation** | | | |
|---|---|---|---|
| **Age** | **Amplitude** | **Age** | **Amplitude** |
| 10 | 14.00 | 45 | 3.50 |
| 15 | 12.00 | 50 | 2.50 |
| 20 | 10.00 | 55 | 1.75 |
| 25 | 8.50 | 60 | 1.00 |
| 30 | 7.00 | 65 | 0.50 |
| 35 | 5.50 | 70 | 0.25 |
| 40 | 4.50 | 75 | 0.00 |

## Notes
- The amplitude of accommodation of the two eyes should be within 1 D of each other.
- Presbyopic patients should be tested while wearing their add. To accurately record the absolute amplitude of accommodation, subtract the numerical value of the add from the measured amps.
- An alternative method of testing young children who may not understand the concept of blur is to start the test with the target close to the patient and move it away until the patient is able to read the letters. This is called the pull-away method and should be denoted in the chart when recording.

## 4.9 FUSED CROSS CYLINDER (FCC)

### Purpose
This is a subjective test used to determine the accuracy of accommodation in non-presbyopes and to find the tentative add for a presbyope. In non-presbyopes, FCC determines over/under accommodation at near under binocular conditions. For an objective test of accommodation accuracy, see Procedure 4.12 on the monocular estimation method (MEM).

### Equipment
- Phoropter with Jackson Cross Cylinders (JCC)
- Cross cylinder target (**Figure 4-8**) and phoropter near rod

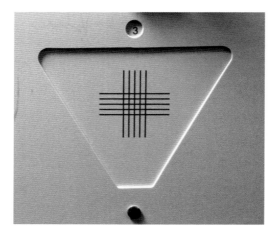

**FIGURE 4-8.** | FCC target.

## Setup

- *Non-presbyopic testing* should be performed with the patient's habitual correction for distance and the patient's near PD dialed into the phoropter. Depending on the patient, it may be appropriate to perform FCC with updated subjective findings or a modified Rx.
- *Presbyopic testing* should be performed with the patient's habitual correction as well but you should confirm with the patient that they can see the cross cylinder target. If the patient cannot see the target, plus sphere should be dialed into the phoropter until the cross cylinder target is visible.
- The cross cylinder target is set on the near point rod at 40 cm in *dim* illumination.
- The JCC is inserted in front of both eyes with the minus cylinder axis set to 90° (red dots vertical). Be sure *not* to change the axis of the correcting cylinder in the phoropter when making this adjustment (**see Figure 4-9**).

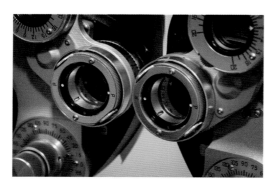

**FIGURE 4-9.** | JCC set at 90°; note that the patient's refractive axis of 15° is unchanged while the JCC is manipulated to 90°.

## Procedure

*Non-Presbyopes*

The FCC procedure is used in non-presbyopes to determine the accuracy of accommodation, i.e., if the patient is under or over accommodating.

1. Ask the patient to report which lines are sharper or clearer, the lines going up and down, side-to-side, or if the lines are equal.

2. If initially the patient reports the vertical lines are sharper (**Figure 4-10A**), reduce the illumination. If the patient then reports the horizontal lines are sharper or equal, proceed to step 3. If the patient reports the vertical lines are still sharper, proceed to step 4.

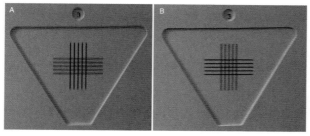

**FIGURE 4-10.** │ FCC from the patient's perspective with (A) the vertical lines appearing clearer and (B) the horizontal lines appearing clearer.

3. For a response of equal (**Figure 4-8**) or horizontal (**Figure 4-10**B) lines as being sharper, add plus lenses binocularly, +0.25 D at a time, until the patient reports that the vertical lines are sharper. Once vertical clarity is achieved, reduce the plus power binocularly until the lines are both equally sharp; this is your endpoint. If equality is not achieved, stop at the last lens before the patient reported the vertical lines sharper.

4. If the patient continues to report that the vertical lines are sharper with reduced illumination, flip the JCC axes so that the minus cylinder axis is at 180° (red dots horizontal).

   a. If the patient then reports that the vertical lines are still sharper, stop the procedure and record "vertical preference."

   b. If the patient reports that the horizontal lines are sharper, record "lead of accommodation." It is highly recommended to measure the lead of accommodation by returning the minus cyl axis of the JCC to 90° and adding minus lenses until the horizontal lines are clearer.

*Tentative Add for Presbyopes*
The procedure for performing FCC in a presbyope is the same for a non-presbyope but testing is performed for a different purpose. Presbyopes are expected to have a lag of accommodation when the test is performed over the distance Rx. For presbyopes, the FCC test is used to determine the tentative add, which is then used during the NRA/PRA procedure (see Procedure 4.10) to determine the final add.

1. Follow procedure steps 1 through 4 as listed above for FCC testing in a non-presbyope. As mentioned previously in setup, it may be necessary for a little plus power to be introduced over the distance Rx in order for the patient to see the cross target initially. Remember to include the added plus to the final FCC value if it had to be introduced to begin the test.

## Recording
- Record the name of the test and the Rx used for testing, e.g., habitual, subjective, or modified.
- Record the total amount of plus added over the distance Rx at the endpoint of the test.
- If an orientation preference is found record the preference, e.g., vertical preference.
- Record if a lead or lag of accommodation was found.

## Examples
- FCC (habitual): +1.00 (lag)
- FCC (subjective): −1.00 (lead)
- FCC (habitual): vertical preference

## Expected Findings
- Non-presbyopes: +0.50 (±0.50); any lead is considered abnormal.
- Presbyopes: Lag of accommodation is expected to increase as a function of age.

## Notes

- Studies have shown that FCC testing in non-presbyopes is not as accurate as other methods such as MEM retinoscopy or open field optometer.
- While any lead of accommodation is considered abnormal, clinically a larger lead is considered more concerning than a smaller lead. Thus, it is highly recommended to measure any lead of accommodation if found.
- Alternative methods have been proposed in which +1.00 to +3.00 sphere is introduced over the distance Rx to reduce the accommodative response and then the test is performed. In this alternative method it is expected that a non-presbyopic patient would prefer the vertical lines and minus lenses would be added until equality is reached at a net of +0.50 (±0.50).
- It is possible to have a horizontal orientation preference. This should be suspected when a relatively large amount of plus does not create a reversal in the clarity of the lines. This is tested similarly to vertical orientation preference (step 4), but the patient will continue to report the horizontal lines as clearer with the change in JCC axis.

## 4.10 NEGATIVE RELATIVE ACCOMMODATION/POSITIVE RELATIVE ACCOMMODATION (NRA/PRA)

### Purpose

In non-presbyopes, NRA/PRA is a subjective test used to determine the patient's ability to increase and decrease accommodation, using lenses, while maintaining single binocular vision. NRA/PRA directly tests accommodation while also indirectly evaluating fusional vergence. In presbyopes, the test is used to balance a tentative add when determining the near add prescription (see section "Balancing an Add" below).

### Equipment

- Phoropter with near point rod and near point card

### Setup

- *Non-presbyopic patients:* The patient's habitual distance correction, distance subjective refraction, or modified distance Rx is dialed into the phoropter along with the patient's near pupillary distance.
- *Presbyopic patients:* The tentative near Rx, determined from any method, is dialed into the phoropter along with the patient's near pupillary distance.
- Near point card set at 40 cm under bright illumination with the patient viewing an isolated line 1–2 lines above the BCVA in the poorer seeing eye.

### Procedure

1. Perform the NRA test first by adding plus lenses binocularly +0.25 D at a time, until the patient reports the first sustained blur. First sustained blur is when the patient reports that the letters are no longer clear, even if the patient can still read them. *Note:* Relaxation of accommodation (NRA) should always be performed prior to stimulation of accommodation (PRA). The patient should also be asked to report if/when any diplopia occurs.
2. Keep track of the total amount of plus added to the starting point in the phoropter. *Note:* The number of "clicks" needed to reach sustained blur can be used for ease of remembering and then converted to diopters for recording.
3. Return the lenses to the initial value used before starting NRA, either the patient's distance prescription or the tentative near prescription.
4. Perform PRA by adding minus lenses binocularly, −0.25 D at a time, until the patient reports the first sustained blur. Note the total amount of minus added.

## Recording

- Record the name of the test and the correction used for testing, e.g., habitual, subjective, or modified.
- Record the total amount of plus and minus, relative to the starting point of either the distance refraction or the tentative near prescription. This should be recorded in diopters and separated by a slash.
- When using NRA/PRA to balance a near add in a presbyope, record the tentative add separately from the NRA/PRA findings. The tentative add will need to be balanced to determine the final add. (See section "Balancing an Add" below).
- If diplopia occurs at any point make note of it in the recording section.

## Examples

- NRA/PRA (habitual): +2.25/−2.50
- NRA/PRA (subjective): +1.00/−1.00 (tentative add +1.25)
- NRA/PRA (habitual): +2.25/−1.00 (diplopia during PRA testing)

## Expected Findings

- *Non-presbyope:* NRA: +2.00 (±0.50); PRA −2.37 (±1.00).
- *Presbyope:* NRA and PRA vary widely but the net plus (tentative add and NRA) should not exceed +2.50 D.
- Diplopia is always considered abnormal.

## Balancing an Add Using NRA/PRA

- Record the tentative add.
- Record the findings of NRA/PRA.
- Add the findings of NRA/PRA algebraically and divide by two. Then add this to the tentative add to get the refined add. *Note:* This method is for the standard distance of 40 cm. The final add may still need to be modified based on the patient's needs and preferred working distance.

*Example*
- Tentative add: +1.00
  NRA/PRA: +1.00/−1.50
  $+1.00 - 1.50 = -0.50$ and $-0.50/2 = -0.25$
  Refined add: +0.75

## Notes

- NRA directly tests relaxation of accommodation and indirectly tests convergence, while PRA directly tests stimulation of accommodation and indirectly tests divergence. Abnormal values on NRA, PRA, or both can indicate a problem with accommodation, vergences, or both. Further testing is required to differentiate. Any diplopia noted during testing is highly suggestive of a vergence problem.
- NRA findings greater than +2.50 (the demand at 40 cm) can indicate that the patient is over-minused or an under-corrected hyperope at distance.

## 4.11 BINOCULAR ACCOMMODATIVE FACILITY (BAF) & MONOCULAR ACCOMMODATIVE FACILITY (MAF)

## Purpose

This is a subjective test used to measure the patient's ability to make rapid accommodative changes under monocular or binocular conditions. The findings can help distinguish between accommodative and binocular disorders.

## Equipment

- Flippers:
  - +2.00/−2.00 lenses for children
  - Amplitude scaled facility lenses (**see Table 4-6**)
- Suppression technique for BAF, see Notes below
- Eye patch for MAF
- Watch, clock, or timer accurate to the second

| TABLE 4-6. Recommended Lenses for Amplitude Scaled Facility | | |
|---|---|---|
| **Amplitude of Accommodation (D)** | **Test Distance (cm)** | **Flipper Lens Power (D)** |
| 22.25 | 10.00 | +/− 3.25 |
| 20.00 | 11.00 | +/− 3.00 |
| 18.25 | 12.00 | +/− 2.75 |
| 16.75 | 13.50 | +/− 2.50 |
| 15.50 | 14.5 | +/− 2.25 |
| 14.25 | 15.5 | +/− 2.25 |
| 13.25 | 16.5 | +/− 2.00 |
| 12.50 | 18.0 | +/− 2.00 |
| 11.75 | 19.0 | +/− 1.75 |
| 11.00 | 20.0 | +/− 1.75 |
| 10.50 | 21.0 | +/− 1.50 |
| 10.00 | 22.0 | +/− 1.50 |
| 9.50 | 23.5 | +/− 1.50 |
| 9.00 | 24.5 | +/− 1.50 |
| 8.75 | 25.5 | +/− 1.25 |
| 8.25 | 26.5 | +/− 1.25 |
| 8.00 | 28.0 | +/− 1.25 |
| 7.75 | 29.0 | +/− 1.25 |
| 7.50 | 30.0 | +/− 1.00 |
| 7.25 | 31.0 | +/− 1.00 |
| 7.00 | 32.0 | +/− 1.00 |
| 6.75 | 33.5 | +/− 1.00 |
| 6.50 | 34.0 | +/− 1.00 |
| 6.25 | 35.5 | +/− 1.00 |
| 6.00 | 37.0 | +/− 1.00 |
| 5.75 | 38.5 | +/− 1.00 |
| 5.50 | 40.5 | +/− 0.75 |
| 5.25 | 42.5 | +/− 0.75 |
| 5.00 | 44.5 | +/− 0.75 |
| 4.75 | 47.0 | +/− 0.75 |
| 4.50 | 49.5 | +/− 0.75 |

*Adapted with permission from Scheiman M, Wick B. *Clinical Management of Binocular Vision: Heterophoric, Accommodative, and Eye Movement Disorders*. 5th ed. Philadelphia: Lippincott Williams & Wilkins; 2020.

## Setup
- The patient wears their habitual correction for near.
- The patient holds a visual acuity card at 40 cm in good illumination.
- See section "Notes" for details on BAF suppression techniques.

## Procedure

*Binocular Accommodative Facility*

BAF is most commonly performed first, as the procedure tests for both accommodative and binocular vision disorders. Many providers advocate for BAF first as a facility screening test followed by MAF only if BAF findings are abnormal.

1. While the patient holds the near card at 40 cm, instruct the patient to let you know when the text is clear. Use a target (line of letters) 1–2 lines larger than BCVA in the poorer seeing eye. Make sure that both of the patient's eyes are unoccluded.
2. Place the plus side of the flipper, e.g., +2.00 in front of the patient's eyes and ask them to report when the print is clear.
3. As soon as the print clears, flip the lenses to the minus side, e.g., −2.00 and ask them to report when the print clears.
4. Continue to repeat steps 2 and 3 while timing the patient for one minute. Make note of how many cycles the patient completes. A full cycle includes clearing both the plus and minus side of the flipper.
   a. It is recommended that a technique to check for suppression is utilized during BAF testing (see BAF Suppression Check below). The test should be ended if the patient suppresses.

*Monocular Accommodative Facility*

This test should be used when an accommodative disorder is suspected or when the patient fails BAF.

1. Occlude the patient's left eye with the eye patch.
2. Perform steps 2 through 4 from the BAF procedure above in the right eye. Then, shift the eye patch to the right eye and repeat steps 2 through 4 from the BAF procedure again for the left eye. Make note of how many cycles the patient completes for each eye.

## Recording
- Record the name of the test and if it was performed with or without correction.
- Record the number of cycles completed in 60 seconds for both eyes together and, if applicable, for each eye monocularly.
- If a patient struggles more with one side of the flipper, e.g., plus, record whether they had greater difficulty clearing the plus or minus lenses, even if the cycles per minute (cpm) were within norms.
- If the patient was unable to clear one side of the flipper, e.g., minus, record "failed minus."
- If suppression occurred during the binocular portion of the test, record which eye suppressed.

## Examples
- BAF sc: 4 cpm, slow on plus; MAF sc: OD 12 cpm and OS 11 cpm
- BAF cc: 3 cpm, failed minus; MAF sc: OD 3 cpm (failed minus) and OS 2 cpm (failed minus)
- BAF cc: 14 cpm
- BAF cc: suppression OD

## Expected Findings

- See expected findings in **Table 4-7**.
- The monocular findings should be within 4 cpm of one another for each eye.

| TABLE 4-7. BAF/MAF Expected Findings | | |
|---|---|---|
| Age | BAF | MAF |
| 8–12 | 5 cpm | 7 cpm |
| 13–30 | 10 cpm | 11 cpm |

## Notes

- It may be preferable to use reading material instead of a near card for children who may not be able to reliably report when text has cleared.

## BAF Suppression Check

Research has shown the importance of checking for suppression during the BAF procedure. Two common methods of suppression testing are described here. However, there are a variety of techniques available.

*Finger Method*

- Intermittently during testing, a finger is placed behind the near card. If the patient is using both eyes, i.e., not suppressing, the patient will have a physiological diplopia response and report two fingers.

*Polaroid Bar Reader Method*

- Polaroid glasses are worn over the patient's habitual correction for near. A polaroid bar reader (**Figure 4-11**) is introduced over the near card (or reading material). If the patient suppresses during the BAF procedure, text will disappear behind the polarized bars coinciding with the eye that is suppressing.

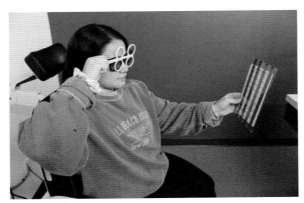

**FIGURE 4-11.** | Polaroid bar reader over the near card as a suppression check in BAF.

## 4.12 DYNAMIC RETINOSCOPY: MONOCULAR ESTIMATION METHOD (MEM)

### Purpose

This test is an objective technique used to measure the accuracy of the accommodative response to a near target. Due to the linkage between accommodation and vergence, this technique can be useful in the diagnosis of vergence and other binocular anomalies. The technique can also be used for predicting the efficacy of some forms of therapeutic intervention. *Note:* Performance of this procedure assumes that the reader is familiar with retinoscopy (see Procedure 3.5).

## Equipment
- Retinoscope
- MEM retinoscopy card(s)
- Loose lenses or lens rack

## Setup
- The MEM card is attached to the retinoscope (see specific manufacturer instructions). Versions for both adults and children are included in most diagnostic equipment kits. Select the card most appropriate for the patient's age and reading ability.
- The test is performed under normal room illumination.
- The patient wears the most plus distance correction, which gives the best corrected visual acuity. Depending on the patient, it may be appropriate to use the subjective or modified Rx.
- The test is performed with both eyes of the patient open.
- The practitioner sits across from the patient with the retinoscope and MEM card, generally at 40 cm. In children, the patient's customary working distance is used.

## Procedure
1. The patient is asked to read the letters/symbols/words on the MEM card. It is recommended for children to call out the symbols/words on the card to ensure attention.
2. While the patient is reading the MEM card, *quickly* scope the horizontal meridian and evaluate the retinoscopy reflex. Be sure to observe the reflex in the center of the pupil rather than at the edge.
3. Estimate the value in diopters required to neutralize the observed motion. (With—plus; Against—minus).
4. Confirm the estimate by quickly (<1 second) interjecting a lens of the estimated power into the patient's line of sight while evaluating the reflex for neutrality. Repeat with other lenses as needed to achieve reflex neutrality. *Note:* To avoid changes in accommodation that will result in invalid data, it is important that the interjection of the lens and evaluation of the reflex be performed quickly.
5. Repeat steps 1 through 4 for the left eye.

## Recording
- Record the technique used (MEM) and the type of correction used, if any.
- Record the lens power, in diopters, required to attain neutrality for the OD and the OS separately.

## Examples
- MEM (habitual): OD +0.50 and OS +0.75
- MEM (subjective): OD −0.50 and OS −0.25
- MEM (sc): OD +0.50 and OS plano

## Expected Findings
- +0.25 to +0.50 (± 0.25) lag.
- Any minus found (lead of accommodation) is abnormal.

## Notes
- MEM represents the dioptric difference between the accommodative stimulus (AS) and the accommodative response (AR). In normal binocular vision, the AR is expected to lag a little behind the exact demand of the AS.

- Due to the linkage between accommodation and vergence, MEM can also be useful in assessing vergence in addition to accommodative disorders.
- MEM can be difficult in young children who are inattentive. For these patients either Bell Retinoscopy or Modified Bell Retinoscopy (procedures outside the scope of this text) may be considered.

## 4.13 MODIFIED THORINGTON (MT)

### Purpose
This test is a subjective, free-space, measurement of the lateral and vertical deviation of the patient at distance and near.

### Equipment
- Transilluminator
- Occluder with Maddox rod (MR)
- Modified Thorington (MT) Card calibrated for the desired testing distance (distance or near)

### Setup
- The patient wears their habitual, subjective, or modified correction for either distance or near depending on the distance at which the MT test is being performed.
- The patient holds the MR over their right eye.
- The MT card is attached to the transilluminator and held by the provider at distance or near. This is typically 10 ft and 40 cm, respectively. Check the manufacturers' guidelines to confirm the distance that your MT Card is calibrated for. See **Figure 4-12**.
  - The grooves of the MR are oriented horizontally to measure the lateral deviation. The patient sees a vertical streak.
  - The grooves of the MR are oriented vertically to measure the vertical deviation. The patient sees a horizontal streak.

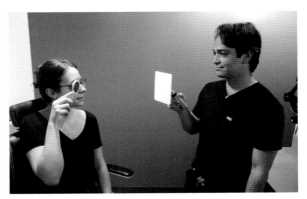

**FIGURE 4-12.** | MT setup.

### Procedure
1. Instruct the patient to look at the light in the center of the card but have an awareness of the red line. Next, instruct the patient to tell you the location of the red line relative to the central light: to the left, to the right, or through the light for the lateral deviation (**see Figure 4-13A and B**); above, below, or through the light for the vertical deviation (**see Figure 4-14**).

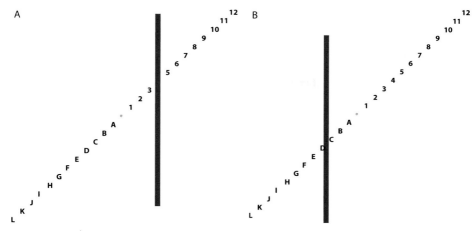

**FIGURE 4-13.** │ MT views from the patient's perspective demonstrating a lateral phoria. (A) The red line is passing through the 4 or to the right of the 0. This is an uncrossed diplopia response indicating a 4Δ esophoria. (B) The red line is passing in between the C and D, to the left of the 0. This is a crossed diplopia response indicating a 3.5Δ exophoria.

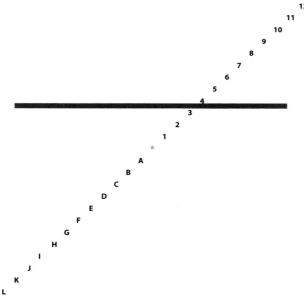

**FIGURE 4-14.** │ MT view from the patient's perspective demonstrating a vertical phoria. The red line is between the 3 and the 4, above the 0, indicating a 3.5Δ left hyperphoria.

2. Perform the lateral phoria first by having the patient hold the grooves of the MR oriented horizontally and proceeding to step 3. After determining the lateral deviation, have the patient rotate the MR so that the grooves are oriented vertically to measure the vertical deviation and repeat steps 3 and 4.

3. To determine the magnitude and direction of the deviation ask the patient to tell you which symbol, e.g., number or letter, is closest to the red line. The targets are each separated by 1Δ when used at the appropriate testing distance. *Note:* Be sure to consult the manufacturer's instructions for your particular MT Card to determine the symbols for your test.

4. Interpretation of the findings for step 3 is outlined in **Table 4-8**.

| TABLE 4-8. Interpretation of Modified Thorington Responses | |
|---|---|
| Lateral | Red line to the left of the light (crossed → exo) |
| | Red line to the right of the light (uncrossed → eso) |
| | Red line through the light (ortho) |
| Vertical | Red line below the light (right hyper) |
| | Red line above the light (right hypo/left hyper) |
| | Red line through the light (ortho) |

*Assuming the Maddox rod is placed over the right eye.

## Recording
- Record the distance at which the test was done, the correction status of the patient, and the name of the test.
- Record the size and the direction of the deviation.
- Record the findings for the lateral deviation followed by the vertical deviation.
- By convention, the hyper eye is always recorded for any vertical deviations, e.g., right hypo is recorded as a left hyper.

## Examples
- Dist. MT (sc): ortho/ortho
- Near MT (cc subjective): 6Δ exo/2Δ left hyper

## Expected Findings
- Distance: 1Δ exo (±2 Δ); no vertical deviation
- Near: 3Δ exo (±3 Δ); no vertical deviation

## Notes
- The patient may report that the red line moves during the test. In this case have the patient close their eyes and tell you through which symbol the red line falls initially.
- Instead of reporting where the red line falls verbally, the patient may be asked to point to the symbol where the red line falls.

## 4.14 MADDOX ROD (MR)

### Purpose
This test is a subjective measurement of the lateral and vertical deviation of a patient at distance and near. This test can be performed in either free space or behind the phoropter.

### Equipment
- Transilluminator
- MR (red or white); can be handheld or dialed into the phoropter
- Prisms (phoropter Risley prisms, prism bars, or loose prism)
- Trial frame if using modified Rx in free space

## Setup

*Phoropter*

- The transilluminator is held at either distance (10 ft) or near (40 cm). The habitual Rx or the correction through which more information is needed, e.g., subjective or modified is dialed into the phoropter along with the appropriate pupillary distance for either distance or near.
- The MR, either red or white, is dialed into the phoropter over the patient's right eye.
- Prism will be introduced using the Risley prisms of the phoropter in the right eye.

*Free-Space*

- The transilluminator is held at either distance (10 ft) or near (40 cm). The habitual Rx or the correction through which more information is needed, e.g., subjective or modified is worn by the patient; along with the appropriate PD for either distance or near if using a trial frame.
- The MR, either red or white, is held over the patient's right eye.
- Prism will be introduced using either loose prisms or prism bars held over the right eye.
  For both the phoropter and free-space techniques, the lateral deviation is measured with the grooves of the Maddox Rod oriented horizontally and the vertical deviation with the grooves oriented vertically. **Table 4-9** outlines which prism orientation should be used to measure the corresponding ocular deviation.

| TABLE 4-9. Prism Orientation for the Measurement of Maddox Rod Phoria | | |
|---|---|---|
| **Prism Orientation** | **Deviation** | **Line Orientation in Space** |
| Base-out | Eso | Line to the right of the light |
| Base-in | Exo | Line to the left of the light |
| Base-down | Right hyper | Line below the light |
| Base-up | Right hypo | Line above the light |

*Assuming the Maddox rod is placed over the right eye.

## Procedure

1. Instruct the patient to look at the light but have an awareness of the red line. Next, instruct the patient to tell you the location of the red line relative to the light: to the left, to the right, or through the light for the lateral deviation and above, below, or through the light for the vertical deviation.

2. To measure the magnitude of the deviation, prism must be used for MR testing. Slowly increase the amount of prism until the line (red if using red MR and white if using white MR) is in alignment with the light from the transilluminator. The amount of prism needed to move the line into alignment with the light is the magnitude of the deviation.

   a. The direction in which the prism should be moved (phoropter) or oriented (free space) is outlined in **Table 4-9**.

## Recording

- Record the distance at which the test was performed, the name of the test, and the correction status of the patient.
- Record the magnitude and direction of the deviation.
- Record the findings for the lateral deviation followed by the vertical deviation.
- By convention the hyper eye is always recorded for vertical phorias, e.g., right hypo is recorded as a left hyper.

**Examples**
- Dist. Maddox Rod (cc habitual): ortho/2Δ right hyper
- Near Maddox Rod (cc subjective): 4Δ eso/ortho

**Expected Findings**
- Distance: 1Δ exo (±2Δ).
- Near: 3Δ exo (±3Δ).

## 4.15 GRADIENT ACCOMMODATIVE CONVERGENCE TO ACCOMMODATION (AC/A) RATIO

**Purpose**

This test is a subjective measurement of the relationship between accommodation and convergence in response to a change of the accommodative stimulus response. This technique is used in the diagnosis and management of binocular vision disorders.

**Equipment**
- Flippers, loose lenses, or phoropter lenses of +/−1.00 D
- Materials for heterophoria measurement
  - von Graefe (phoropter with near rod and near card)
  - Modified Thorington (MT) card with transilluminator

**Procedure**
1. The near heterophoria should first be measured according to the chosen method. See either Procedure 4.3 for von Graefe or Procedure 4.13 for MT.
2. After performing near heterophoria testing introduce the +1.00 D lenses binocularly, either in free space or in the phoropter, and re-measure the heterophoria position. The difference between the phoria position from step 1 and step 2 gives you the AC portion of the AC/A ratio. The stimulus to accommodation is the power of the lens used for testing and represents the A portion of the AC/A ratio. In this case it is +1.00.
3. The test is then repeated with −1.00 D lenses. It is recommended to always test the plus lenses of the AC/A ratio first in order to avoid overstimulating the accommodative response, particularly in younger individuals.

**Recording**
- Record the name of the test, the method of testing, e.g., VG, MT, CT, and if the test was performed with or without correction.
- If the results of testing differed between the plus and minus powers record the power of the lens and the AC/A ratio obtained with that lens.

**Examples**
- Gradient AC/A Ratio (MT) sc: 4/1
- Gradient AC/A Ratio (VG) cc: 2/1
- Gradient AC/A Ratio (MT) cc: with +1.00 (2/1) and −1.00 (5/1)

**Expected Findings**
- Various expected norms have been reported in the literature depending on the method of testing. Generally, AC/A findings outside of 2/1 and 6/1 are considered suspect for a binocular vision disorder.

## Notes

- In addition to the gradient method of AC/A measurement, a method for calculating the AC/A ratio using the patient's interpupillary distance (IPD), near fixation distance (NFD) and prism cover test (PCT) findings can also be used. The formula to calculate the AC/A ratio by this method is as follows:

$$AC/A = IPD\ (cm) + NFD\ (m)\ (PCT\ near - PCT\ far)$$

For this formula, esophoria is recorded as plus and exophoria as minus. It is important to note that the results from the calculated AC/A ratio will be approximately 10% higher than that of the gradient AC/A ratio due to the lag of accommodation that naturally occurs during the gradient AC/A procedure.

- The results from the AC/A ratio with the +/− 1.00 D lenses should be equivalent, if not the patient may have a vergence and/or accommodative dysfunction and further investigation is needed.

- If a +/− 1.00 D flipper is not available a +/− 2.00 D flipper may be used, but the fraction should be reduced when recording, e.g., 4/2 → 2/1. Research has indicated that the response to the AC/A accommodative stimulus behaves non-linearly and thus it is not recommended to use higher powers until this relationship is better understood.

- The main source of error in the measurement of the AC/A ratio is failure to control the accommodative response. The practitioner should remind the patient to keep the target clear at all times in order to control the accommodative response.

## 4.16 ASSOCIATED PHORIA

### Purpose

Fixation disparity is the small misalignment of the visual axes when both eyes are open in patients with normal fusion. The associated phoria is the measurement of the misalignment of the visual axes that appears when the fixation disparity is corrected with prism, i.e., it is the measure of the underlying phoria present during binocular viewing. It can be a valuable diagnostic procedure for binocular disorders, particularly in presbyopes. Additionally, the associated phoria can be used to determine the amount of prism to prescribe for patients with vertical imbalances.

### Equipment

- Associated phoria target (produced in a variety of designs)
- Phoropter with polarizing filters and Risley prisms, or polarized glasses worn over habitual correction
- Risley prisms (phoropter) or hand-held prism bars

### Setup

- The test can be performed at distance and/or near, and both vertical and horizontal fixation disparity can be measured. The patient should wear the habitual correction for the distance being tested. Depending on the patient, it may be appropriate to use the findings from the subjective refraction or a modified Rx.
- The polarizing filters are dialed into the phoropter or polarizing filters are worn over the patient's glasses. Both eyes should be open for the procedure.
- There are a variety of associated phoria targets, which is not limited to the following: Mallett Unit, AO Slides, Saladin Card, Sheedy Disparometer, Wesson Card, two Pola cross tests, two Pola pointer tests, and two Pola double pointer tests. It is recommended to consult the manufacturer's guidelines for specific details recommended for setup.

## Procedure

The general steps outlined for this procedure are described for the Wesson Card. The authors make no specific recommendations for the target used for the measurement of fixation disparity and associated phoria. It is recommended to consult the manufacturer guidelines for procedure details of the specific associated phoria target used.

1. The general procedure is to use a target consisting of vernier offset test (nonius) lines of fixed size, usually polarized so one line is seen by each eye. The patient is then asked to report when the offset line is directly aligned with a reference line. The amount of prism needed to bring the offset line into alignment with the reference line (fixation disparity of zero) is the associated phoria.

2. It is important to check for suppression during associated phoria testing. Depending on the specific target used, there will be a suppression check seen only by the right eye and only by the left eye. The patient should be asked to report if either suppression check disappears during testing. If suppression occurs during testing, end the test, determine which eye is suppressing, and record the results.

   *Note:* Associated phoria has been used as a method to determine the appropriate amount of vertical prism correction to prescribe. It is typically not recommended to use associated phoria findings to prescribe for lateral prism as there is a tendency to overestimate the needed prism correction for patients with eso deviations.

### Vertical Associated Phoria

1. The Wesson Card is rotated 90° so that the lines are oriented horizontally. If the arrow is aligned with the reference line, the patient has an associated phoria of ortho. If the arrow falls above the reference line, the patient has a right hyper fixation disparity and if the arrow falls below the reference line, the patient has a right hypo fixation disparity.

2. Measure the amount of vertical associated phoria by introducing prism in the right eye, e.g., if the reference line falls below the arrow (right hyper fixation disparity) use BD prism on the right eye to bring the reference line into alignment with the arrow. **Table 4-10** outlines prism orientation and interpretation for the associated phoria.

| TABLE 4-10. Prism Orientation and Interpretation for the Measurement of the Associated Phoria | | |
| --- | --- | --- |
| Arrow (In Relation to Reference Line) | Associated Phoria | Measuring Prism |
| Above | Right Hyper | BD on right eye |
| Below | Right Hypo (left hyper) | BU on right eye |
| Right | Crossed (exo) | BI on right eye |
| Left | Uncrossed (eso) | BO on right eye |

BD, base down; BI, base in; BO, base out; BU, base up

### Horizontal Associated Phoria

1. The Wesson Card is rotated back to the horizontal position so that the lines are now oriented vertically. If the arrow is aligned with the reference line, the patient has an associated phoria of ortho. If the reference line falls to the left of the arrow, the patient has a crossed or exo deviation and if the reference line falls to the right of the arrow the patient has an uncrossed or eso deviation.

2. Measure the amount of horizontal associated phoria by introducing prism in the right eye, e.g., use BI prism in an exo deviation to move the reference line into alignment with the arrow.

### Recording
- Record the name of the test, the target used, the distance at which the test was done, and the correction status.
- Record the amount and direction of the prism required to achieve alignment.
- If the phoria is ortho denote horizontal and vertical phoria with an H and V.
- If a vertical associated phoria exists, specify the eye over which the prism was placed.

### Examples
- Associated phoria (Wesson Card) habitual: Near H ortho and V ortho
- Associated phoria (Wesson Card) subjective: Near 2Δ BO and 2Δ BD OD
- Associated phoria (AO slides) sc: suppression OS

### Expected Findings
- Associated phoria: ortho at distance and near.

### Notes
- Free space testing with a trial frame and polarizing lenses allows the clinician to test associated phoria in different positions of gaze. Testing vertical associated phoria in downgaze is frequently useful in clinical practice.
- The magnitude of the associated phoria is influenced by a variety of factors including, proximal vergence, vergence adaptation, suppression, and reduced peripheral fusion.
- While typically the fixation disparity is in the same direction as the heterophoria, it is possible for patients to have a paradoxical response in which the fixation disparity is opposite the direction of the heterophoria. Patients with this pattern are usually exo.

## 4.17 WORTH FOUR DOT (W4D)

### Purpose
This is a subjective test used to determine the patient's sensory fusion at distance and near, or to check for a central suppression scotoma.

### Equipment
- W4D target attachment or flashlight
- Red-green glasses
- Transilluminator if using the W4D attachment

### Setup
- The patient wears their habitual correction for the distance being tested with the red-green glasses over their correction. The red lens goes over the right eye and green lens over the left eye.
- If using the W4D attachment, place the attachment on the end of the transilluminator with the white dot located at the bottom and red dot at the top (**see Figure 4-15**).
- Near W4D is performed at 40 cm (16 in) and distance W4D at 6 m (20 ft). *Note:* It has been suggested that using a test distance of 4 m under dark conditions may be more accurate. Some near W4D tests are calibrated for 33 cm; consult the manufacturer's specific instructions.

### Procedure
1. Hold the W4D target at the appropriate distance with the target pointed at the patient's face. Confirm that the patient can see the red dots with the right eye and the green dots with the left by alternately occluding each eye.

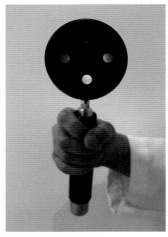

**FIGURE 4-15.** | The W4D as held by the examiner.

2. Ask the patient how many spots of light they see.
   a. Four dots → fusion
   b. Two red dots → suppression OS
   c. Three green dots → suppression OD
   d. Five dots → diplopia
3. If the patient sees five dots, ask the patient to describe their orientation using the green dots as the reference point (**see Figure 4-16**).
   a. Red dots to the right → eso (uncrossed) deviation
   b. Red dots to the left → exo (crossed) deviation
   c. Red dots above → Right hypo deviation (record as left hyper)
   d. Red dots below → Right hyper deviation
4. Record the interpretation of the patient's response.

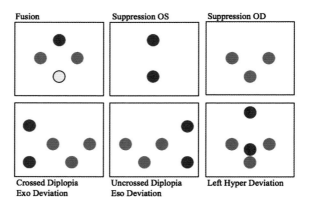

**FIGURE 4-16.** | Examples of the appearance of the W4D as seen by the patient. In this example, the red lens is over the patient's right eye and the green lens is over the patient's left eye.

*Testing for a Central Suppression Scotoma*

1. Perform the W4D test at near as outlined above. If the patient has fusion at 40 cm, slowly begin to move away from the patient.

2. Ask the patient to report any changes in the number of dots. If either the red or the green dots disappear, record the eye that is suppressing and at what distance. Distances of <2 m are considered distinctly abnormal.

3. If the patient still reports seeing four dots at a distance of 3 m (10 ft), stop the test and record "no suppression to 3 m."

## Recording

- Record the name of the test and the distance at which the test was done.
- Interpret the findings (**see Figure 4-16**) and record as appropriate, e.g., W4D @ 40 cm fusion or W4D @ 20 cm suppression OS.
- If the patient sees five dots record "diplopia" and the orientation, e.g., W4D @ 40 cm diplopia eso.
- Vertical deviations are recorded noting the hyper eye by convention, e.g., W4D @ 40 cm diplopia L hyper.
- Record the distance at which suppression occurred when testing for a central suppression scotoma, e.g., W4D @ 2 m suppression OS.

## Examples

- W4D @ 40 cm fusion
- W4D @ 2 m suppression OS
- W4D @ 40 cm diplopia L hyper

## Notes

- W4D cannot determine with certainty which eye is deviating, only the relationship between the eyes. Therefore, it is incorrect to record an eye with the horizontal deviation, e.g., eso OS. The exception to this is vertical deviations where the hyper eye is recorded by convention.
- A combination of both horizontal and vertical deviations can occur. Ask the patient to describe the orientation of the five dots (displaced obliquely) and record both findings, e.g., W4D @ 40 cm diplopia exo, R hyper.
- Prisms can be used to measure the magnitude of the deviation or when considering prescribing prism to promote fusion.
- The W4D test can be performed in both light and dark conditions. Dark conditions may lessen the effects of peripheral fusion and detect instances of suppression more readily.
- Individuals with red/green color vision defects can still perform the W4D test.
- Modifications to the W4D for children, who do not have reliable verbal responses, have been suggested, e.g., "touching four dots" but these have been shown to be unreliable and could only be used to determine left or right suppression and not fusion.

## 4.18 FOUR PRISM DIOPTER BASE OUT TEST (4Δ BO TEST)

## Purpose

An objective test used to determine the presence or absence of a small central suppression scotoma or mictrotropia. Patients with a slight reduction in best corrected visual acuity (20/25 to 20/40) in one eye and mildly reduced stereopsis (30 to 80 seconds of arc) should undergo 4Δ BO testing. Macular diseases affecting the foveal area will create a similar clinical presentation and must be ruled out.

## Equipment
- Loose 4Δ prism
- Isolated single letter, one line above the VA in the poorer seeing eye, at distance

## Setup
- The patient wears their habitual distance correction and views an isolated single letter one line above the VA in the worse seeing eye on the distance visual acuity chart.

## Procedure
1. Instruct the patient to fixate on the distance target and try to keep it clear and single, even if the target appears to move.
2. Hold the 4Δ prism between your thumb and forefinger so it will be positioned base out when placed in front of the patient's better seeing eye (**see Figures 4-17 and 4-18**).
3. Quickly insert the prism in front of the better seeing eye while watching the opposite eye for movement. A normal response is a concomitant movement outward, then an inward refixation movement. Keep the prism in front of the eye for several seconds to allow time

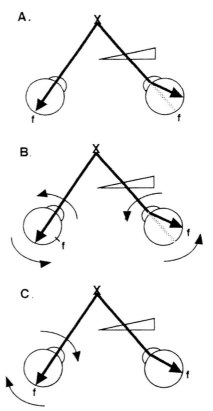

**FIGURE 4-17.** Movement of the eyes during the 4Δ BO test when the patient does not have a suppression scotoma. (A) The prism placed over the patient's right eye, shifting the retinal image and causing the patient to see double. (B) To avoid diplopia, the right eye moves inward to regain foveal fixation. The left eye makes a concomitant outward movement. (C) To avoid diplopia, the left eye makes an inward refixation movement to regain foveal fixation.

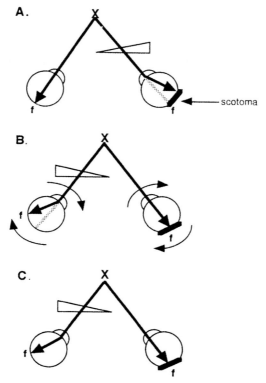

**FIGURE 4-18.** │ Movement of the eyes during the 4Δ BO test when the patient has a suppression scotoma in their right eye. (A) When the prism is placed over the patient's right eye, the retinal image shifts but is still located within the suppression zone. The patient does not see double so neither eye moves. (B) When the prism is placed over the patient's left eye, the retinal image shifts and the left eye moves inward to regain foveal fixation. The right eye makes a concomitant outward movement. (C) The retinal image in the right eye is still located within the suppression zone, so there is no refixation movement of the right eye.

for the refixation movement. Step 3 may be repeated as often as necessary to ascertain the movement of the poorer seeing eye.

4. After determining a refixation movement of the better seeing eye, repeat the test in the poorer seeing eye. Remember to adjust the prism so it continues to be in the BO position in the poorer seeing eye. A normal response is a concomitant movement outward, then an inward refixation movement. Keep the prism in front of the eye for several seconds to allow time for the refixation movement.

## Recording
- Record the name of the test and if the test was performed with or without correction.
- An abnormal response, i.e., no concomitant movement outward followed by refixation of the eye without the prism, is recorded as a "positive" test result and indicates suppression. If suppression occurs, indicate which eye is suppressing. See **Table 4-11** for further description of test results.
- Record "negative" if the test results do not indicate suppression.

**TABLE 4-11.  4Δ BO Test Interpretation**

| 4Δ BO Interpretation | | |
|---|---|---|
| Normal | Eye with prism will move inward | Eye without prism will move outward and then inward to refixate |
| Abnormal | Eye with prism will not move | Eye without prism will not move outward and then inward to refixate |

### Examples
- 4Δ BO (sc): (+) suppression OD
- 4Δ BO (cc): (−)

### Notes
- It is recommended to perform other tests of central suppression, such as the W4D or Bagolini lenses, when results of the 4ΔBO test are variable or atypical to correlate findings.

## 4.19 PURSUITS AND SACCADES

### Purpose
The aim of this procedure is to assess the quality of both refixation (saccade) and smooth (pursuit) eye movements.

### Indications
This test is used to further assess patients who show abnormalities with eye movements during extraocular motility testing. This test should be performed on patients who are symptomatic when reading and their symptoms are not explained by a refractive or binocular problem.

### Equipment
- Two fixation targets. Ideally, this is a red and green bead for adults or two small pictures for children.

### Setup
- The patient and examiner should be standing in front of each other about 1 meter apart. The patient should have their legs slightly apart and standing comfortably.
- The examiner will hold the fixation target(s) about 40 cm from the patient.
- This test is performed binocularly.

### Procedure
The procedure described below is adapted from the NSUCO oculomotor test. Consult the NSUCO Oculomotor Test Manual for further details.

*Pursuits*
1. Instruct the patient to follow a single fixation target as it is moved around. Ask the patient to keep their eyes on the target at all times. Do not give any specific instructions regarding head and body movement, as this should be observed during testing.
2. The target should be held such that the midline of the circle is in line with the patient's eyes.
3. Smoothly move the fixation target in a 20 cm circle not going beyond 40 cm from the patient's eyes in any position.
4. Perform this circle movement two times in the clockwise (CW) direction, and two times in the counterclockwise direction (CCW).
5. Observe the patient's eye, head, and body movements.

*Saccades*

1. Hold two fixation targets about 20 cm apart at eye level of the patient. The targets should be not more than 40 cm from the patient. It is best to have two targets that are identifiably different, e.g., a red bead or sticker and a green bead or sticker, for ease of instruction (**see Figure 4-19**).

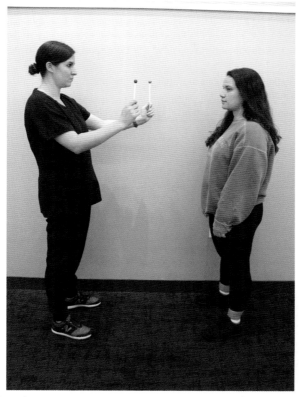

**FIGURE 4-19.** | Saccade test setup.

2. Do not give specific instructions on head or body movement during the test, as this should be observed throughout the procedure.

3. Instruct the patient to look at one target and hold their fixation on the target. Tell the patient not to look at the other target until instructed to do so. Then, tell the patient to look at the other target and fixate on that target. Repeat five round trip cycles asking the patient to look from one target to the next.

## Recording
- Include the name of the test.
- Both pursuits and saccades are evaluated using four criteria:
  - Ability
  - Accuracy
  - Head Movement
  - Body Movement
- Each criterion is graded on a five-point scale, **see Table 4-12**.

**TABLE 4-12. Pursuit and Saccade Scoring for Ability, Accuracy, and Head and Body Movement**

**a. Ability**

| Pursuits | Saccades |
|---|---|
| 1. Completes less than one-half rotation in either the clockwise (CW) or counterclockwise (CCW) direction. | 1. Completes less than two round trips. |
| 2. Completes at least one-half, but not one full rotation in either the CW or CCW direction. | 2. Completes two round trips. |
| 3. Completes one rotation in either the CW or CCW direction, but not two full rotations. | 3. Completes three round trips. |
| 4. Completes two rotations in either direction, but not two rotations in the other. | 4. Completes four round trips. |
| 5. Completes two rotations in both directions. | 5. Completes five round trips. |

**b. Accuracy**

| Pursuits | Saccades |
|---|---|
| 1. No attempt to follow the target or refixates >10 times. | 1. Gross overshooting or undershooting is observed. |
| 2. Refixates 5–10 times. | 2. Moderate to large overshooting or undershooting is observed. |
| 3. Refixates 3–4 times. | 3. Constant slight overshooting or undershooting is observed. |
| 4. Refixates 2 or less times. | 4. Intermittent slight overshooting or undershooting is observed. |
| 5. No refixations. | 5. No overshooting or undershooting is observed. |

**c. Head Movement and d. Body Movement;**

**Both use the same movement scale and are used for both pursuits and saccades**

| |
|---|
| 1. Gross movement of head/body. |
| 2. Moderate to large movement of head/body. |
| 3. Constant slight movement of head/body. |
| 4. Intermittent slight movement of head/body. |
| 5. No movement of head/body. |

• Recording is documented with the numerical score of each criterion in the following format: Pursuits: Ability / Accuracy / Head Movement / Body Movement, Saccades: Ability / Accuracy / Head Movement / Body Movement.

## Examples
• NSUCO Oculomotor Test: Pursuits 4 / 3 / 3 / 4, Saccades 3 / 3 / 2 / 2

## Expected Findings
• The norms for the NSUCO oculomotor test have been determined for males and females aged 5–14. The minimum acceptable scores for saccades and pursuits by age and sex are included in **Tables 4-13** and **4-14**, respectively.

**TABLE 4-13.  Saccade Minimal Acceptable Score by Age and Sex**

| Age | Ability | | Accuracy | | Head Movement | | Body Movement | |
| --- | --- | --- | --- | --- | --- | --- | --- | --- |
| | Male | Female | Male | Female | Male | Female | Male | Female |
| 5 | 5 | 5 | 3 | 3 | 2 | 2 | 3 | 4 |
| 6 | 5 | 5 | 3 | 3 | 2 | 3 | 3 | 4 |
| 7 | 5 | 5 | 3 | 3 | 3 | 3 | 3 | 4 |
| 8 | 5 | 5 | 3 | 3 | 3 | 3 | 4 | 4 |
| 9 | 5 | 5 | 3 | 3 | 3 | 3 | 4 | 4 |
| 10 | 5 | 5 | 3 | 3 | 3 | 4 | 4 | 4 |
| 11 | 5 | 5 | 3 | 3 | 3 | 4 | 4 | 5 |
| 12 | 5 | 5 | 3 | 3 | 3 | 4 | 4 | 5 |
| 13 | 5 | 5 | 3 | 3 | 3 | 4 | 5 | 5 |
| ≥14 | 5 | 5 | 4 | 3 | 3 | 4 | 5 | 5 |

**TABLE 4-14.  Pursuit Minimal Acceptable Score by Age and Sex**

| Age | Ability | | Accuracy | | Head Movement | | Body Movement | |
| --- | --- | --- | --- | --- | --- | --- | --- | --- |
| | Male | Female | Male | Female | Male | Female | Male | Female |
| 5 | 4 | 5 | 2 | 3 | 2 | 3 | 3 | 4 |
| 6 | 4 | 5 | 2 | 3 | 2 | 3 | 3 | 4 |
| 7 | 5 | 5 | 3 | 3 | 3 | 3 | 3 | 4 |
| 8 | 5 | 5 | 3 | 3 | 3 | 3 | 4 | 4 |
| 9 | 5 | 5 | 3 | 4 | 3 | 3 | 4 | 4 |
| 10 | 5 | 5 | 4 | 4 | 4 | 4 | 4 | 5 |
| 11 | 5 | 5 | 4 | 4 | 4 | 4 | 4 | 5 |
| 12 | 5 | 5 | 4 | 4 | 4 | 4 | 5 | 5 |
| 13 | 5 | 5 | 4 | 4 | 4 | 4 | 5 | 5 |
| ≥14 | 5 | 5 | 5 | 4 | 4 | 4 | 5 | 5 |

- The test is failed if the patient scores below the minimum acceptable score for their age and sex.

# 5

# Ocular Health Assessment

Benjamin Young, OD, FAAO / Jennifer Reilly, OD, MSc, FAAO / Maureen Hanley, OD

## 5.1 INTRODUCTION TO OCULAR HEALTH ASSESSMENT

Ocular health assessment is critical to both developing and paring down the primary eye care provider's differential diagnosis. By listening carefully to the patient's chief complaint, taking a comprehensive case history, and performing entrance and refractive testing, a keen clinician will be able to tailor their ocular health assessment to efficiently reach the most accurate diagnosis. Since several of the procedures listed below require pupillary dilation or very bright illumination, the ocular health assessment is typically performed at the end of the examination to avoid adversely affecting other test results (e.g., visual acuity, pupils, subjective refraction). By this point in the examination, the examiner should have a fairly clear indication of the patient's ocular health status in addition to a well-developed differential diagnosis.

Symptoms such as transient monocular vision loss, flashes of light, or ocular pain warrant a thorough ocular health assessment, as potentially sight-threatening or even life-threatening disease may be present. The patient may also have a medical condition with serious potential ocular manifestations, such as diabetes or hypertension, or they may be taking medication such as prednisone or hydroxychloroquine that put them at risk of toxicity which may permanently damage ocular structures such as the retina or lens. While many of the entrance tests, such as pupillary testing, color vision testing, and extraocular motility testing screen for health problems, the ocular health assessment is pivotal in determining a much more specific cause for the abnormalities in previous testing. The patient's best-corrected visual acuity (BCVA) in particular is an excellent indicator of ocular health status, as visual acuity of 20/20 or better indicates that the macula is functioning well, and the media along the visual axis are clear. If visual acuity is not 20/20 and functional etiologies such as amblyopia have been ruled out, an ocular health problem is the likely cause.

The core testing portion of the ocular health examination is designed to effectively and efficiently screen for disease or potential problems in each of three major areas:

1. The anterior segment of the eye;

2. the posterior segment of the eye; and

3. the neurological elements of the eyes and the visual system. To enhance examination of the neurological status of the patient, see also Chapter 8, "Cranial Nerve Screening."

If the main route for assessment uncovers unusual findings or if the patient's symptoms or case history suggest a health problem, side trips or problem-specific testing are incorporated into the examination (see **Figure 5-1**). There are numerous problem-specific tests available, and that number continues to grow as new technology and instrumentation advance (Chapters 9 and 10 detail a number of these more advanced techniques); but, the techniques chosen for inclusion in this chapter allow the examiner to assess a wide range of common health problems without the need for additional equipment outside the standard of care diagnostic equipment found in the vast majority of primary eye care provider exam rooms.

The main route suggested in this section is not meant to be rigidly defined. Individual examiners may prefer to modify this portion of the examination based on their own professional judgment or patient population. For instance, an examiner whose patient population is primarily elderly may include the Amsler grid test in their main flow to routinely screen for macular disease.

When contemplating the tests to include in the core examination, it is important to determine whether or not the patient's eyes will be dilated. Pupillary dilation greatly enhances the examiner's ability to observe certain ocular structures, such as the crystalline lens, the vitreous, the optic nerve head (ONH), and the peripheral retina. Procedures such as binocular indirect ophthalmoscopy (BIO) allow for examination of the retina beyond the region of the

## Flow of Ocular Health Assessment

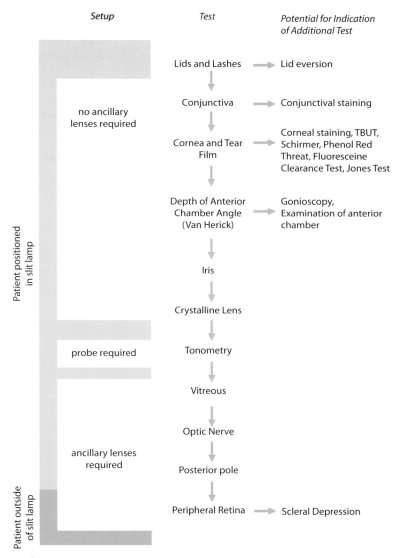

**FIGURE 5-1.** | This diagram illustrates the relationship between the main route or core procedures within the ocular health assessment examination and side trips or problem-specific procedures. The main route procedures are down the center and the side trips are on the right.

posterior pole. The standard of optometric care now recommends that comprehensive ocular examinations include examination of the ocular fundus including the peripheral retina.

When incorporating dilation into the examination, careful consideration must be given to the sequence of testing. For instance, all tests requiring accurate accommodation (e.g., negative relative accommodation/positive relative accommodation, amplitude of accommodation, binocular accommodative facility and monocular accommodative facility), must be completed prior to instillation of dilating drops. Pupillary testing must also be completed before dilation, as the drops will keep the pupils from adequately constricting. Slit lamp biomicroscopy should be performed prior to dilation to evaluate the integrity of the anterior segment of the eye, and the anterior chamber angle depth must be estimated via the Van Herick technique to determine if it is safe to dilate. If the angle depth is equal to or less than 1/4:1 according to the Van Herick method, then gonioscopy should be performed to more accurately assess the angle and the safety of dilation. Finally, the patient's intraocular pressure (IOP) must be measured prior to dilation.

All techniques that are enhanced by pupillary dilation should be deferred until after dilation occurs. These include evaluation of the crystalline lens and anterior vitreous with the biomicroscope and assessment of the posterior segment. **Figure 5-2** presents a suggested

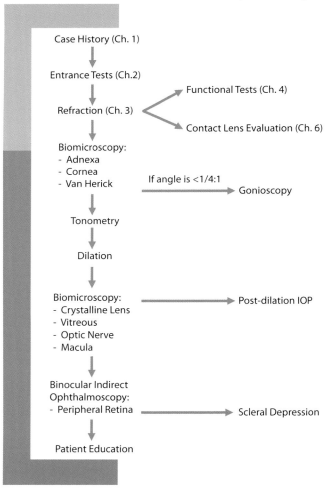

**Flow of the Ocular Health Assessment within a Comprehensive Eye Exam**

**FIGURE 5-2.** │ Flow diagram illustrating a suggested sequence of tests for the ocular health assessment when the patient's pupils are being dilated. The first three groups are not solely part of the health assessment but are included to remind the examiner that these tests must be completed prior to dilating the patient's pupils. The procedures on the right are problem-specific techniques that are performed only when indicated.

examination sequence for a comprehensive examination when the patient's pupils are to be dilated.

A number of techniques described in this section involve instruments that are placed in direct contact with ocular surfaces or fluids. It is critical that these instruments be disinfected following the guidelines set forth by the Centers for Disease Control and Prevention (CDC) (or other local legal requirements if outside the United States), see Procedure 2.2, "Infection Control." The examiner should also observe Standard Precautions whenever a procedure involves touching a patient, e.g., vigorous hand washing with soap and water or an alcohol-based hand sanitizer before and after every patient encounter to prevent the spread of infection. Clear instructions given to the patient are also crucial in maximizing safety and accuracy.

The procedures presented in this chapter are grouped according to their primary purpose. Techniques for evaluating the anterior segment of the eye are presented first. Procedures for observing the posterior segment are next. Tests used to assess the neurological elements of the eye, including screening for optic nerve dysfunction, are at the end of the chapter and in Chapter 8.

## 5.2 BIOMICROSCOPY (SLIT LAMP)

### Purpose
The aim of this procedure is to evaluate the health of the anterior segment of the eye as far posterior as the anterior portion of the vitreous humor. The slit lamp is particularly important for evaluating the fit of a contact lens on the eye (see Chapter 6 for more details). Auxiliary lenses are often used with the slit lamp to visualize structures otherwise obscured, such as a gonioscopy lens to view deep angle structures, or a 90 D lens to view the ocular fundus.

### Equipment
- Biomicroscope (slit lamp)

### Basic Components of the Slit Lamp
Though there are different variations of the slit lamp depending on the manufacturer, there are a number of components common to all slit lamps:
- **Microscope Arm**
  The microscope arm houses the viewing system, composed of the objective and ocular lenses. The angle of the microscope arm can be varied, although it is typically kept in the center pointed straight ahead at the eye (otherwise known as 0°). The following components are located on the microscope arm:
  - *Oculars:* The eyepieces the examiner looks through to visualize the image. The lenses within the oculars can compensate for the examiner's refractive error, and the distance between the oculars can be adjusted to match the examiner's PD.
  - *Magnification changer:* A dial or knob which can either increase or decrease the image seen through the oculars.
- **Illumination Arm**
  The illumination arm houses the light source. The angle of the arm can be varied from 0° to 90° from center. The following components are located on the illumination arm:
  - *Reflecting mirror:* Directs light from the illumination source toward the eye.
  - *Slit controls:* Changes the focus of the beam from diffuse to focal illumination. There are two size controls: one to vary the slit width and another to vary the slit height. There is also a control that varies the orientation (rotation) of the slit beam.
  - *Click stop:* The position of the reflecting mirror relative to the viewing system. When the mirror is "in click stop," the focus of the slit will be coincident with the focus of the viewing system; this setup is also referred to as "confocal," as the focus of slit beam aligned

with the focus of the oculars. When the mirror is "out of click stop," the focus of the slit beam is not coincident with the focus of the viewing system (i.e., no longer confocal).
- *Filters:* Used to vary the appearance of the slit beam. Most slit lamps include a cobalt blue filter, a green or red-free filter, and at least one neutral density filter.
• **Slit Lamp Position Controls**
- *Joystick/elevation knob:* Typically, a single control found on the instrument base which moves the slit lamp closer and further away from the eye, allowing for focus on more anterior or posterior structures. The joystick also controls the left-to-right movement of the slit lamp, and typically is twisted to control the elevation, allowing for viewing of more superior or inferior structures.

## Setup

• Hand hygiene should be performed by the examiner at the start of any slit lamp procedure.
• The patient removes their spectacles and may or may not remove their contact lenses, depending on the purpose of the examination.
• The room illumination is dim.
• The examiner disinfects the forehead rest and the chin rest by wiping with alcohol and drying with a tissue.
• The examiner adjusts the height of the instrument table to a comfortable position for both the patient and the examiner.
• The reflecting mirror is set in the click stop position.
• The patient places their chin in the chin rest and forehead gently against the forehead rest.
• The examiner adjusts the chin rest to align the patient's outer canthus with the demarcation line on the upright support of the headrest.
• The patient closes their eyes before the examiner turns the instrument on.
• The examiner sets the magnification on a low setting (6× or 10×) and removes all filters.
• If not wearing any correction, the examiner adjusts the individual eyepieces to align with their distance spectacle prescription. If wearing an updated pair of glasses, the examiner sets the power of the oculars to plano in both eyes.
• The examiner adjusts the horizontal separation of the oculars to align with their PD. If the PD and focus is set properly, the examiner should obtain a fused binocular view when looking through the oculars.
• The examiner places one hand on the joystick to align and focus the microscope. The other hand is used to operate the slit controls on the illumination arm, to vary the angle of the illumination arm, or to manipulate the patient's eyelids (**Table 5-1**).

**TABLE 5-1. Type of Slit Beam, Angle of the Illumination Arm from the Straight-Ahead Position, and Magnification Used to Evaluate Various Ocular Structures During the Routine Slit Lamp Examination**

| Ocular Structure | Type of Slit Lamp Beam | Angle of Illumination Arm | Magnification |
|---|---|---|---|
| Lids/lashes | Diffuse | 30° | Low |
| Conjunctiva | Wide parallelepiped | 30° | Low |
| Cornea | Narrow parallelepiped | 30°–45° | Medium |
| Anterior chamber angle depth | Optic section | 60° | Medium |
| Aqueous | Conical beam | 30°–45° | High |
| Iris | Wide parallelepiped | 30°–45° | Medium |
| Lens | Narrow parallelepiped | 20°–30° | Medium |

## Procedure

The anterior segment of the eye is typically examined in an anterior-to-posterior sequence in the following order: lids/lashes, conjunctiva, tear film, cornea, anterior chamber angle, iris, lens, anterior vitreous humor. By convention, the right eye is typically examined first, followed by the left eye.

### Lids and Lashes

1. Use low and diffuse illumination with the illumination arm set approximately 30° from center.
2. Set the magnification to a low setting (6× or 10×).
3. Instruct the patient to close their eyes. Starting at the temporal canthus, scan from temporal to nasal across the upper lid and lashes (see **Figure 5-3**).
4. Instruct the patient to open their eyes and to look up. Scan from nasal to temporal across the lower lid and lashes, observing the tear meniscus, the lid apposition to the globe, and structures within the lid margin (e.g., the openings of the meibomian glands).

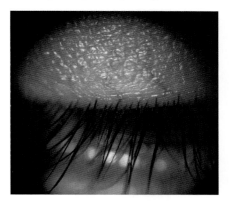

**FIGURE 5-3.** │ Photograph of diffuse illumination on the upper lid margin in downgaze.

### Conjunctiva

1. Narrow the beam to a wide parallelepiped, with the illumination arm set approximately 30° from center.
2. Keep the magnification on a low setting (6× or 10×).
3. Instruct the patient to open their eyes and to look up.
4. Evert the lower lid by pressing your index finger or thumb just below the lid margin. Scan from temporal to nasal, observing the inferior palpebral and bulbar conjunctiva. Look for elevations/depressions, discolorations, and evaluate the openness of the inferior punctum.
5. Instruct the patient to look down.
6. Place your thumb close to the upper lash margin and gently push the lid upwards. Scan from nasal to temporal across the superior bulbar conjunctiva.
7. Instruct the patient to look first to the left and then to the right, while you scan the temporal and nasal bulbar conjunctiva.
8. If indicated, evert the upper lid at this time (see Procedure 5.6).

### Cornea and Tear Film

1. Decrease the beam to a narrow parallelepiped, approximately 1–2 mm wide. Set the illumination arm approximately 30° to 45° from center (see **Figures 5-4** and **5-5**).

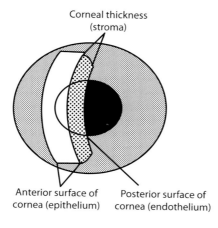

Corneal thickness
(stroma)

Anterior surface of
cornea (epithelium)

Posterior surface of
cornea (endothelium)

**FIGURE 5-4.** | Diagram of a corneal parallelepiped. Note the three-dimensional effect obtained when the parallelepiped is properly focused.

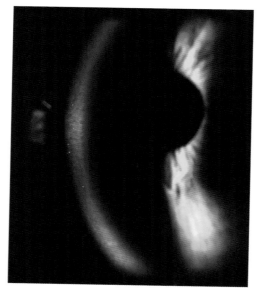

**FIGURE 5-5.** | Photograph of a corneal parallelepiped.

2. Set the magnification to a medium setting (16× or 20×).

3. Instruct the patient to look straight ahead. At this point the illumination arm is angled temporally, so it is often convenient to estimate the depth of the temporal anterior chamber by the Van Herick technique now (see steps 1 through 7 in section "Depth of the Anterior Chamber Angle by the Van Herick Technique"). Then, scan across the central portion of the cornea looking for any opacities or irregularities. When you reach the apex of the cornea, swing the illumination arm to the other side, set it at the proper angle, and continue scanning. It may be necessary to back up slightly after shifting the illumination arm, so you do not miss scanning part of the cornea. If appropriate, when you have scanned to the nasal aspect of the cornea, measure the nasal anterior chamber by the Van Herick method.

4. Instruct the patient to look down. Elevate the upper lid with your thumb, and scan across the superior one-third of the cornea. Remember to swing the illumination arm to the other side when you reach the corneal apex.

5. Instruct the patient to look up. Pull down the lower lid with your index finger if necessary, and scan across the inferior one-third of the cornea. Remember to shift the illumination arm when you reach the corneal apex.

*Depth of the Anterior Chamber Angle by the Van Herick Technique*

If you have not done so already, measure the depth of the anterior chamber angle at this time.

1. Set the illumination arm 60° to the temporal or nasal side of the patient's line of fixation (on the same side that you are assessing).
2. The magnification should remain on a medium setting (16× or 20×).
3. Narrow the beam to an optic section (see **Figures 5-6** and **5-7**).

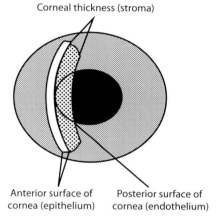

Corneal thickness (stroma)

Anterior surface of cornea (epithelium)    Posterior surface of cornea (endothelium)

**FIGURE 5-6.** | Diagram of a corneal optic section.

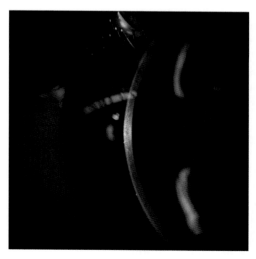

**FIGURE 5-7.** | Photograph of a corneal optic section. *Note:* this image demonstrates the proper width and focus of an optic section beam on the cornea, but is not yet placed at the limbus which would be the necessary positioning to estimate the anterior chamber angle by Van Herick.

4. Instruct the patient to look straight ahead.

5. Focus the light sharply on the cornea at the very edge of the temporal or nasal limbus (on the same side that you are assessing).

6. Compare the width of the "shadow" formed on the iris (representing the depth of the anterior chamber) to the width of the optic section (representing the thickness of the cornea) (see **Figure 5-8**).

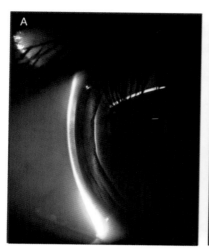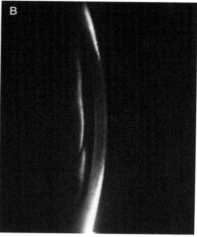

**FIGURE 5-8.** | Photograph of the Van Herick technique. An optic section is positioned at the temporal limbus. (A) The width of the "shadow" is greater than the width of the optic section, so the anterior chamber angle is estimated as >1:1. (B) The width of the "shadow" is equal to the width of the optic section, so the anterior chamber angle is estimated as 1:1.

> *Note*: The shadow is actually a dark interval between the light on the cornea and the light on the iris that represents the optically empty aqueous in the anterior chamber.

> *Note*: When estimating the depth of the nasal angle, it may be necessary to have the patient look temporally in order to attain a 60° angle between the lamp and the microscope.

7. If the angle width is equal to or less than 1/4:1, gonioscopy is indicated to evaluate the angle more thoroughly (see Procedure 5.18) *Note*: If the microscope arm was moved for this procedure (see Notes below), return it to center before proceeding.

*Iris*

1. Increase the slit width to a wide parallelepiped (approximately 3mm) and set the illumination arm 30° to 45° from center.

2. Keep the magnification on a medium setting (16× or 20×).

3. Instruct the patient to look straight ahead.

4. Scan across the iris surface, looking for irregularities. Note the pupillary light reflex. The pupil should constrict when the slit lamp beam reaches the pupillary margin.

*Crystalline Lens*

1. Narrow the angle of the illumination arm to about 10–20° from center.

2. Keep the magnification on a medium setting (16× or 20×).

3. Reduce the slit beam to a narrow parallelepiped (about 1 to 1/2 mm).

4. Slowly move the slit lamp closer to the patient until the light is directed through the pupil and becomes sharply focused on the anterior surface of the lens. Scan the front of the lens. Then move the biomicroscope closer to the patient to examine the deeper layers of the lens (see **Figure 5-9**). Focus on the posterior surface of the lens. Look for any opacities, irregularities, or discolorations within the lens. Swing the illumination arm to the opposite side, set to 10° to 20° from straight ahead, and again examine the lens from the anterior to the posterior surface. If any opacity is noted, narrow the beam to an optic section to locate its depth within the crystalline lens.

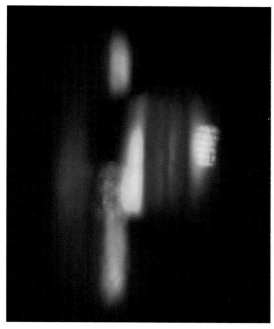

**FIGURE 5-9.** | Photograph showing a parallelepiped of the lens through an undilated pupil. The beam is focused at the plane of the posterior Y suture.

## Recording
- Record each eye separately.
- List each structure evaluated and record your observations.
- Record any abnormalities or pertinent negatives.
- Photographs are recommended in cases where they enhance descriptions.

## Examples
- Lids/Lashes:    OD: Clean and clear    OS: Collarettes at base of lashes, few capped glands
- Conjunctiva:    OD: White and quiet    OS: Concretions inf palpebral
- Cornea:    OD: Clear    OS: 2+ SPK inf
- Angle:    OD: >1:1 N and T    OS: 1/4:1 N and 1/8:1 T
- Iris:    OD: Clear and flat    OS: Flat; 1mm round nevus at 3:00 mid-periphery
- Lens:    OD: Clear    OS: Epicapsular stars

| BIOMICROSCOPY at a glance | |
|---|---|
| **Purpose** | **Technique** |
| Prepare the slit lamp | Clean and disinfect patient contact surfaces<br>Focus the oculars<br>Adjust the pupillary distance (PD)<br>Check click stop, set mirror to click stop<br>Magnification on low |
| Prepare the patient | Adjust table height so patient is comfortable<br>Adjust chin rest to proper height |
| Scan the lids and lashes | Diffuse beam<br>Illumination arm at 30°<br>Low magnification |
| Scan the conjunctiva | Wide parallelepiped<br>Illumination arm at 30°<br>Low magnification<br>Hold lids and direct the patient's gaze as needed |
| Scan the cornea | Narrow parallelepiped<br>Illumination arm at 30°–45°<br>Medium magnification<br>Scan three times—superior, central, inferior cornea—<br>holding lids and directing patient's gaze as needed |
| Estimate the depth of the anterior chamber angle | Optic section<br>Illumination arm at 60°<br>Medium magnification<br>Focus at the temporal and nasal limbus<br>Compare depth of anterior chamber to thickness of cornea |
| Scan the iris | Wide parallelepiped<br>Illumination arm at 30°–45°<br>Medium magnification |
| Scan the lens | Narrow parallelepiped<br>Illumination arm at 10°–20°<br>Medium magnification |

## Notes

- As an alternative for the Van Herick estimation to assess the anterior chamber angle, the illumination arm can be set 30° to one side and the microscope 30° to the other side, yielding a 60° angle between the lamp and the microscope.

## SPECIAL SLIT LAMP PROCEDURES

The following procedures (5.3 through 5.6) are not considered to be part of the routine slit lamp evaluation but are incorporated into the examination when indicated. For the special slit lamp procedures, the setup is the same as that outlined for routine biomicroscopy.

## 5.3 EXAMINATION OF THE ANTERIOR CHAMBER

### Purpose

The aim of this procedure is to check for the presence of cells and/or flare in the aqueous humor.

## Indications

The procedure intends to rule out an active iritis or anterior uveitis.

## Equipment and Setup

- See Procedure 5.2

## Procedure

1. Reduce all room illumination. Wait a few minutes until the examiner's eyes are dark adapted.
2. Set the illumination arm 30° from center.
3. Adjust the magnification to a high setting (25× or 40×).
4. Create a *conical beam* by adjusting the width of the beam to a narrow parallelepiped and adjusting the vertical slit control to the shortest setting. Increase the brightness of the beam to the maximum setting.
5. Instruct the patient to look straight ahead and to blink whenever they need to.
6. Direct the beam into the pupil. Slowly move the slit lamp forward and back, alternately focusing from the posterior cornea to the anterior surface of the lens. Whenever the slit lamp is focused in between the cornea and the lens, direct your attention to the anterior chamber to look for the presence of cells and/or flare in the aqueous.

## Recording

- The results of this procedure are included in the slit lamp recording section, under "anterior chamber."
- Record for each eye separately.
- If the anterior chamber is clear, record "no cells or flare."
- If the anterior chamber is not clear, record your observations. The number of cells and the amount of flare may be graded on a scale of 1 to 4, or as minimal, moderate, or severe. You may also indicate the number of cells seen.

## Examples

- Anterior Chamber:       OD: No cells or flare       OS: Moderate flare, no cells
- Anterior Chamber:       OD: Clear, (−)c/f       OS: 2+ cells, tr flare

## Notes

- This procedure is usually done at the completion of the routine slit lamp examination because of the need to adjust a number of controls on the slit lamp.
- The vertical size of the slit beam may be increased to aid in detection of cells if the suspected uveitis is mild.
- The conical beam can be created on medium magnification and then increased to high magnification once setup and focus have been achieved; the actual assessment for cell and flare should be performed on high magnification.

## 5.4 SPECULAR REFLECTION TECHNIQUE

## Purpose

The aim of this procedure is to evaluate the corneal endothelium.

## Indications

The procedure intends to investigate for corneal endothelial dysfunction (e.g., suspected Fuchs' Dystrophy).

## Equipment and Setup
- See Procedure 5.2

## Procedure
1. Adjust the slit beam to a narrow to medium width parallelepiped.
2. Begin with the magnification on low or medium (10× or 16×).
3. Focus the parallelepiped on the cornea with the illumination arm set approximately 30° from center.
4. Using the joystick, adjust the position of the microscope or change the angle of the illumination arm until the slit beam intersects the reflection of the light filament on the cornea. This is the point at which the angle of reflection is equal to the incident angle of the light. When properly set up, you will see an area of bright glare from the front surface of the cornea. This will be visible through one ocular only. The endothelial cells will be visible adjacent to the reflection of the filament, on the side of the pupil.
5. Without moving the slit lamp, increase the magnification to the highest setting (25× or 40×).
6. Adjust the focus of the slit lamp so that it is sharply focused on the corneal endothelium. Observe the mosaic pattern of the endothelial cells (see **Figure 5-10**).
7. Move the entire slit lamp and readjust the illumination arm to observe other areas of the endothelium as needed.

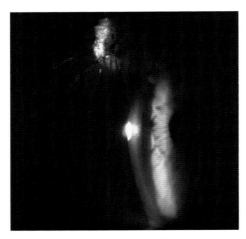

**FIGURE 5-10.** | Photograph showing the use of specular reflection for observing the corneal endothelium. When high magnification (25× or 40×) is used, the mosaic pattern of the endothelial cells can be visualized within the reflected light on the posterior aspect (right side as imaged above) of the parallelepiped beam.

## Recording
- The results of this procedure are listed in the slit lamp recording section under "cornea." It is not necessary to indicate that specular reflection was performed.
- Record your observations for each eye separately.

## Examples
- Cornea:    OD: normal endothelium    OS: normal endothelium
- Cornea:    OD: guttata present    OS: guttata present

## Notes
- Exact focus is critical.

## 5.5 SCLEROTIC SCATTER TECHNIQUE

### Purpose
The aim of this procedure is to evaluate the cornea for areas of localized corneal edema within the stroma.

### Indications
This procedure intends to investigate for corneal edema when edema is suspected.

### Equipment and Setup
- See Procedure 5.2

### Procedure
1. Adjust the slit beam to a narrow parallelepiped.
2. Push the entire microscope to one side so you are able to directly observe the cornea along the patient's line of sight without looking through the oculars of the slit lamp.
3. Set the illumination arm approximately 45° from the patient's line of sight.
4. Focus the slit beam at the patient's temporal limbus. When the beam is properly positioned, you will see a halo of light at the nasal limbus (see **Figures 5-11** and **5-12**).
5. Observe the patient's cornea against the dark background of the pupil, looking for haziness.

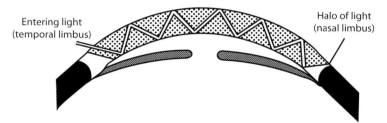

**FIGURE 5-11.** | Diagram of sclerotic scatter, showing the path of the light as it travels through the cornea. If the cornea is clear, the light entering at the temporal limbus will be totally internally reflected and emerge at the nasal limbus, producing a limbal glow. If the cornea is edematous or opacified, the light will be scattered rather than reflected, and haziness or a grayish appearance will be observed.

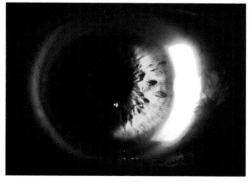

**FIGURE 5-12.** | Photograph of the setup for the sclerotic scatter technique. The parallelepiped is focused on the temporal limbus, to the right in the photograph, creating a halo of light at the nasal limbus, to the left in the photograph. If edema were present, it would appear as a gray cloudiness within the stroma of the central cornea.

## Recording

- The results of this procedure are listed in the slit lamp recording section under "cornea." It is not necessary to indicate that sclerotic scatter was performed.
- Record your observations for each eye separately.
- The haziness caused by localized corneal edema is also sometimes referred to as central corneal clouding (CCC). It is usually graded on a scale of 1 to 4, or qualified as mild, moderate, or severe.

## Example

- Cornea:    OD: no edema    OS: grade 1+ CCC

**Notes**

- In patients who wear gas permeable lenses, this technique should be performed immediately after the lenses have been removed, as corneal edema may dissipate quickly.

## 5.6 EVERSION OF THE UPPER EYELID

### Purpose

The aim of this procedure is to observe the palpebral conjunctiva of the upper lid.

### Indications

There are several indications for eversion of the upper lid including, investigation for a suspected foreign body underneath the upper lid, to establish the baseline condition of the palpebral conjunctiva prior to dispensing a contact lens prescription and/or monitoring during contact lens wear, or to investigate for palpebral inflammation during evaluation of a red eye.

### Equipment and Setup

- See Procedure 5.2
- Sterile cotton-tipped applicator

### Procedure

1. With the patient positioned in the slit lamp, instruct the patient to look down.
2. Grasp the patient's eyelashes or upper lid at the lid margin or base of the lashes between your thumb and index finger. Gently pull the lid down and away from the globe.
3. With your free hand, insert the cotton tip of the cotton-tipped applicator at the posterior (upper) margin of the tarsal plate in the center of the lid.
4. Gently press down on the applicator while pulling the lid margin anteriorly and upward. Be sure not to push down on the tarsal plate, but just past it's posterior edge. Once the lid is everted, tether it by firmly holding the patient's eyelashes against the superior orbital rim with your thumb or index finger.
5. Remove the cotton-tipped applicator and reposition the slit lamp to view the superior palpebral conjunctiva. The illumination arm should be set approximately 30° from the straight-ahead position and the beam should be adjusted to a wide parallelepiped. Set the magnification to the low or medium setting (10× or 16×).
6. Scan the superior palpebral conjunctiva, looking for elevations, depressions, foreign bodies, or injection.

### Recording

- The results for this procedure are recorded in the slit lamp recording section under "palpebral conjunctiva" or "tarsal plate."

- Record each eye separately.
- A papillary response of the palpebral conjunctiva may be observed as papillary conjunctivitis or giant papillary conjunctivitis (GPC) and can be graded on a scale of 1 to 4, or qualified as mild, moderate, or severe.
- There is no need to indicate that lid eversion was performed. It is implied that the patient's upper lid was everted when the upper palpebral conjunctiva is recorded.

### Example
- Sup palpebral conjunctiva:          OD: Clear                    OS: 1+ follicles
- Tarsal plate:                       OD: Clear                    OS: 2+ papillae

### Notes
- The tip of the examiners index or middle finger of either hand may be used in place of a sterile cotton-tipped applicator to push down and evert the lid.
- Many standardized scales and standardized sets of photographs now exist for assessing and grading the degree of findings such as follicles or papillae. It is recommended that the reader select one such scale and use it consistently in clinical practice so as to make evaluation of these findings consistent upon repeated measures on the same patient or between patients.

## 5.7 INSTILLATION OF DROPS

### Purpose
The aim of this procedure is to instill proper dosages of eyedrops onto the surface of the eye while maintaining sterility. Pharmaceutical agents in the form of eyedrops are routinely instilled in a patient's eye or eyes to anesthetize the cornea, to dilate the pupil, and for other diagnostic purposes. Many ocular therapeutic pharmaceutical agents are in drop form and may be instilled in the same manner. *Note:* Any use of drugs, including eyedrops, requires the examiner to have an awareness of the contraindications and side effects of the selected drug. If performing this procedure on a child, parental consent must be obtained for the use of diagnostic or therapeutic drugs.

### Equipment
- Bottle containing eye drops
- Tissues

### Setup
- Hand hygiene should be performed by the examiner before the instillation of eyedrops.
- The patient is seated and given a tissue.
- Dim room illumination may prevent excess lacrimation.
- If you plan to instill dilating drops, the patient should be informed of the adverse effects of dilation, and consent should be obtained before proceeding. Visual acuity, appropriate entrance testing, assessment of the anterior segment and anterior chamber angle of both eyes, assessment of IOP should be performed prior to any mydriatic drop instillation.
- Medications, allergies, and pregnancy/breastfeeding should be reviewed prior to any drop instillation.

## Procedure

1. Inform the patient that you are going to instill drops in their eyes and that the drops may cause temporary stinging.
2. Remove the bottle cap and hold it in the palm of your hand or in-between the base of your fingers without touching the inside surface. Hold the bottle between the thumb and index finger of your dominant hand.
3. Instruct the patient to lean their head back and look up to the ceiling. Provide a fixation target if necessary.
4. Using the middle finger of the hand holding the bottle or the index finger of your opposite hand, gently pull down or evert the lower lid of the patient's right eye, as shown in **Figure 5-13**. This creates a pocket in the inferior cul-de-sac to hold the drop immediately following its instillation. It is often necessary to hold the patient's upper lid in addition to everting their lower lid. Then, it is appropriate to use one hand to hold the upper lid and the other hand to hold the bottle and evert the lower lid.

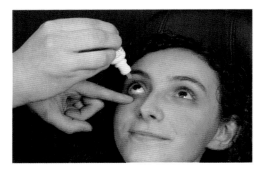

**FIGURE 5-13.** | Instillation of drops into the patient's right eye. While the patient looks up, the examiner pulls down the inferior lid to form a pocket where the drop is instilled.

5. Position the bottle tip close to the patient's eye, but far enough away that the patient's lashes will not touch the tip even if they blink (1–2 cm above the lashes).
6. Squeeze the bottle to allow a single drop to fall into the patient's inferior cul-de-sac.
7. Repeat steps 3 through 6 for the left eye if indicated.
8. Instruct the patient to close their eyes and gently wipe the excess fluid from their eyes with a tissue.
9. If you experience great difficulty in controlling the eyelids sufficiently to permit instillation of drops (e.g., in small children), you may use the following technique:
    a. Do not attempt to open the patient's eyes but allow them to keep their eyes gently shut.
    b. Recline the patient into a supine position.
    c. Place two drops of the agent on the inner canthus where the upper and lower lids meet.
    d. Instruct the patient to open their eyes slowly. The hydrostatic pressure of the patient's tears will pull the drops into the eye in sufficient quantity to work.

## Recording

- Record the name of the pharmaceutical agent used including its concentration, how many drops were instilled into each eye, and the time of day.

## Examples

- Dilated with one drop 1% tropicamide and one drop 2.5% phenylephrine OD only @ 9:45 AM
- 1 gtt cyclopentolate 1% at 2:14pm OD & OS

## LACRIMAL AND DRY EYE ASSESSMENT

The following procedures (5.8 through 5.13) are not considered to be part of the routine slit lamp evaluation but are incorporated into the examination when indicated. For the lacrimal and dry eye assessment procedures, the setup is the same as that outlined for routine biomicroscopy. Some of the following procedures also serve a purpose outside of the lacrimal and dry eye assessment as outlined in indications below.

## 5.8 CORNEAL OR CONJUNCTIVAL STAINING

### Purpose
The aim of this procedure is to evaluate the integrity of the corneal or conjunctival epithelium.

### Indications
This procedure intends to investigate for epithelial disruption in conditions such as dry eye syndrome, bacterial keratitis, and corneal abrasion, or to investigate the depth and size of corneal or conjunctival lacerations.

### Equipment and Setup
- See Procedure 5.2
- Sodium fluorescein (NaFl) strips. *Note*: Fluorescein is the most commonly used vital dye to evaluate corneal integrity
- Rose Bengal or lissamine green strips
- Sterile saline solution
  *Note*: the use of dyes requires the examiner to have an understanding of any contraindications. The examiner should observe the same precautions as discussed in Procedure 5.7.

### Procedure
1. Over a sink or trash can, wet the end of the strip with a drop of sterile saline solution.
2. Instruct the patient to look up and away from you. As shown in **Figure 5-14**, pull down the lower lid and touch the moistened end of the strip to the patient's temporal bulbar conjunctiva, such that if the patient blinks when the strip touches their eye, the strip will not rub across their cornea.

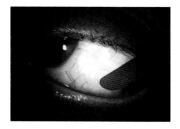

FIGURE 5-14. | Instillation of fluorescein into the patient's eye. As the patient looks superior-nasally, the examiner supports the upper lid, pulls down the lower lid, and touches the moist end of the fluorescein strip to the temporal bulbar conjunctiva.

3. Instruct the patient to blink several times to spread the dye over the corneal and conjunctival surfaces.
4. Properly position the patient in the slit lamp.
5. Set the illumination arm 30° from center. Adjust the slit to a wide parallelepiped and set the magnification to the medium setting (16× or 20×).

6. Insert the cobalt blue filter if using fluorescein dye. *Note*: Rose Bengal or lissamine green staining is observed without the use of filters.

7. Scan the cornea and conjunctiva and look for staining. Fluorescein staining appears bright green when viewed with the cobalt blue filter (see **Figure 5-15**). Rose Bengal staining appears deep pink in white light. Lissamine green staining appears pale green in white light.

8. Carefully note the location and the pattern of staining.

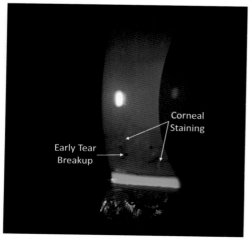

Corneal Staining

Early Tear Breakup

**FIGURE 5-15.** | Photograph showing mild staining of the inferior cornea and early break-up of the tear film.

## Recording

- The results for this procedure are recorded in the slit lamp recording section under "cornea" or "conjunctiva."
- Record for each eye separately.
- Indicate the ophthalmic dye used.
- If the results are normal, record "no staining." If there is staining, indicate the amount and the pattern of the staining. Photographs of the staining pattern are extremely helpful.

## Examples

- Cornea          OD: No staining with RB     OS: Mild punctate staining with NaFl inf
- Conjunctiva   OD: No staining with NaFl   OS: Large area of coalesced staining sup

## Notes

- Corneal staining may be evaluated after instillation of liquid fluorescein combined with a topical anesthetic for techniques such as Goldmann applanation tonometry (GAT; see Procedure 5.14)
- Lissamine green and Rose Bengal reveal similar staining patterns, but lissamine green produces less stinging or irritation upon instillation and is tolerated better than Rose Bengal by most patients.
- Many standardized scales and standardized sets of photographs now exist for assessing and grading the degree and location of staining in the eye. It is recommended that the reader select one such scale and use it consistently in clinical practice so as to make evaluation of staining consistent upon repeated measures on the same patient or between patients.

## 5.9 TEAR BREAKUP TIME (TBUT)

### Purpose
The aim of this procedure is to measure the stability of the tear film.

### Indications
TBUT should be measured when you suspect dry eye disease or a lacrimal deficiency based on the patient's symptoms and/or the slit lamp evaluation. In addition, a baseline TBUT should be measured prior to fitting a patient with contact lenses. The TBUT must be performed prior to instillation of a topical anesthetic or dilating agent because these may alter the quantity and composition of the tear film. This procedure is also called fluorescein breakup time in the literature. *Note:* Fluorescein should not be instilled when a patient is wearing *soft* contact lenses, as it will stain the lenses. Soft lenses should be removed prior to performing this procedure. Fluorescein will also stain clothing, so be careful on instillation.

### Equipment
- Slit lamp (biomicroscope)
- Sodium fluorescein (NaFl) strips
  *Note:* This procedure can be performed with a standard fluorescein strip or a low volume (1 μl/1 mm) fluorescein strip. The norms for both are listed below.
- Sterile saline solution

### Setup
- See Procedure 5.2.
- Adjust the slit lamp so it is comfortable for both the patient and the examiner.
- Focus the oculars, adjust the PD, and set the magnification on the lowest setting (6× or 10×).
- Insert the cobalt blue filter and set the illumination arm approximately 30° from the straight-ahead position. Open the slit to a wide parallelepiped beam.

### Procedure
1. Over a sink or trash can, moisten the end of a fluorescein strip with one drop of sterile saline.
2. Instruct the patient to look up. Pull down the lower lid of the right eye and touch the moistened end of the strip flat against the patient's temporal bulbar conjunctiva or inferior palpebral conjunctiva, such that if the patient blinks when the strip touches their eye, the strip will not be dragged across their cornea. Repeat for the left eye.
3. Position the patient in the slit lamp and focus on the patient's cornea. The tear film will appear bright green due to the fluorescein.
4. Measure the TBUT on the right eye first.
5. Instruct the patient to blink several times to spread the dye over the corneal and conjunctival surfaces and then to keep their eyes open looking straight ahead without blinking.
6. Scan the entire cornea looking for dry areas, which will appear as dark spots or streaks. Count the number of seconds between the last blink and the first appearance of one or more of these dry spot formations (tear film breakup). See **Figure 5-16** for a photograph showing the appearance of breakup of the tear film.
7. Repeat steps 5 and 6 two more times and average the results. Note the position of the first dry spots. Observe if the tear film consistently breaks up in a specific location.
8. Repeat steps 5 through 7 on the patient's left eye. Steps 1 and 2 may have to be repeated if the dye drained quickly.

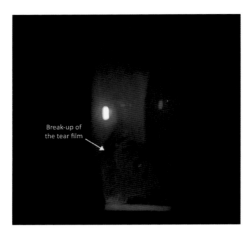

**FIGURE 5-16.** | Photograph showing breakup of the tear film (dark patches within the green fluorescein).

## Recording
- Record the results for each eye separately.
- Record the average of the three trials in seconds.

## Example
- TBUT: OD 6 seconds, OS 7 seconds
- TBUT: OD >10 seconds, OS >10 seconds

## Expected Findings
- The normal TBUT is between 10 and 45 seconds when using standard fluorescein strips. A TBUT greater than 5 seconds is considered normal when using a smaller volume fluorescein strip, and the use of such strips should be indicated when recording.
- A breakup time longer than 10–20 seconds is not diagnostically significant. It is acceptable to record ">10 seconds" for measurements beyond that timed interval.
- A TBUT less than 10 seconds is indicative of an unstable tear film for a standard fluorescein strip, and less than 5 seconds for a low volume fluorescein strip.
- If the tear film consistently breaks up in the same location, it may indicate a defect in the corneal epithelium rather than a tear deficiency and staining should be examined (see Procedure 5.8).

## Notes
- Noninvasive breakup time (NIBUT) is another method to assess tear film stability and does not disrupt the tear film prior to assessment. This procedure involves projecting an image onto the tear film such as keratometry mires or a grid generated by a corneal topographer and observing the reflection for first image disruption. The time is counted in seconds from last blink to first image disruption and is recorded in the same manner as mentioned above, ensuring to record the name of the procedure or method used. The normative values for NIBUT measurements are longer (in seconds) than TBUT norms.

## 5.10 SCHIRMER TESTS: SCHIRMER #1 TEST AND BASIC LACRIMATION TEST

### Purpose
The aim of this procedure is to evaluate the integrity of the lacrimal secretion system. The Schirmer #1 test correlates with the amount of total tear secretion within a 5-minute period.

Total tear secretion is the sum of basal secretion and reflex secretion; a topical anesthetic is not used. In the basic lacrimation test, a topical anesthetic is used to eliminate reflex secretion, so only the amount of basal secretion within a 5-minute period is assessed.

## Indications

The Schirmer tests are indicated when a lacrimal deficiency is suspected based on the patient's symptoms or slit lamp findings. These measurements may also be important baseline data before refractive surgery.

## Equipment

- Two Schirmer test strips
- Topical anesthetic (e.g., 0.5% proparacaine)
- Millimeter ruler (or millimeter scale on the Schirmer box or strip)
- Watch or clock

## Setup

- Perform hand hygiene.
- Before removing the Schirmer strips from their cellophane wrapping, fold the rounded ends of the strips so they will be creased at the notch.
- Remove the strips from the cellophane wrapper, taking care not to touch the rounded ends.
- Dim the room illumination.
- Perform the test with the patient in the upright, seated position.

## Procedure

*Schirmer #1 Test*

1. Instruct the patient to look up.
2. Gently pull down the lower lid of the right eye.
3. Place the folded, notched end of a Schirmer strip over the lower lid margin within its temporal third. Avoid touching the cornea with the Schirmer strip (see **Figure 5-17**).

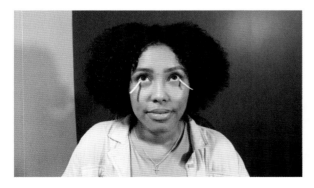

**FIGURE 5-17.** | Schirmer strips positioned in the lateral one third of the patient's lower lid. The patient is instructed to look up to avoid contact between the strips and the cornea.

4. Insert the second Schirmer strip in the left eye in the same manner.
5. Instruct the patient to keep their eyes open and continue to look up. The patient may blink freely, although excessive blinking may result in significant reflex tearing.
   a. The patient may close their eyes for improved comfort, but it is important that they do not squeeze their eyes shut.
6. Remove the Schirmer test strips from each eye after 5 minutes, unless the entire strip wets before the end of the time period.
7. Mark the end of the wet portion of the strips. Measure the amount of wetting from the notch in millimeters.

*Basic Lacrimation Test*

1. Instill one drop of topical anesthetic in each of the patient's eyes (see Procedure 5.7).
2. Wait for the reactive hyperemia and reflex tearing to subside, then gently blot the excess fluid from the patient's inferior cul-de-sac.
3. Repeat steps 1 through 7 under Schirmer #1 test (see above).

## Recording
- Record the data for each eye separately.
- Record the test used (Schirmer #1 or basic lacrimation).
- Record the amount of wetting (in mm) on the Schirmer strip and the amount of time (in minutes) the strip was left in the eye.

## Examples
- Schirmer #1 test: OD 30 mm/3 min., OS 30 mm/3 min.
- Basic lacrimation test: OD 10 mm/5 min., OS 12 mm/5 min.

## Expected Findings
- Although there is some disagreement about the interpretation of Schirmer tests, it is generally believed that wetting less than 10 mm in 5 minutes on either the Schirmer #1 test or the basic lacrimation test is significant. Wetting less than 5 mm in 5 minutes is considered diagnostic of lacrimal insufficiency or severe dry eye.
- If there is 25 mm of wetting or more in a 5-minute period on the Schirmer #1 test, it indicates excessive reflex tearing. The basic lacrimation test should be performed.

## 5.11 PHENOL RED THREAD TEST (COTTON THREAD TEST)

### Purpose
The aim of this procedure is to evaluate the integrity of the lacrimal secretion system.

### Indications
The phenol red thread (PRT) test is indicated when a lacrimal deficiency is suspected based on the patient's symptoms and/or the slit lamp findings.

### Equipment
- Phenol red thread designed for lacrimal testing; one thread is needed for each eye being tested
- Millimeter ruler (or millimeter scale on the box that the threads come in)
- Watch or clock accurate to the second

### Setup
- This test should be performed before manipulation of the eyelids, or before any drops or dyes have been instilled into the eyes. Anesthetic is not needed to perform this test. Hand hygiene is performed at the start of the procedure.
- Remove the threads from their cellophane wrapper, taking care to preserve their sterility by not allowing them to touch anything. The examiner will hold the thread far enough from the bent end which will contact the patient's eye.
- The eyes are tested one at a time with the right eye tested first by convention.
- Perform the test with the patient in the upright, seated position.

### Procedure
1. Instruct the patient to look up and gently pull down the lower lid.
2. Place the bent end of one thread over the lower lid margin within the lateral third of the lower lid (see **Figure 5-18**). Avoid touching the cornea with the thread.

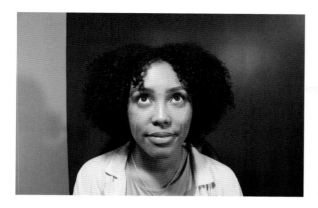

FIGURE 5-18. | Phenol red thread positioned in the lateral one third of the patient's lower lid. The patient is instructed to look up to avoid contact between the thread and the cornea.

3. Instruct the patient to keep their eyes open, to look straight ahead, and to blink normally.
4. After exactly 15 seconds, remove the test thread by pulling down the lower eyelid and gently lifting upward on the thread.
5. Measure the full length of the wet portion of the thread from its very tip, in millimeters, disregarding the bend. The thread will change colors in areas that were moistened (typically from a yellow to light red color when wet).
6. Repeat steps 1 through 5 for the left eye.

### Recording
- Record the data for each eye separately.
- Record "PRT test" or "cotton thread test."
- Record the amount of wetting (in mm) on the thread. If a length of time other than 15 seconds was used, also record the duration of the test.

### Examples
- PRT test: OD 14 mm/15 seconds, OS 11 mm/15 seconds

### Expected Findings
- Wetting <10 mm in 15 seconds is considered significant for aqueous deficient dry eye.
- Wetting of 10–19 mm in 15 seconds is considered borderline for dry eye.
- Wetting of ≥20 mm in 15 seconds is considered normal.
- Wetting approaching 30 mm and >30 mm in 15 seconds is indicative of increased reflex tearing and re-testing should be considered.

## 5.12 FLUORESCEIN CLEARANCE TEST (OR "FLUORESCEIN DYE DISAPPEARANCE TEST")

### Purpose
The aim of this procedure is to evaluate the rate at which new tears replace existing tears in the eye.

### Indications
The fluorescein clearance test is indicated when a lacrimal deficiency or possible blockage of the lacrimal drainage system is suspected based on the patient's symptoms and/or the slit lamp findings.

### Equipment
- Slit lamp

- Sterile saline solution
- Fluorescein strips
- Watch or clock

## Setup
- See Procedure 5.2.
- Adjust the slit lamp so it is comfortable for both the patient and the examiner.
- Focus the oculars, adjust the PD, and set the magnification on the lowest setting (6× or 10×).
- Dim the room illumination.

## Procedure
1. Over a sink or trash can, moisten the end of a fluorescein strip with one drop of sterile saline.
2. Instruct the patient to look up. Pull down the lower lid of the right eye and touch the moistened end of the strip flat against the patient's temporal bulbar conjunctiva or inferior palpebral conjunctiva, such that if the patient blinks when the strip touches their eye, the strip will not be dragged across their cornea. Repeat for the left eye. The patient may wipe away excess dye that is tearing down their cheek but should not blot dye from the lid margin or ocular surface.
3. Position the patient in the slit lamp, insert the cobalt blue filter, and focus on the patient's cornea with a wide parallelepiped beam. The tear film will appear green due to the fluorescein. Assess the appearance (color intensity) of the fluorescein on the cornea of each eye. The patient may then sit back and relax while being careful not to blot dye away from the lid margin or ocular surface.
4. Once 5 minutes have elapsed after dye instillation, again position the patient comfortably in the slit lamp with the same setup above.
5. Assess the color intensity or amount of dye still present in the tear film, compared to the initial assessment, using a 0 to 4+ grading scale (initially developed by Zappia and Milder in 1972), see section "Recording" below.

## Recording
- Record the grade of fluorescein presence or color intensity at five minutes for each eye separately. A grade of 0 indicates that no dye remains in the tear film, 1+ indicates trace or minimal dye remains, 2+ indicates moderate change in color intensity, 3+ indicates minimal change in color intensity, and 4+ indicates no change in color intensity of the dye in the tear film.  It may be helpful to include the time elapsed as well, particularly if a time other than 5 minutes was used.

## Examples
- Fluorescein clearance test: OD 3+, OS 4+ / 5 minutes
- Fluorescein clearance test: OD 1+, OS 1+ / 5 minutes

## Expected Findings
- In patients with normal tear production and turnover, only trace (1+) or no fluorescein should be detectable at the 5-minute interval.
- A grade of 2+ to 4+ after five minutes is indicative of aqueous tear deficiency. Similarly, an asymmetric grade ≥2 points between the eyes, (e.g., OD: 2+, OS: 4+) may indicate a lacrimal drain blockage in the eye with more remaining fluorescein (OS in the example provided). Re-testing or further investigation may be necessary if a blockage is suspected, see Procedure 5.13 Jones #1 Test.

# 5.13 JONES #1 (PRIMARY DYE) TEST

## Purpose
The aim if this procedure is to determine the patency of the lacrimal excretory system, from the punctum to the inferior meatus of the nose.

## Indications
The Jones #1 test should be performed when the patient complains of tearing, particularly unilateral tearing, or if the slit lamp evaluation shows pooling of the tears or punctal stenosis. This test can only be performed on one eye at each visit and must be done prior to Goldmann tonometry or any other tests requiring instillation of fluorescein.

## Equipment
- Sterile saline solution
- Sodium fluorescein strips
- Sterile cotton-tipped applicator
- Tissues
- Burton lamp or other UV light source

## Setup
- Perform hand hygiene.
- Over a sink or trash can, wet a fluorescein strip with a couple of drops of sterile saline.
- Instruct the patient to look up, gently pull down their lower lid and instill a moderate amount of fluorescein into the inferior cul-de-sac. The equivalent of one to two drops of liquid is required. Instill fluorescein into the symptomatic or suspect eye only.
- Instruct the patient to blink firmly three or four times.

## Procedure
*Method #1 (Traditional Jones #1 Test)*
1. Wait 2 minutes after instillation of the fluorescein.
2. Insert a sterile cotton-tipped applicator into the nose under the inferior meatus, located approximately 2-3 cm into the nose along the floor of the nasal canal.
3. Remove the applicator and check the cotton tip for the presence of fluorescein. If fluorescein is not grossly visible, observe the cotton tip under the UV light for fluorescence.

*Method #2 (Modified Jones #1 Test)*
1. After instilling the fluorescein and having the patient blink, wipe away the excess fluorescein.
2. Wait approximately 6 minutes, then instruct the patient to gently blow their nose on a tissue.
3. Examine the tissue for the presence of fluorescein. If fluorescein is not grossly visible, examine the tissue under the UV light.

*Method #3 (Fluorescein Appearance Test)*
1. After instilling the fluorescein and having the patient blink, wipe away the excess fluorescein.
2. Wait 15–30 minutes and examine the back of the patient's throat with the UV light for the presence of fluorescein.
3. If fluorescein is not present, continue checking for up to 90 minutes after instillation of the fluorescein. In the large majority of patients, fluorescein will be present within 30–60 minutes.

## Recording

- Indicate which testing method was used (Jones #1, modified Jones #1, or fluorescein appearance test) and which eye was tested.
- The Jones test is recorded as "positive" if fluorescein appears on the cotton applicator, tissue, or in the throat. A positive result indicates that the lacrimal excretory system is not obstructed.
- The Jones test is recorded as "negative" if fluorescein is not present. A negative result indicates a potential blockage of the lacrimal excretory system in the eye tested. The test may be repeated on the examined eye ensuring that enough fluorescein was used in the assessment. If the result is again negative and a blockage is suspected, dilation and irrigation may be considered (see Procedure 10.3).
  Note: The above terminology may be confusing because for most tests "positive" indicates that an abnormality is present. It may be less confusing to simply record the presence or absence of fluorescein.

## Examples

- Jones #1 test: OD negative
- Modified Jones #1 test: OS positive
- Fluorescein appearance test: OD no fluorescein after 90 min

## 5.14 GOLDMANN APPLANATION TONOMETRY (GAT)

### Purpose

The aim of this procedure is to measure the intraocular pressure (IOP).

### Indications

GAT is the gold standard of IOP measurement and should be used when an accurate measurement of the IOP is critical, such as in patients with glaucoma, patients who have been identified as at high risk for developing glaucoma, and in patients using oral or topical steroid medication.

### Equipment

- Slit lamp (biomicroscope)
- Goldmann tonometer probe
- Liquid fluorescein combined with a topical anesthetic or 0.5% proparacaine, a fluorescein strip, and sterile saline

### Setup

- Slit lamp setup is the same as Procedure 5.2 with the following specifications.

*Patient Preparation*

- The patient removes their glasses and/or contact lenses.
- The examiner evaluates the patient's anterior segment, especially the cornea, to rule out conditions that contraindicate applanation tonometry (e.g., red eye of infectious origin or severely traumatized cornea).
- Prepare the cornea by instilling one drop of anesthetic with liquid fluorescein in the patient's lower cul-de-sac (see Procedure 5.7). *Note:* If you choose to use a topical anesthetic with fluorescein strips, instill a single drop of anesthetic first. Then, wet the fluorescein strip with a drop of sterile saline, instruct the patient to look to the side, control the upper and lower lids so as to limit blinking, and touch the moistened end of the strip to the temporal bulbar or inferior palpebral conjunctiva.

- Insert the cobalt blue filter. Scan across the cornea, checking for corneal staining that is present prior to performing tonometry (see Procedure 5.8).

*Tonometer Preparation*

- Disinfect the tonometer probe according to manufacturer and CDC guidelines (or other local legal requirements if outside the United States).
- Place the probe within the holder. *Note*: The holder is typically found at the top of the microscope arm or on a separate housing unit that swings from the bottom.
- Rotate the tonometer probe to align the zero with the white marking on the prism holder. *Note*: If the patient's corneal astigmatism exceeds 3.00 D, rotate the prism until the red marking on the prism holder is aligned with the axis mark that corresponds to the patient's minus cylinder axis.
- Position the tonometer arm so the applanation prism is properly aligned in the center of an ocular. *Note*: The image of the probe is typically only viewed in the center of one ocular. Depth perception is not necessary for this procedure.
- Open the slit beam to its widest setting. Adjust the illumination arm so the tip of the applanation prism is brightly illuminated with the blue light. The angle of the illumination arm should be 45–60° from center. Set the magnification on a low or medium setting (6× to 16×).
- Set the measurement drum between 10 and 20 (corresponding to pressure readings of 10–20 mmHg). The measurement drum is typically found at the base of the Goldmann tonometer probe holder.

## Procedure

1. Ensure the patient is positioned comfortably in the slit lamp and instruct the patient to keep their eyes open and to look straight ahead. If the patient has difficulty keeping their eyes open, it may be necessary to hold the patient's upper lid. The upper lid should be held firmly against the patient's orbital rim to avoid pressing against the globe.
2. With the tonometer prism positioned slightly inferior to the visual axis, move the tonometer toward the cornea. When the prism is 2–3 mm from the cornea, elevate the tonometer to align the prism with the corneal apex, look through the oculars and slowly move the joystick forward until the prism is in contact with the cornea (see **Figure 5-19**). The initial positioning of the probe 2–3 mm from the cornea is performed with the examiner looking outside of the slit lamp oculars to ensure safe and proper alignment.

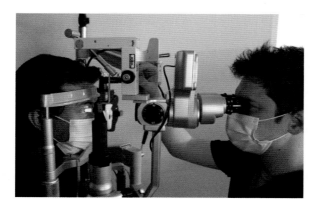

**FIGURE 5-19.** | GAT setup with applanation prism in contact with the patient's cornea.

*Note:* As an alternative for the initial alignment, center the prism on the corneal apex to the extent possible and position it approximately 1–3 mm from the corneal surface. With the prism in this position, when you look in through the slit lamp oculars, you should see a pair of blue or whitish reflections in the shape of the tonometer mires; these are referred to as "ghost mires." Adjust the position of the prism until these reflections are equal mirror images of one another and centered in the field of view (as if you were aligning the tonometer mires themselves). Then gradually bring the prism into contact with the cornea by moving it forward with the joystick. The tonometer mires should be visible and nearly properly aligned.

3. Once the prism is in contact with the cornea, looking through the oculars, center the semicircles horizontally and vertically, as shown in **Figure 5-20A–C,** by moving the slit lamp up and down and/or left and right with the joystick. *Note:* If the mires are too far from center, adjustments should be made off cornea by pulling the probe back and adjusting the slit lamp position before re-applanating; *minor* adjustments may be made while making contact with the cornea.

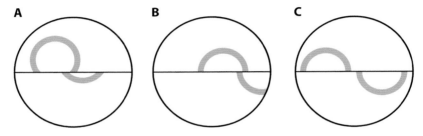

**FIGURE 5-20.** | (A) The upper semicircle is larger than the lower semicircle, indicating that the applanation prism is misaligned vertically on the patient's cornea. The prism must be moved up to center the semicircles. (B) The lower semicircle is missing its right half, indicating that the applanation prism is misaligned horizontally on the patient's cornea. The prism must be moved to the right to center the semicircles. (C) The semicircles are full and equal in size, indicating that the applanation prism is properly centered on the patient's cornea, but the pressure dial is not properly set. The pressure drum should be increased for an accurate reading to be obtained.

4. Observe the thickness of the mires to ensure that they are neither too thick nor too thin. Ideal thickness is 1/10 the diameter of the semicircles.

*Note:* Thick mires are an indication of too much fluorescein or excess tearing and will create a false high reading. If you observe excessively thick mires, withdraw the tonometer prism and correct the problem by blotting the excess fluid from the patient's eye with a tissue. Wipe the tonometer tip with a tissue to remove any residual fluorescein before attempting to take a to-nometer reading again. Thin mires indicate too little fluorescein and will give a false low reading. If too thin mires are observed, withdraw the tonometer prism and instill more fluorescein in the patient's eye before repeating tonometry (see **Figure 5-21A–B**).

5. When the mires are of proper thickness and the semicircles are equal in size and centered, turn the pressure drum to obtain the correct reading. The correct position for a pressure reading is when the inner edge of the superior semicircle meets the inner edge of the inferior semicircle (see **Figure 5-22A–D**). When the mires are properly aligned and the pressure on the cornea is appropriate for a pressure reading, it is often possible to observe the pulsation of the IOP.

A                              B

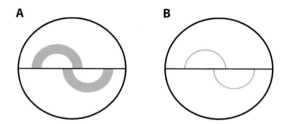

**FIGURE 5-21.** | (A) These mires are too thick, indicating that there is too much fluorescein or excess lacrimation. The pressure reading will be too high if the problem is not corrected. (B) These mires are too thin, indicating that there is not enough fluorescein in the patient's eye. The pressure reading will be too low if this is not corrected.

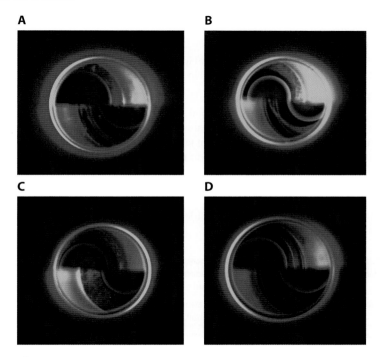

**FIGURE 5-22.** | When the semicircles are of proper width, equal in size, and centered, the pressure dial is adjusted. (A) The semicircles are too thin and are overlapping too much, indicating that the pressure dial is set too high and there is not enough fluorescein. (B) The semicircles are of an appropriate width but not overlapping and positioned slightly to the right, indicating that the pressure dial is set too low. Move the joystick slightly to the right and increase the reading on the pressure dial. (C) The semicircles of an appropriate width and are nearly in the correct position. The prism should be moved slightly to the right. The inner ring of the upper semicircle is just touching the inner ring of the lower semicircle as it should be to capture the patient's IOP accurately. (D) The mires are nearly perfect mirror images of one another, and the inner edges of the mires are aligned, indicating that the pressure dial is set appropriately. This will yield an accurate measurement of the IOP.

6. As soon as you have obtained an accurate reading of the IOP, withdraw the tonometer prism from the cornea. Immediately wipe the tonometer tip with a tissue to remove any fluorescein. Look at the pressure dial and note the pressure reading.

*Note*: If the pressure reading is high or if there is a difference of greater than 2 mm between the eyes, consider obtaining a second reading.

7. Repeat steps 1 through 6 on the other eye.
8. When all necessary measures have been taken, re-examine the cornea for significant corneal staining or abrasions.

## Recording

- Write "T$_A$" or "GAT" to indicate that the IOP was obtained by the technique of applanation tonometry.
- The reading for the right eye is recorded first (or above) and the reading for the left eye is recorded after (or below).
- Record the time of day the test was performed.

## Examples

- T$_A$ 18/23 10:30 am
- GAT @ 12:05pm: 12/13
- GAT @ 9:25am OD 15 mmHg, OS 15 mmHg
- IOP @ 2:30pm (GAT): 20 mmHg/16 mmHg

## Expected Findings

- The average IOP is 15.5 mmHg. The normal range is considered to be 8–21 mmHg.
- Pressure readings greater than 21 mmHg are not automatically assumed to be indicative of glaucoma. Likewise, pressure readings that fall within the normal range do not rule out the possibility of glaucoma. Other examination results must be considered (e.g., pachymetry, ONH appearance, visual field results).
- A difference in pressure readings of more than 2 mmHg between the two eyes is considered significant.
- Diurnal variations of 3–4 mmHg are considered normal, and IOP is expected to be higher in the morning.

| GOLDMANN APPLANATION TONOMETRY at a glance | |
| --- | --- |
| **Purpose** | **Technique** |
| Prepare slit lamp | Magnification low or medium<br>Insert cobalt filter |
| Prepare patient | Scan anterior segment to rule out contraindications<br>Instill topical anesthetic and fluorescein and rescan the cornea |
| Prepare tonometer | Position applanation prism<br>Rotate prism to compensate for corneal astigmatism (as needed)<br>Brightly illuminate tonometer tip<br>Measuring dial set between 10 and 20 mmHg |
| Properly position prism on cornea | Ensure contact with cornea by looking for limbal glow<br>Use joystick to move prism until semicircles are equal in size and centered<br>Check the thickness of mires, correct if necessary |
| Obtain correct IOP reading | Turn pressure dial until inner rings of the semicircles meet<br>Withdraw prism from the cornea<br>Read pressure reading from dial<br>Recheck cornea for staining |

*Note:* There are portable versions of applanation tonometry that allow the examiner to obtain IOP readings outside of the slit lamp. With these instruments, the examiner performs the GAT procedure as outlined above but stabilizes themselves and the patient in free space using either the integrated forehead rest or their hands resting against the patient's face and head.

## 5.15 NONCONTACT TONOMETRY (NCT)

### Purpose
The aim of this procedure is to measure the intraocular pressure (IOP.)

### Indications
When applanation tonometry is contraindicated, as in the case of a red eye of infectious origin, or to screen for IOP abnormalities during routine eye exams.

*Note:* Several NCTs are available, and many are automated. The reader is advised to review the documentation that comes with their particular NCT before attempting the procedure.

### Equipment
- Noncontact tonometer

### Setup
- Disinfect the forehead rest and the chin rest by wiping them with alcohol and drying them with a tissue.
- Turn on the instrument.
- Adjust the level of the table so both the patient and the examiner are comfortable.
- Adjust the height of the chin rest to align the patient's outer canthus with the notch on the upright support of the headrest.

### Procedure
1. Inform the patient that the instrument is used to measure the pressure in the eye and reassure them that it will not be painful or harmful.
2. Instruct the patient to place their chin in the chinrest, press their forehead firmly against the forehead rests, and to look straight ahead.
3. Instruct the patient to open both eyes.
4. Align the center of the pupil with the on-screen target. Some models begin IOP acquisition automatically, while others require a button to be pressed.

   *Note*: If the patient blinks or if the machine is unable to record the result, repeat steps 3 through 4. It may be helpful to ask the patient to blink once or twice then hold their eyes wide open as you press the button for acquisition.
5. Repeat steps 3–4 for the other eye.

### Recording
- Write "NCT."
- Record the reading for the right eye followed by the reading for the left eye. *Note*: some instruments will report multiple readings per measurement, while others will report an average. Record all reported readings.
- Record the time of day the measurements were taken.

### Examples
- NCT @ 9:53am: 15, 16, 16 OD; 12, 11, 13 OS
- NCT @1:30pm: OD 16 mmHg, OS 17 mmHg

### Expected Findings
- IOP norms are the same for GAT as NCT (see Procedure 5.14).
- There is some evidence to suggest that NCT may over-estimate IOP at higher readings.

### Notes
- NCT should not be used to manage or determine treatment protocol changes in glaucoma patients or patients at high risk for developing glaucoma.
- If there is suspicion for glaucoma, or if NCT reveals an IOP above 21 mmHg, GAT should be performed unless otherwise contraindicated.

## 5.16 REBOUND TONOMETRY

### Purpose
The aim of this procedure is to measure the intraocular pressure (IOP.)

### Indications
This procedure intends to screen for IOP abnormalities in patients who cannot tolerate GAT.

### Equipment
- Rebound tonometer
- Rebound tonometer probe

### Setup
- The patient removes their glasses and/or contact lenses.
- The examiner disinfects the forehead rest of the tonometer by wiping it with alcohol and drying with a tissue. The examiner performs hand hygiene.
- The examiner turns on the tonometer and places the rebound tonometer probe into the front of the rebound tonometer housing unit.
- The examiner holds the rebound tonometer in their dominant hand.

### Procedure
1. Inform the patient that the instrument is used to measure the pressure in the eye and that you would like to demonstrate how it works. Reassure the patient that it will not be painful or harmful.
2. Instruct the patient to look straight ahead at a large optotype (e.g., 20/400 E).
3. Bring the tonometer probe about 2 cm away from the center of the patient's right cornea.

   *Note*: to increase stabilization, consider resting the hand holding the probe against the patient's cheek.
4. Using your free hand, extend the forehead rest at the top of the rebound tonometer until it makes contact with the patient's forehead.
5. Press the large button on the tonometer to acquire a reading and look to ensure that the probe is making contact with the cornea.

   *Note*: You may hear a short beep if a successful reading has been taken. If you hear two beeps, check to ensure that the tonometer is perpendicular to and at the proper distance from the cornea. The tonometer may also direct you to move the forehead rest further back or closer to the patient to ensure proper contact of the probe on the cornea.
6. Repeat step 5 five to six times as indicated by the particular instrument used. Record the average.

*Note:* You may hear a long beep indicating that enough successful readings have been acquired, and the average will be given on the tonometer display. The tonometer may ask you to repeat the measurements if needed.

7. Repeat steps 2 through 6 with the left eye.

## Recording

- Write "$T_R$" or "Tonomtery (rebound)" to indicate that the IOP was obtained by the technique of rebound tonometry. The type of rebound tonometer used may also be recorded.
- The reading for the right eye is recorded first, followed by the left eye.
- Record the time of day the test was performed.

## Examples

- $T_R$ 18/19 10:30 am
- Tonometry (rebound) @ 12:05 pm: 12/12
- IOP @ 2:30 pm (iCare): 20 mmHg/18 mmHg

## Expected Findings

- IOP norms are the same as those for GAT and NCT (see Procedure 5.14).
- Rebound tonometry has been found to result in very similar readings to GAT. However, rebound tonometry is not the current gold standard for IOP measurement.

## Notes

- Rebound tonometry should not be used to manage or determine treatment protocol changes in glaucoma patients or patients at high risk for developing glaucoma.
- If there is suspicion for glaucoma, or if rebound tonometry reveals an IOP above 21 mmHg, GAT should be performed unless otherwise contraindicated.

## 5.17 PACHYMETRY

### Purpose

The aim of this procedure is to measure the central corneal thickness (CCT).

### Indications

This procedure intends to further investigate a patient identified as high risk for glaucoma (see section "Notes" below), or when disease such as Fuchs' Dystrophy is suspected, as corneal endothelial dysfunction may lead to corneal edema.

### Equipment

- Pachymeter with probe
- Anesthetic e.g., 0.5% proparacaine

### Setup

The following procedure describes the measurement of CCT with a handheld instrument commonly available in many practices.

- Evaluate the patient's anterior segment, especially the cornea, to rule out conditions that contraindicate touching the cornea with the pachymeter probe (e.g., red eye of infectious origin or severely traumatized cornea).
- Turn on the instrument.

*Pachymeter Probe Preparation*

- Disinfect the pachymeter probe according to manufacturer and CDC guidelines (or other local legal requirements if outside the United States). Perform hand hygiene.

### Procedure

1. Instill one drop of anesthetic into both of the patient's eyes (see Procedure 5.7).
2. Hold the pachymeter with your dominant hand. Instruct the patient to fixate on a distant target (e.g., 20/400 optotype) and to keep both eyes open.
3. Place the end of the probe gently against the patient's right cornea perpendicular to the surface and in the center of the cornea. The instrument will indicate when a valid reading has been registered, usually by a beeping noise.
4. Take three to five readings depending on the specific instrument used.
5. Repeat steps 2 through 4 for the left cornea.

### Recording

- Record the pachymetry readings in microns.
- Record the readings provided on the screen of the device: either three to five readings and the calculated average, or occasionally only the average is provided.

### Example

- CCT  OD 578, OS 582
- CCT  OD 536, 540, 537    OS 542, 540, 546

### Expected Finding

- Normal, healthy corneas are approximately $555 \pm 35$ microns thick and symmetrical to the other eye.

### Notes

- Pachymetry has been identified as an independent risk factor for the conversion of ocular hypertension to primary open-angle glaucoma according to the Ocular Hypertension Treatment Study in 2002.
- Corneal thickness may affect the measurement of IOP (see Procedure 5.14).

## 5.18 GONIOSCOPY

### Purpose

The aim of this procedure is to observe and evaluate the anterior chamber angle.

### Indications

Gonioscopy is used to determine if the patient is at risk of angle closure prior to pupillary dilation, such as when the anterior chamber angle is less than 1/4:1 by the Van Herick technique (see Procedure 5.2). The technique is also used to investigate anterior chamber angle structures in patients with glaucoma of either the open-angle or closed-angle variety, suspected iris neovascularization, syndromes associated with glaucoma (e.g., pigment dispersion or pseudoexfoliation), a history of blunt trauma to the eye, or any suspicious iris lesions.

*Note*: Gonioscopy is contraindicated in the presence of corneal penetrating injury or hyphema.

### Equipment

- Gonioscopy lens
- Slit lamp (biomicroscope)
- Highly viscous lubricant
- Topical anesthetic (e.g., 0.5% proparacaine)
- Tissues
- Sterile saline irrigating solution (*optional*)

> *Note:* Numerous indirect (mirrored) gonioscopic lenses are available, varying in size, shape, and number of mirrors. The Goldmann three-mirror lens is commonly used because it is versatile, allowing for observation of the retina as well as the anterior chamber angle. The procedure described here assumes use of the three-mirror lens but, with minor modifications, will apply to all indirect gonioscopy lenses.

## Setup

Slit lamp setup is the same as Procedure 5.2 with the following specifications:

- Disinfect the gonioscopy lens according to manufacturer and CDC guidelines (or other local legal requirements if outside the United States). Perform hand hygiene.
- Adjust the slit beam to a medium width parallelepiped and set the illumination arm of the biomicroscope centered at 0°. Magnification should start at 6× to 10×.
- Fill the concave face of the gonioscopy lens with two to three drops of highly viscous lubricant, taking care to avoid bubbles in the solution. Set the lens face down (i.e., concave side up) on top of a sterile tissue nearby.
- Instill a drop of a topical anesthetic into the eye to be examined. If both eyes are to be examined, instill the anesthetic into both eyes (see Procedure 5.7).

## Procedure

*Insertion of the Lens*

1. Properly position the patient in the slit lamp. It is helpful to lower the chin rest slightly, so the patient's lateral canthus falls slightly below the alignment mark. This ensures that the slit beam can reach the gonioscopy mirror when the mirror is in the superior position.

2. Grasp the gonioscopy lens in your dominant hand between your thumb and index finger. Hold it in such a way that when it comes to rest on the patient's eye, the thumbnail-shaped mirror will be located at the 12 o'clock position. *Note:* Insertion of the lens is performed with the examiner looking outside of the slit lamp oculars.

3. Instruct the patient to look down and grasp their upper lid and lashes firmly with your nondominant hand. Tether the upper lid by firmly pressing the patient's upper lashes against the superior rim of their orbit (see **Figure 5-23**).

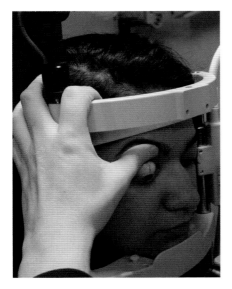

**FIGURE 5-23.** | Photograph showing the tethering of the lashes of the upper eyelid and eyelashes against the patient's brow to prevent eye closure. This technique is useful for a variety of procedures.

4. Instruct the patient to look up and pull down the patient's lower lid with the middle or fourth finger of the hand holding the lens or use the lower lip of the gonioscopy lens to carefully push down on the lower lid.

5. Insert the lower edge of the lens into the inferior cul-de-sac (see **Figure 5-24**). Rock the lens toward the patient until the entire lens is firmly in contact with the globe, as shown in **Figure 5-25**. Look through the central lens of the Goldmann 3-mirror to tell when the lens is in contact with the globe.

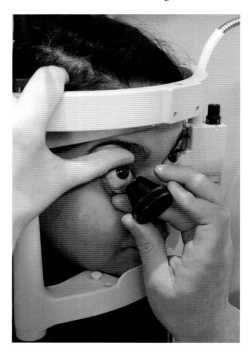

FIGURE 5-24. | Insertion of the gonioscopy lens. The examiner's left hand is holding the patient's upper lid. The patient's lower lid is being retracted with the fourth finger of the examiner's right hand (the hand holding the lens).

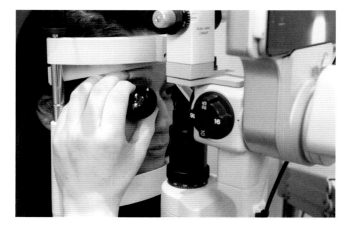

FIGURE 5-25. | Gonioscopy lens inserted and positioned for examination. The lens is held parallel to the patient's face, with the gonioscopy (thumbnail-shaped) mirror in the 12 o'clock position for observation of the inferior quadrant.

6. Instruct the patient to *slowly* look down until they are fixating straight ahead. Then slowly release the patient's lids. Continue holding the lens throughout the entire procedure, but do not apply too much forward pressure. Tell the patient to blink normally but to avoid hard blinks, which are more likely to dislodge the gonioscopy lens than normal blinks.

7. Check that the thumbnail-shaped mirror is located at the 12 o'clock position. If it is not, rotate the lens until this mirror comes to that position.

*Observation of the Anterior Chamber Angle*

1. Looking outside the oculars, position the vertical slit beam in the gonioscopy mirror located at the 12 o'clock position.

2. Look through the oculars and focus on the angle structures. Once the angle is in focus, increase the width of the slit beam or increase the magnification to enhance your view. If glare from the mirror or lens surface interferes with your view, it can be eliminated by altering the angle of the illumination arm slightly (5° to 10°), or by very slightly altering the tilt of the gonioscopy lens.

3. Begin evaluating the anterior chamber angle at the pupil. Direct your gaze gradually across the iris, noting any elevations or abnormalities. Note where the iris inserts. This is the posterior border of the anterior chamber angle. Identify the structures visible in the angle and note any unusual or abnormal findings (see **Figure 5-26**).

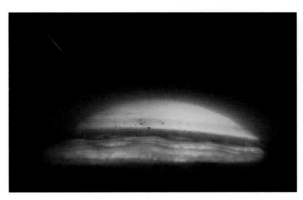

**FIGURE 5-26.** | Photograph showing the anterior chamber angle as viewed through the gonioscopy mirror (the beam is widened for full view). The trabecular meshwork is lightly pigmented. The ciliary body band is the most posterior structure visible, indicating a wide-open angle.

4. If you have difficulty identifying the structures, narrow your beam to an optic section and increase the angle of the illumination arm to approximately 20°. The beam should appear as two focal lines along the corneal dome, intersecting and merging into one at Schwalbe's line. Since Schwalbe's line is actually a ledge, you should also appreciate that the optic section curves out slightly as it passes over this structure.

5. If using the three-mirror lens, rotate it 90° to observe one of the lateral angles. Use two hands to rotate the lens. One hand is used to hold the lens gently but firmly against the globe to maintain contact, while the other hand turns the lens. *Note:* If using the four-mirror lens, it is not necessary to rotate the lens, but only to move the biomicroscope to be able to observe through the appropriate mirror.

6. Rotate the slit beam to the horizontal position and repeat steps 2 through 4.

7. If using the three-mirror lens, rotate it two more times, turning it 90° each time, to observe the entire 360° angle. Each time the lens is rotated, the slit beam is also rotated to

correspond to the position of the mirror. The beam should be oriented vertically when the mirror is in the superior or inferior positions and oriented horizontally when the mirror is in the nasal or temporal positions. *Note*: If using the four-mirror lens, it is only necessary to move the slit lamp and beam to the appropriate mirror.

### Removal of the Gonioscopy Lens

1. Remind the patient to keep their forehead pressed firmly against the forehead rest and instruct them to look up.

2. To remove the gonioscopy lens, apply firm but gentle pressure against the lower lid margin at the central edge of the lens, slightly indenting the sclera to break the suction between the lens and the cornea (see **Figure 5-27**). *Note*: If using a lens that is not held to the eye by any suction forces, the lens may simply be removed directly off the eye.

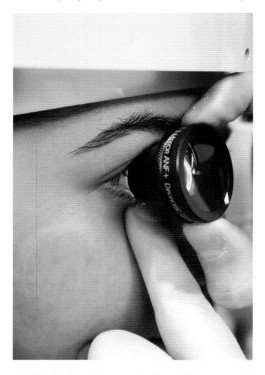

**FIGURE 5-27.** | Removal of the gonioscopy lens. While the patient looks up, the examiner presses the lower lid against the patient's inferior sclera at the edge of the lens.

3. If a highly viscous solution with preservatives was used, gently irrigate the patient's eye with sterile saline as the residual solution may cause irritation. Otherwise, the patient may dab excess solution from their eyes with a tissue.

## Recording

- Draw a large "X." Each compartment within the X represents an anatomical quadrant of the angle. In each compartment, record the most posterior angle structure observed, using the following abbreviations:
  - "CBB" ciliary body band
  - "SS" scleral spur
  - "TM" trabecular meshwork, "ATM" anterior trabecular meshwork, or "PTM" posterior trabecular meshwork
  - "SL" Schwalbe's line

*Note*: If unable to draw a large X because of limitations with the electronic medical record system, record the most posterior angle structure observed in list form for each eye.

- Record any unusual or abnormal findings for each quadrant. Pigmentation of the trabecular meshwork may be graded on a scale of 0 to 4, where 0 is no pigment and 4 is darkly pigmented.
- Remember that your view through the gonioscopy mirror is reversed. Recording should be anatomically correct. For example, when the mirror is placed at 12 o'clock, the inferior anterior chamber angle is being observed and should be recorded at the bottom of the X.

## Example

An example of recording the findings of gonioscopy is shown in **Figure 5-28**.

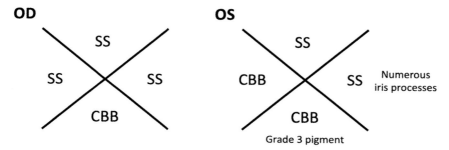

FIGURE 5-28. | Recording of gonioscopy findings. The initials indicate the most posterior structure visible in each quadrant of the angle. Abnormal or unusual variations (pigment, iris processes) are also indicated in the appropriate quadrant.

| GONIOSCOPY at a glance | |
|---|---|
| **Purpose** | **Technique** |
| Prepare slit lamp | Adjust oculars, set PD<br>Low magnification<br>Illumination arm at 0°<br>Medium width parallelepiped |
| Prepare gonio lens | Fill the disinfected gonio lens meniscus with two to three drops of lubrication fluid |
| Prepare patient | Scan anterior segment<br>Instill topical anesthetic |
| Insert gonio lens | Hold lens in dominant hand<br>Hold the patient's upper and lower lids<br>Insert lower edge of lens in cul-de-sac, rotate lens to contact the cornea<br>The patient slowly directs gaze to the straight-ahead position<br>Release lids and tell the patient to blink normally |
| Observe anterior chamber angle | Position gonio mirror at 12 o'clock<br>Position slit beam in mirror<br>Focus on angle structures, increase magnification if needed<br>Rotate lens 90°, rotate slit, and focus<br>Rotate lens through 360°, focusing on all four quadrants |
| Remove gonio lens | The patient looks up<br>Apply pressure against lower lid at edge of lens to break suction<br>Clean and disinfect lens<br>Irrigate patient's eye with sterile saline solution as needed |

## Notes

- Positioning the thumbnail mirror superiorly at the beginning of the procedure permits you to observe the inferior angle first. The inferior angle is usually the most open and the most pigmented, so it is easier to identify the angle structures.
- Systems are available that grade the angle from 0 to 4 based on the openness of the angle. However, these grading systems are not standardized and can be confusing.

> *Note:* A gonioscopy lens such as the Goldmann 3-mirror may also be used to observe and evaluate specific areas of the retina with a magnified, stereoscopic image. The procedure of using the gonioscopy lens in this way is the same as what is outlined above in Procedure 5.18, with careful attention drawn to a retinal lesion or unusual variation previously detected with another procedure such as BIO (Procedure 5.20) or fundus biomicroscopy (Procedure 5.22). The examiner should move the slit lamp towards the patient to visualize these more posterior structures and use one of the three ancillary lenses on the gonioscopy lens: the trapezoid mirror for the equator, the square mirror for the mid-periphery, and the thumbnail mirror for the peripheral retina.

## 5.19 DIRECT OPHTHALMOSCOPY

### Purpose

The aim of this procedure is to evaluate the health of the posterior segment of the eye. The direct ophthalmoscope is also useful to detect certain anomalies in the anterior segment of the eye.

### Equipment

- Monocular direct ophthalmoscope

### Setup

- Perform hand hygiene.
- Dim the room illumination.
- The examiner stands during this procedure.
- Adjust the examation chair so the patient's eyes are about at your eye level.
- Instruct the patient to remove their corrective lenses and to look at a nonaccommodative fixation target straight ahead or slightly above the horizontal plane at distance.
- For patients with a high myopic or high hyperopic prescription if the examiner is unable to obtain a good view of the disc, have the patient put on their glasses and see if this helps the examiner's view of the fundus.

### Procedure

1. Hold the handle of the ophthalmoscope in your right hand and align the aperture in front of your right eye. Start by examining the patient's right eye. Brace the head of the ophthalmoscope against your face or glasses. Use your index finger to turn the lens wheel.

2. Position the ophthalmoscope about 10 inches from the patient's eye, about 5–15° temporal to their line of sight. Use the spot beam with about a +4.00 lens to focus on the patient's iris. Check the optical clarity of the media by moving the ophthalmoscope about 30° in each direction (back and forth and up and down). Observe the orange (red) reflex of the fundus within the pupil for dark areas indicative of media opacities. If you need more magnification (e.g., to look at a corneal scar) then move closer and increase the dioptric power of the lens wheel.

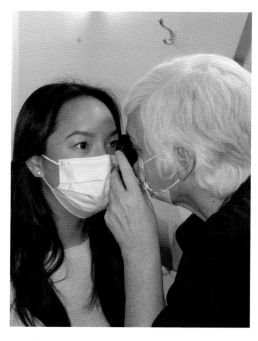

FIGURE 5-29. | Proper position of the examiner to perform direct ophthalmoscopy.

3. Slowly reduce the plus power and move closer to the patient until your hand holding the ophthalmoscope touches their face (see **Figure 5-29**). Continue reducing plus power slowly until the features of the ocular fundus come into focus. On your journey to the retina, you may observe lenticular opacities and floaters. When you reach the retina the power on the lens wheel should be approximately the examiners spectacle Rx and the patient's spectacle Rx added together, e.g., if the examiner is a −2.00 (and not wearing their glasses) and patient is a −3.00 then the wheel should read about −5.00.

4. Locate the optic nerve head (ONH or "disc"). The ONH should be visible when you are positioned approximately 15° temporal to the patient's visual axis.

5. Examine the ONH: margins, rim tissue (color and contour), cup size, and depth. Determine the cup-to-disc (C/D) ratio for both its horizontal and vertical dimensions; this step is critical. Examine the veins as they exit from the cup for spontaneous venous pulsation (SVP).

6. Examine the peripapillary retina, which is the region adjacent to the disc.

7. Examine the fundus out to the midperiphery by following blood vessels from the ONH in each of four directions: superior, nasal, inferior, and temporal. Instruct the patient to look up, down, right, and left while examining the corresponding quadrant. Evaluate the vasculature, looking carefully at arteriovenous crossings. Estimate the ratio of the thickness of the arteries to the thickness of the veins (A/V ratio). Evaluate the retinal background, noting the color and evenness of the pigmentation. Some examiners evaluate the optic nerve then go straight to the macula region, and then view superior, nasally, and then temporally.

8. Move so you are positioned along the patient's line of sight and examine the macula. It is preferred that the examiner reposition themselves to see the macular region but as an alternative, instruct the patient to look directly at the middle of the ophthalmoscope

light in order to examine the macula. The former method is preferred, because the latter method may introduce constriction of the pupil due to the pupillary near response. Determine if the color of the macula is homogenous and look for the presence of a foveal reflex.

*Note:* If, at any time during steps 4 through 8, you observe possible or probable hemorrhages or microaneurysms, reexamine those areas through the "red-free" or green filter to enhance the contrast. The red-free filter may also help you with estimating cup to disc ratios.

9. Repeat steps 2 through 8 on the patient's left eye, holding the ophthalmoscope in your left hand and using your left eye.

### Recording
- Record the observations for each eye separately.
- Observations should be noted for each of the following: media, disc margins, disc color, C/D ratio (indicating the horizontal and vertical measurements separately), vasculature (including A/V ratio and presence or absence of SVP), macula (including presence or absence of foveal reflex), and background. Abnormalities and pertinent negatives should be noted.
- Photographs of what you have seen are recommended when they will enhance descriptions.
- The magnification produced by a direct ophthalmoscope is the (power of the eye)/4. So, an emmetropic eye would be 15x. It gives a virtual erect image.

### Example
- Direct ophthalmoscopy:
  Media: clear OD, clear OS
  C/D: 0.30 round OD, 0.10 V/0.15 H OS
  Color: pink OD, pink OS
  Margins: distinct, flat OD, indistinct edematous margins superiorly, inferiorly distinct OS
  Vasculature: A/V 2/3, +SVP OD, A/V 2/3, -SVP OS
  Macula: clear, +FR OD, pigment mottling, -FR OS
  Background: clear OD, clear, tessellated OS

## 5.20 BINOCULAR INDIRECT OPHTHALMOSCOPY (BIO)

### Purpose
The aim of this procedure is to evaluate the health of the posterior segment of the eye through a dilated pupil. BIO allows examination of the entire ocular fundus through a dilated pupil and is the instrument of choice for screening of the peripheral retina.

### Indications
This procedure intends to screen the peripheral retina for pathology during routine eye examinations, to investigate for a retinal etiology of a patient's symptoms or clinical signs, or to monitor patients with known peripheral retinal pathology.

### Equipment
- BIO with power supply.
- Handheld condensing lens. Lens powers range from +14 D to +33 D. The +20 D lens is one of the most commonly used.
- Dilating pharmacologic agents (e.g., 0.5% or 1% tropicamide and 2.5% phenylephrine).
  *Note:* see dilating drop precautions in Procedure 5.7 setup or section "Notes" below.

## Setup

*Preparing the Patient*

- Perform hand hygiene and instill dilating drops into the patient's eyes approximately 30 minutes prior to the time of the BIO examination.
- Once the patient's eyes are adequately dilated, position the patient in the exam in chair in either a seated or supine position. If using the supine position, adjust the patient to a reclining position so they are facing upward, and their face is parallel to the floor and slightly below your waist level.

*Preparing the BIO and Condensing Lens*

- Position the BIO on your head, adjusting the headbands to provide an even distribution of weight and a comfortable fit. The forehead strap should be positioned directly above your eyebrows.
- Position the oculars as close to your eyes (or your glasses) as possible. When properly positioned, the oculars should have a slight degree of pantoscopic tilt. Adjusting the pantoscopic tilt of the oculars is accomplished by loosening the set screw(s) on the bracket that attaches the illumination system to the headband.
- Adjust the PD to allow you to achieve binocular viewing. Adjustment of the PD is accomplished either by sliding the individual oculars or by turning a screw located next to or below the oculars. Close your left eye and hold out your thumb at eye level, 40–50 cm away. Adjust the right ocular until your thumb is centered in your field of view. Close your right eye and adjust the left ocular in the same manner. If the PD is properly adjusted for you, you should see a single, fused image when both eyes are open.
- Turn on the power supply and set the intensity of the light by positioning the rheostat at or below the halfway setting. Adjust the position of the light on the BIO by turning the horizontal rod or set screw that controls the mirror angle. The light should be positioned in the upper half of your field of view while looking at your thumb at a 40–50 cm viewing distance.
- Hold the condensing lens in your dominant hand between your thumb and index finger. The lens is held with the more convex surface facing the examiner. Most lenses have a silver ring or dot marking either the more convex or the less convex surface.
- Tilt the lens slightly so it is approximately parallel to your face. The lens may also be tilted slightly along the horizontal or vertical axis to reduce reflections from the lens surface.

## Procedure

*Obtaining a Stationary View*

1. Instruct the patient to fixate in the direction you wish to view (e.g., instruct the patient to look up to examine the superior retina).
2. Use one of your hands to hold the patient's upper lid and the other hand to hold the patient's lower lid. Use the middle finger of your dominant hand (the hand holding the condensing lens) to control one of the patient's lids. This allows you to rest your hand on the patient's face to steady the lens.
3. Position your head so the light from the BIO is centered in the patient's pupil.
4. Holding the condensing lens at arm's length from you and approximately 2 cm from the patient's eye, position the lens so it intersects the beam of light and is centered in front of the patient's pupil. If the lens is properly positioned, you will see a blurred image of the red fundus reflex through the lens.
5. Slowly pull the lens away from the patient's eye, keeping the red reflex centered in the lens, until the entire lens is filled with the image of the retina. If you are using a +20 D lens, it should be approximately 4 to 5 cm away from the eye at this point. You should have a clear view of the retina through the condensing lens (see **Figure 5-30**).

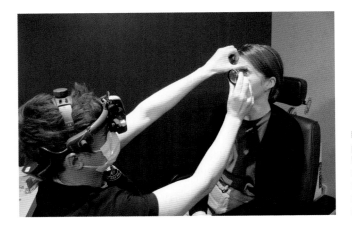

**FIGURE 5-30.** | Proper placement of the condensing lens to achieve a full image in the lens while performing BIO. Note that the hand holding the lens is being steadied against the patient's face.

*Scanning the Retina*

To view the entire retina, you must be able to scan with the BIO in addition to obtaining stationary views. Scanning means that you must move both yourself and the condensing lens while maintaining a view of the ocular fundus.

1. First obtain a stationary view as described in steps 1 through 5.

2. Keeping your waist and hips stationary, move your upper body both back and forth and side to side. As you move, keep all components of the optical system (examiner's line of sight, center of the condensing lens, center of the patient's pupil) aligned. You will lose the retinal image if proper alignment is not maintained. Remember to keep the condensing lens at arm's length and approximately 4–5 cm from the patient's eye. As you move, keep the lens positioned so it is roughly parallel to your face.

*Conducting a Systematic Examination*

It is recommended that you view the peripheral retina first and the posterior pole last to enhance the patient's comfort during the examination. Encourage the patient to blink whenever necessary but to keep their eyes open between blinks. Do not hold the examining light in one place for longer than 8 seconds at a time.

*Note*: The procedure described below assumes the patient is reclined in the supine position but, with minor modifications, may apply to a patient who is seated.

1. To examine the patient's right eye, begin by standing on the patient's right side.

2. Beginning with the superior retina, obtain overlapping views in eight positions: superior, superior nasal, nasal, inferior nasal, inferior, inferior temporal, temporal, and superior temporal. Instruct the patient to look in the direction you wish to view and stand 180° away. For example, to view the nasal retina of the patient's right eye, instruct the patient to look directly to their left while you stand on the patient's right, or temporal, side. You will need to walk clockwise around the patient during examination of the right eye to maintain this relationship. The patient should not look as far to the side as they are able, but only toward the direction you indicate.

3. In each of the eight positions, first obtain a stationary view of the equatorial region. Then, scan toward the peripheral retina, then back toward the posterior pole and then to the left and to the right.

4. After completing the examination of the peripheral retina, instruct the patient to look at your right ear, and obtain a stationary view of the posterior pole. Instruct the patient to look at your left ear when examining the patient's left eye.

*Note*: A green or "red-free" filter may be used throughout the BIO examination to enhance contrast if pathology such as hemorrhages are observed.

5. When you have completed the examination of the right eye, you should be standing on the patient's left side.

6. Examine the patient's left eye by repeating steps 2 through 4, walking counterclockwise around the patient. You will be standing on the patient's right side at the completion of the examination.

## Recording

- Record the presence and size in disc diameters (DD) or clock hours of retinal lesions or other unusual features or variations in the fundus appearance. Indicate the location of the lesions by clock hour and distance (in DD) from the closest retinal landmark. **Figure 5-31** illustrates the normal peripheral retinal landmarks. It is helpful to remember that the field of view through a +20 D condensing lens is roughly 8 DDs.

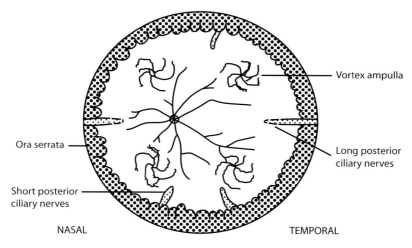

FIGURE 5-31. | Diagram showing peripheral retinal landmarks. The ora serrata is the anterior limit of the retina. The nasal ora serrata is more scalloped in appearance than the temporal portion. The long posterior ciliary nerves, located at 3 and 9 o'clock, divide the retina into superior and inferior halves. The short ciliary nerves, located close to the vertical midline, divide the retina roughly into nasal and temporal halves. The ampullae of the vortex veins mark the equatorial region of the retina. There is one or more ampulla in each quadrant.

- The use of photographs, drawings, or diagrams may be used to enhance your descriptions.
- Remember that your view through the condensing lens is flipped and inverted (i.e., upside down and backward). Illustrations and descriptions should be anatomically correct. Indicate where the lesion is anatomically located on the retina, not where it appears to be located through the condensing lens.
- Record pertinent negatives when applicable, for example, "peripheral retina unremarkable; no holes, tears, lesions, or detachments."

## Examples

- OD: 2DD lattice degeneration at 1:00 o'clock anterior to the vortex ampulla. No holes, tears, or detachments.
  OS: 3DD choroidal nevus with overlying drusen at 4:30, 2DD from the ONH; no elevation or fluid. Periphery clear; no holes, tears, lesions, or detachments.

| BINOCULAR INDIRECT OPHTHALMOSCOPY at a glance | |
|---|---|
| **Purpose** | **Technique** |
| Prepare patient | Wait approximately 30 minutes after instilling dilating drops<br>Position the patient so that they are seated or reclined (provider preference) |
| Prepare BIO | Adjust headband<br>Position oculars<br>Adjust PD<br>Adjust position of the light within your field of view<br>Properly position condensing lens in your dominant hand |
| Obtain stationary view of patient's retina | Hold patient's lids, direct their fixation<br>Position BIO light in center of pupil<br>Position condensing lens close to patient's eye, center to see red reflex<br>Pull lens away from eye until entire lens fills with red reflex<br>Tilt lens if necessary, to reduce reflections and provide a clearer image |
| Systematically scan retina | Begin at the superior retina, obtain overlapping views in eight positions<br>At each position, scan from equator to far periphery, then back toward posterior pole<br>If reclined, walk around patient, always standing opposite area being observed<br>Obtain a stationary view of posterior pole |

## Notes
- Prior to dilating the patient, you must obtain best-corrected visual acuity and IOP, and you must estimate the depth of the anterior chamber angle. In addition, you should perform any other tests whose findings are necessary to understand the patient's problems and that cannot be properly done on the dilated eye (e.g., pupils).

## 5.21 SCLERAL DEPRESSION

### Purpose
The aim of this procedure is to expand the examiner's view of the far peripheral retina in conjunction with BIO and to allow three-dimensional viewing of peripheral retinal lesions.

### Indications
To obtain information about a peripheral retinal lesion noted during BIO, to investigate the etiology of symptoms such as new onset flashes or floaters, or to investigate for sequelae of recent, direct trauma to the eye.

### Equipment
- BIO
- Handheld condensing lens
- Scleral depressor

### Setup
- The setup is the same as for BIO (see Procedure 5.20). The examiner performs hand hygiene and proper disinfection of equipment to be used. The patient is typically reclined to the supine position for scleral depression.
- Hold the scleral depressor between the thumb and the forefinger of your dominant hand. If you are using the thimble type of depressor, put your index finger inside the thimble and use your thumb to stabilize it as necessary.
- Inform the patient that they will feel some pressure from the scleral depressor, but it will not be painful.

## Procedure

1. Precisely localize the lesion or retinal area that you wish to depress with the BIO.
2. Stand 180° from the area you want to observe. Instruct the patient to look toward you.
3. Position the scleral depressor on the patient's lid, tangential to the globe and directly over the area to be depressed, as shown in **Figure 5-32A-B**. It is helpful to remember that the ora serrata is located approximately 8 mm posterior to the limbus, and the equator is about 6 mm posterior to the ora serrata.

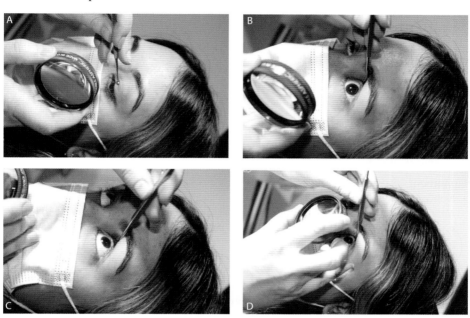

**FIGURE 5-32.** | (A) The examiner is positioning the scleral depressor on the upper lid behind the patient's superior limbus. Note that the depressor is held tangential to the globe. (B) The examiner retracts the lid with the depressor to the desired location of the lesion or area of interest. The scleral depressor is now properly positioned for depression of the patient's superior peripheral retina. (C) When the depressor is in position, the patient will be instructed to look up (or toward the area of interest). (D) The examiner applies tangential pressure to the globe while viewing the desired retinal location through the condensing lens.

4. Instruct the patient to look away from you, in the direction of the depressor. Keep the depressor positioned tangential to the globe (see **Figure 5-32C**).
5. Obtain a view of the retina through the condensing lens. If your scleral depressor is positioned properly, you will see an elevated area slightly paler than the surrounding retina under the tip of the depressor. If you do not observe this elevation, move the depressor more posteriorly or side to side, always maintaining its position tangential to the globe. Do not press inward on the globe. Very little pressure is required for scleral depression.
6. Once you are certain that the scleral depressor is overlying the area you wish to examine, use a massaging motion along the lid to manipulate the retina and obtain different views of the lesion and the surrounding tissue.
7. If you are using scleral depression to extend your peripheral retinal view rather than observing a specific lesion, repeat steps 3 through 6 for each of the eight positions of gaze during your routine BIO examination.

## Recording
- Record your observations in the peripheral retinal evaluation section of the patient's record.
- Indicate that scleral depression was performed.
- Record pertinent negatives as well as abnormal findings.

## Examples
- Periphery OD: Scleral depression 360°—no holes, tears, or detachments.
  Periphery OS: Small retinal hole, 2 DD posterior to ora at 2 o'clock. No subretinal fluid or traction seen with scleral depression.

## 5.22 FUNDUS BIOMICROSCOPY

### Purpose
The aim of this procedure is to evaluate the health of the posterior segment of the eye. A noncontact auxiliary lens is used in conjunction with the biomicroscope to provide an inverted, wide-field, stereoscopic image with excellent resolution. Fundus biomicroscopy is used primarily for viewing the posterior pole. Views of the peripheral retina may be obtained with some lenses using this technique.

### Equipment
- Noncontact auxiliary lens
  *Note:* Numerous auxiliary lenses for fundus biomicroscopy are available, varying in size, power, field of view, and optical design. The procedure that follows applies to any high-plus condensing lens (e.g., 78 D, 90 D, or Superfield) that provides an indirect view of the fundus (an inverted and reversed aerial image).
- Slit lamp (biomicroscope)
- Dilating agents (e.g., 0.5% or 1.0% tropicamide and 2.5% phenylephrine)
  *Note:* See dilating drop precautions in Procedure 5.7 setup or section "Notes" below.

### Setup
Slit lamp setup is the same as Procedure 5.2 with the following specifications:
- Instill dilating drops into the patient's eyes approximately 30 minutes prior to the time of the examination. Although dilation is recommended, it is also possible to perform this procedure without the aid of dilation.
- Adjust the table height and chin rest of the biomicroscope so the patient is comfortable. Set the illumination to a moderate intensity and the illumination arm of the biomicroscope in the center, straight-ahead position (0°). Adjust the beam to a narrow parallelepiped. Set the magnification on the lowest setting (6× or 10×). *Note:* some examiners prefer to have the height of the beam fit within the patient's pupil, while others prefer a tall beam.
- Hold the auxiliary lens vertically between the thumb and index finger of your left hand to examine the patient's right eye. Hold the lens in your right hand to examine the patient's left eye.

### Procedure
It is recommended that the posterior segment is examined systematically in the following order: optic nerve, retinal arcades, nasal retina, macula, and posterior vitreous. By convention, the right eye is typically examined first, followed by the left eye.
1. Instruct the patient to fixate straight ahead. Alternatively, you can instruct the patient to look across at your opposite ear, e.g., if examining the patient's right eye, the patient can fixate on your right ear.

2. Center the slit lamp beam in the patient's right pupil and focus on the cornea.

3. Place the lens in front of the patient's eye so the back surface just clears the lashes (approximately 1 cm from the patient's cornea). The distance between the lens and the cornea will vary depending on the power of the auxiliary lens used (see **Figure 5-33**). If the lens is properly positioned, you will see a blurred red fundus reflex when looking through the oculars of the slit lamp.

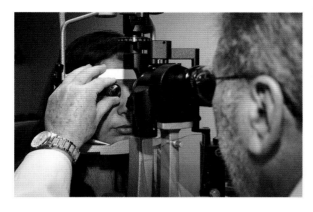

**FIGURE 5-33.** | Proper positioning of the auxiliary lens for observation of the posterior pole during fundus biomicroscopy.

4. Using the joystick, focus on the fundus image by slowly moving the slit lamp away from the cornea, keeping the beam centered in the pupil.

5. Once the retinal image is focused, widen the slit lamp beam to observe a greater area of the ocular fundus. The magnification can be changed to the medium or high setting at this time.

### Optic Nerve

1. Use the joystick and the vertical adjustment knob on the slit lamp to scan across the posterior ocular structures until the optic nerve comes into view.

2. Increase the width and height of the slit beam so the optic nerve is fully illuminated, observing the C/D ratio, neural rim tissue appearance, and noting any abnormalities, elevation or excavation.

### Posterior Pole

1. Use the joystick and the vertical adjustment to scan across the superior arcade until the terminal end of the main central retinal vein and artery branches.

2. Scan from superior to inferior until you observe the inferior terminal end of the retinal arcade.

3. Scan from temporal to nasal along the inferior arcade until you see the optic nerve again.

4. Scan the retina nasal to the optic nerve, using the vertical adjustment to observe the nasal arcades.

5. Return to the optic nerve.

### Macula

1. Use the rheostat to lower the intensity of the slit lamp illumination.

2. Scan the macula from nasal to temporal, looking for the foveal light reflex (FR) and taking note of any fluid/edema, thickening, or any other irregularities in appearance.

3. Return to the optic nerve.

*Posterior vitreous*

1. Use the joystick to pull the slit lamp away from the patient. Your view of the optic nerve will be blurry.

2. Scan the posterior vitreous and look for any irregularities (e.g., vitreal fragments, hemorrhaging, asteroid hyalosis).

## Recording

- Record each eye separately.
- Note in the record which auxiliary lens was used because the view obtained with one lens may appear different than the view obtained with other methods of retinal evaluation.
- Remember that your retinal view is inverted. Descriptions and illustrations should be anatomically correct. If an anomaly is observed, indicate where the lesion is located on the retina, not where it appears through the lens.
- Photographs are recommended in cases where they enhance descriptions.

## Examples

- Vitreous:       OD: Clear                          OS: Asteroid Hyalosis
- Optic Nerve:  OD: 0.30H/0.35V; Pink and    OS: 0.80H/0.70 V; Focal notching
                           healthy 360                         sup with drance hemorrhage
- Posterior Pole:  OD: Clear                       OS: Hemorrhages and exudates at
                                                                  inf a/v bifurcation
- Macula:          OD: Clear and flat, (+)FR    OS: Several soft drusen with mod
                                                                  thickening, blunted foveal reflex

## Notes

- As an alternative you may use a lens holder mounted on the upright support of the head rest or an adapter that rests against the patient's eyelids. These are not available for all lenses.
- To check for possible irregularities of the macula, narrow the beam to a slit and focus it in the macular area first oriented vertically and then oriented horizontally. Check the slit on the macula for gaps and/or curves and ask the patient if they see a break or thinning of the slit lamp beam. Checking the macula this way is known as the "Watzke-Allen slit beam test," and a positive finding is called a "Watzke sign."
- If the reflections from the surface of the lens are interfering with your view, tilt the lens slightly or increase the angle of the illumination arm to approximately 10° from center to reduce the glare.
- If at any time during your fundus biomicroscopy examination you observe possible or probable hemorrhages or microaneurysms, reexamining those areas through the "red-free" or green filter may enhance the contrast.

> *Note*: To increase the visibility of the retinal nerve fiber layer (NFL) surrounding the ONH, increasing the illumination with the rheostat and using the red-free filter may enhance contrast and highlight any focal defects or diffuse loss of fibers. This procedure may be incorporated into the fundus biomicroscopy examination of glaucoma suspects, as damage to the NFL may be the first clinical sign of glaucoma.

## 5.23 AMSLER GRID

## Purpose

The aim of this procedure is to assess the integrity of the visual field corresponding to the macular region of the retina.

## Indications

This procedure is used to investigate the visual impact of suspected or confirmed macular disease. Some examiners use the Amsler grid to screen for macular pathology in all elderly patients as part of their routine comprehensive eye exam.

## Equipment

- Amsler grid book
- Amsler grid recording sheets (*optional*)
- Occluder
- Illumination source

## Setup

- The patient wears their best near correction and holds the occluder.
- The examiner holds the chart at a distance of 28 to 30 cm from the patient under bright illumination.

  Note: the technical distance is 28.7 cm, but most practitioners use 28 to 30 cm in the clinical setting.

## Procedure

1. Begin testing the better seeing eye and instruct the patient to cover up the poorer seeing eye with the occluder.

   Note: Starting with the better seeing eye will enhance the patient's understanding and thus the reliability of their responses.

2. Confirm that the patient can see the white dot in the center of the grid. If the white dot is visible to the patient, tell them to look at the white dot throughout the test but to pay attention to the rest of the grid with their peripheral vision.

   Note: if the patient is unable to see the central white dot, another form of Amsler grid with intersecting diagonal lines is recommended to direct the patient toward the center of the grid.

3. Say to the patient, "While looking at the white dot and without moving your eyes":
   a. "Can you see all four corners of the grid?"
   b. "Are any of the horizontal or vertical lines missing or distorted?"
   c. "Are all the squares the same size?"

4. If the patient reports any abnormalities in grid appearance, ask them to point to the location of the anomaly and describe what they see.

5. Watch the patient. Make sure that the non-tested eye remains occluded and that the patient maintains fixation on the white dot. Throughout the test maintain the testing distance at 28 to 30 cm.

6. Repeat steps 2 through 5 with the other eye occluded.

## Recording

- If there are no problems, record "Amsler" and the eye tested, followed by "normal, no scotoma, no metamorphopsia" or WNL, which means "within normal limits."
- If there is a problem, record the eye, the nature of the problem, and its location on the grid.
- If possible, ask the patient to draw what they see on an Amsler recording chart or draw on the grid for the patient according to their description (see **Figure 5-34**).

## Examples

- Amsler: OD normal, no scotoma, no metamorphopsia, OS normal, no scotoma, no metamorphopsia

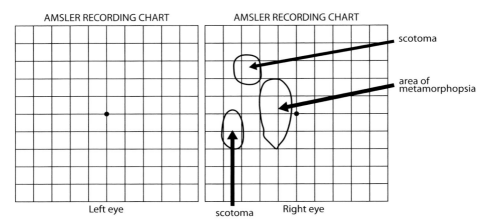

**FIGURE 5-34.** | The Amsler grid recording sheet. A blank form is shown for the left eye. For the right eye, the chart shows positive findings.

- Amsler: OD WNL, OS upper left corner not seen
- Amsler: OD metamorphopsia centrally, OS scotoma 2° round, 5° superior-temporal to fixation

### Notes
- The Amsler grid booklet contains an account of the theory of the test, lists and explains the questions to ask, and briefly gives the indications for the use of all six test plates. The procedure described here pertains only to the first plate. The complete Amsler grid book is available commercially.

## 5.24 TANGENT SCREEN

### Purpose
The aim of this procedure is to assess the integrity of the central 30° of the patient's field of vision. The tangent screen is *not* considered standard of care for glaucoma management. The tangent screen is, however, the procedure of choice for some patients. Patients with suspected hysterical fields, patients with severe arthritis (who are incapable of placing their chin in the holder of an automated perimeter or who cannot depress the buzzer), patients who are claustrophobic in a bowl setting may respond better with a tangent screen. Some patients with markedly reduced central vision may only respond to mapping the visual field with a tangent screen field. The tangent screen is also useful when an automated device or Goldman field device is not available.

### Equipment
- Tangent screen: a flat, nonreflective, black screen, usually made of feltlike cloth, with a small white object attached to the center of the screen to serve as a fixation target. On most tangent screens, the fixation target is surrounded by concentric circles, stitched into the surface of the screen at intervals of 5° when viewed from 1 meter.
- Thirty to fifty 1.0 to 2.0 mm diameter nonglossy, short black pins.
- The test targets (1-, 2-, 3-, 4-, 6- and 10-mm diameter). Usually, white test objects are used but occasionally red targets or blue targets (3 mm or 6 mm diameter) can be used to access optic nerve disorders.

- Black, nonglossy wand
- Eye patch
- Recording paper

## Setup
- The tangent screen should be moderately and evenly illuminated (standard illumination is 7 foot-candles). This level of illumination is achieved by having the room lights on and the overhead lamp from the stand aimed at the tangent screen providing equally diffused light over the tangent screen.
- Usually, the patient wears their habitual distance correction. The Rx should be worn if the patient's distance Rx is over −1.75 or +1.00. Essentially you do not want the patient to be more than 1 diopter out of focus at the one-meter testing distance. If the spectacle frame or the bifocal segment causes interference, the patient may need to hold a metal rimmed trial lens or wear a trial frame with the appropriate Rx.
- Patch the left eye to test the right eye first.
- Have the patient sit with their eye 1 meter from the tangent screen and level with the central fixation target both vertically and horizontally.
- In general, the examiner stands on the side being tested.

## Procedure
*Demonstration Test*
1. The examiner stands on the side of the field being tested. Never cross the wand over the vertical meridian.
2. Instruct the patient to fixate on the central white button.
3. Tell the patient you are going to test their side vision. Instruct them to tell you when they see the test object in their side vision and always to maintain fixation on the central fixation target.
4. Point to the fixation target and tell the patient to respond when the target appears or disappears, depending on the task at the time.
5. Present a large (e.g., 6 mm white) test target in various positions in the field. The patient should indicate that the target is seen.
6. Randomly turn the wand over so the target is hidden to test the patient's reliability and fixation. This step should also be repeated several times during the actual testing procedure.
7. Explain to the patient that the disappearance of the object is normal and that they should not be alarmed if it disappears. Ask them to say "gone" when they no longer see it, and to say "I see it," or "now" when it comes into view.
8. Always observe the patient, not the screen, in order to be sure that the non-tested eye remains occluded and that the patient directs gaze at the fixation target at all times.

*Testing the Visual Field*
1. Determine the size target you wish to use. Most practitioners use a 3-mm diameter white target. However, if you wish to be very precise present the smallest target in your test set (1 mm or 1.5 mm white) statically at 25° temporal to fixation (see **Figure 5-35**).

   Increase the size of the target until the patient responds and use that as your starting target.
2. Plot three to four points on the temporal field with the threshold target. Place a black pin on the screen when the patient responds that they see the white target.

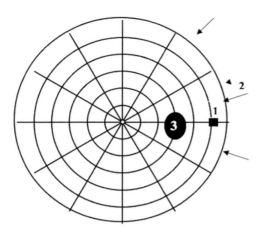

**FIGURE 5-35.** | Presentation of targets temporal to fixation on the tangent screen for the right eye.

3. Plot the blind spot:

   a. Start with the target near the fixation point and move it into the temporal field slightly below the horizontal meridian.

   b. Plot eight points to outline the blind spot going from non-seeing to seeing. Minor changes in the blind spot size are usually non-diagnostic; therefore, a minimal amount of time should be spent on this procedure (see **Figure 5-36**).

   c. Move the target around the outer circumference of the blind spot to verify the border.

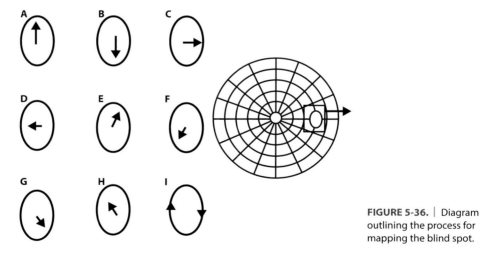

**FIGURE 5-36.** | Diagram outlining the process for mapping the blind spot.

4. Plot the limit of the remainder of the temporal isopter at 15° intervals (see **Figure 5-37**).

   a. If the patient sees the target at the edge of the screen, put a black pin at the edge and move to the next location.

   b. If the patient does not see the target at the edge of the screen, advance it at approximately 2° per second toward the fixation point until the patient reports that they do see it. Put a black pin at the location where it was first seen.

   c. Plot additional points on either side of the horizontal and vertical meridian.

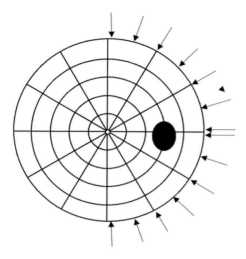

**FIGURE 5-37.** | Diagram outlining the process for mapping the temporal isopter.

5. Scan the temporal field by moving the threshold target along the radial stitch marks on the tangent screen as shown in **Figure 5-38**.

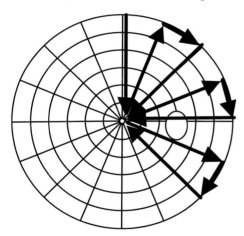

**FIGURE 5-38.** | Diagram outlining the process for scanning the temporal field.

6. The examiner moves to the other side of the tangent screen and plots the isopter for the nasal field at 15° intervals as shown in **Figure 5-39**.
7. Scan the nasal field by moving the threshold target along the radial stitch marks on the tangent screen. Occasionally have the target disappear by turning over the wand to ensure the patient is following the procedure correctly.
8. Patch the patient's right eye and repeat steps 1–7 for the left eye.

## Recording
- Record the results for each eye separately.
- It should be indicated if the test was the baseline exam, or a follow up, and if a follow up, a comparison to previous exams should be included.
- The test target size and color should be recorded.
- The description of the findings should be recorded for each eye and a copy of the field should be saved in the patient's record.

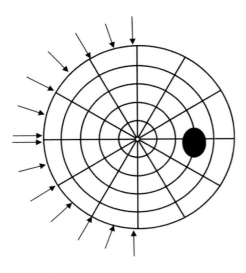

FIGURE 5-39. | Diagram outlining the process for mapping the nasal isopter.

## Examples

- Tangent screen, follow-up test

  OD: superior nasal step with 2/1000 W extending to 10° from fixation with sloping margins. Isopter returns to normal with a 6/1000W

  OS Superiorly large relative paracentral scotoma superiorly with 2/1000 W with sloping margins and inferiorly shallow relative scotoma with 2/1000 W

  Both visual fields consistent with longstanding glaucoma, stable OU. OD with inferior compromise of rim at approximately 7:30 o'clock and OS narrowing of rim tissue at 1:00 and 5:00 o'clock.

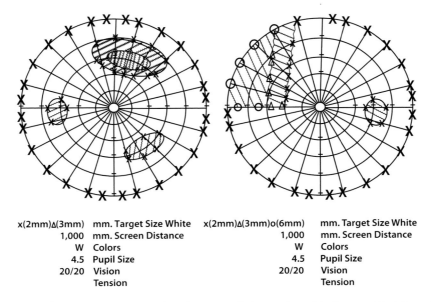

| x(2mm)Δ(3mm) | mm. Target Size White | x(2mm)Δ(3mm)o(6mm) | mm. Target Size White |
|---|---|---|---|
| 1,000 | mm. Screen Distance | 1,000 | mm. Screen Distance |
| W | Colors | W | Colors |
| 4.5 | Pupil Size | 4.5 | Pupil Size |
| 20/20 | Vision | 20/20 | Vision |
| | Tension | | Tension |

FIGURE 5-40. | A tangent screen recording sheet example for a patient with glaucoma. The interpretation of these fields is listed under 'Examples'. The right eye field is on the right and the left eye field is on the left in the example above, which is standard.

## 5.25 D-15 COLOR TEST

### Purpose
The aim of the procedure is to provide in-depth analysis of color vision defects identified through clinical screening tests.

### Indications
A D-15 color vision test is performed when routine color vision testing or the case history indicate the presence of a color vision anomaly. The D-15 is sensitive to red-green and blue-yellow dyschromatopsia in both acquired and congenital color vision deficiencies.

### Equipment
- D-15 Test, including standard scoring sheet
- Proper illuminant (e.g., MacBeth easel lamp)
- Eye patch
- Latex-free gloves (*optional*)

### Setup
- The patient wears their habitual near correction.
- Both the examiner and the patient may wear gloves to protect the colored caps of the test from skin oils.
- Place the caps color up in a random (scattered) order on the lid closer to the examiner.
- To ensure the validity of the test, work under the proper illuminant, with other light sources in the room turned off.

### Procedure
1. Instruct the patient to place the patch over their left eye to test their right eye.
2. Instruct the patient to rearrange the caps in order of similarity, starting with the reference cap which is glued down and to the patient's left. Tell the patient to do the test quickly, allowing 2 minutes per eye (see **Figure 5-41**).

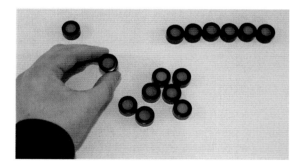

**FIGURE 5-41.** | Photograph of a patient performing the D-15 color vision test.

3. When the patient has rearranged the caps, close the lid, turn the box over, and open it upside down. The number of each cap is printed on the bottom of the cap and will now be visible.
4. Record the order of the caps selected for the right eye.
5. Instruct the patient to place the eye patch over their right eye and test the left eye by repeating steps 2 through 4.
6. Repeat the test if the caps are out of order in either eye.

## Recording
- Use the standard recording sheet, as shown in **Figure 5-42.**
- Write down the numbers of the caps in the patient's order in the space where it says, "subject's order."
- Connect the dots on the chart according to the numerical order of the caps.
- Make a notation if the patient was unusually slow.

## Expected Findings
- See **Figure 5-42,** patient A.

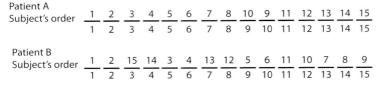

Patient A
Subject's order

| 1 | 2 | 3 | 4 | 5 | 6 | 7 | 8 | 10 | 9 | 11 | 12 | 13 | 14 | 15 |
|---|---|---|---|---|---|---|---|---|---|---|---|---|---|---|
| 1 | 2 | 3 | 4 | 5 | 6 | 7 | 8 | 9 | 10 | 11 | 12 | 13 | 14 | 15 |

Patient B
Subject's order

| 1 | 2 | 15 | 14 | 3 | 4 | 13 | 12 | 5 | 6 | 11 | 10 | 7 | 8 | 9 |
|---|---|----|----|---|---|----|----|---|---|----|----|---|---|---|
| 1 | 2 | 3 | 4 | 5 | 6 | 7 | 8 | 9 | 10 | 11 | 12 | 13 | 14 | 15 |

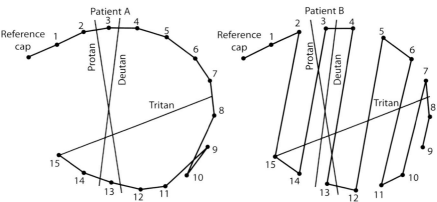

**FIGURE 5-42.** | Recording examples for two patients on the D-15 color vision test. Patient A is normal. The reversal of the order between cap 9 and cap 10 is considered to be within normal limits. Patient B has a strong deuteranomalous color vision defect.

## 5.26 PHOTOSTRESS RECOVERY TIME TEST

### Purpose
The aim of this procedure is to determine the time required for the macula to return to a near-normal level of visual acuity after being exposed to a bright light source for a specified duration of time.

### Indications
This procedure is indicated when the patient has reduced BCVA in one eye due to suspected macular pathology.

### Equipment
- Direct ophthalmoscope with visuscope (fixation) target or transilluminator
- Occluder
- Distance visual acuity chart
- Timer, watch or clock accurate to the second

## Setup

- The examiner measures the best-corrected visual acuity in each eye prior to the start of the test.
- Room illumination should be off or as dim as possible.
- The patient then removes their spectacles but holds onto them in their hand.
- The examiner sits near the patient to one side.

## Procedure

1. Allow the patient to dark adapt both eyes for 1 minute.
2. Have the patient hold the occluder over their left eye.
3. Adjust the dial to the visuscope target in the direct ophthalmoscope and set the rheostat to its brightest position.
4. Look through the ophthalmoscope and direct the light into the patient's unoccluded eye positioned 2 cm away.
5. Instruct the patient to look at the center of the visuscope target. Monitor the patient's fixation to ensure that they are looking in the proper place.
6. Maintain the light on the patient's macula for 10 seconds.
7. Withdraw the light, have the patient put on their best optical correction, and present the distance visual acuity chart.
8. Measure the elapsed time in seconds from the removal of the light until the patient is able to read half or more of the letters on the chart one line above their best-corrected visual acuity for that eye.
9. Repeat steps 1 through 7 on the left eye with the right eye occluded.

## Recording

- Indicate "photostress with ophthalmoscope."
- Record the elapsed time until the endpoint is reached in seconds for the right eye and left eye.

## Examples

- Photostress with ophthalmoscope: OD 20 seconds; OS 25 seconds
- Photostress with ophthalmoscope: OD 30 seconds; OS 120 seconds

## Expected Findings

- Normal: 60 seconds or less in each eye. No greater than 6-second difference between the two eyes.

## Notes

- A delayed photostress recovery time suggests a macular disorder involving the photoreceptors, the retinal pigment epithelium, and/or the choriocapillaris.

## 5.27 RED DESATURATION TEST

## Purpose

The aim of this procedure is to test the integrity of the optic nerve by testing the eye's sensitivity to the color red.

## Indications

This procedure intends to investigate for unilateral or asymmetric optic nerve pathology.

### Equipment
- Red-capped bottle (such as those containing tropicamide or cyclopentolate)
- Occluder

### Setup
- The patient sits comfortably in front of the examiner in a normally illuminated room.

### Procedure
*Comparison Between the Two Eyes*
1. Have the patient occlude the eye suspected of optic neuropathy to test the better-seeing eye first.
2. Hold one of the red-capped bottles 40 cm from the patient and instruct them to look at it.
3. Tell the patient that the red cap represents 100% redness. Ask the patient to confirm that they understand.
4. Now occlude the better-seeing eye and have the patient look at the same object with the eye suspected of having optic neuropathy.
5. Ask the patient to rate the redness perceived by the suspect eye on a scale of 1% to 100%.

### Recording
- Write "Red Desaturation."
- To compare the eyes, record the patient's responses for both the right eye and left eye.

### Examples
- Red Desaturation: OD 100%; OS 100%.
- Red Desaturation: OD 100%; OS 50%.

### Expected Findings
- Normal: No more than 10% difference when the two eyes are compared.

## 5.28 EXOPHTHALMOMETRY

### Purpose
This procedure aims to measure the position of the eyeball in the orbit to rule out protrusion (exophthalmos) or recession (enophthalmos) of the eyes relative to the orbital structures.

### Indications
When the external examination suggests an asymmetry in the size of the palpebral apertures, a bilateral increase in aperture size, or an enophthalmos or exophthalmos of one or both eyes. It is done routinely on patients with Graves' disease to monitor the progress of any exophthalmos associated with their condition.

### Equipment
- Hertel and/or Luedde exophthalmometer
- Distance fixation target located directly in front of the patient

### Setup
- Seat the patient so that their eyes are level with the examiner's eyes. Have the patient remove their spectacles.

### Procedure
*Hertel Exophthalmometer*
1. Ask the patient to close their eyes while the instrument is being positioned.

2. Loosen the set screw on the right side of the exophthalmometer's base. The base should now slide freely.

3. Position the left side of the base so that the curved foot plate is resting firmly against the patient's right lateral orbital rim. The inner edge of the foot plate should be at the lateral canthus.

4. Slide the base in or out to position the right side of the base against the patient's left lateral rim as described in step 3. The foot plates should be symmetrically positioned with respect to each orbit.

5. Once the base is properly positioned, tighten the set screw to prevent the base from sliding.

6. Hold the exophthalmometer in both hands, resting your fingers on the patient's face to stabilize it. The instrument base must be parallel to the floor, as shown in **Figure 5-43**.

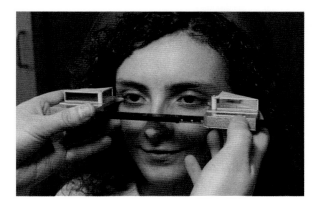

**FIGURE 5-43.** | Hertel exophthalmometer properly positioned for measuring. Note that the base is held parallel to the floor and the patient is instructed to look straight ahead.

7. Instruct the patient to open both eyes wide and to fixate on the distance target.

8. To measure the proptosis of the patient's right eye, close your left eye, look into the instrument's mirror that is to your left with your right eye, and move your head from side to side until you are at the measuring position. The measuring position is determined in one of two ways, depending on the particular instrument:

   a. If there are two red vertical lines in the mirror, the measuring point is the position at which the two red lines coincide (see **Figure 5-44A-B**).

   b. If there are no red lines, the measuring point is the position at which the zero edge of the scale is aligned with the inside edge of the mirror.

9. Determine where the patient's corneal apex intersects the scale. This is the exophthalmometry reading in millimeters.

10. To measure the patient's left eye, close your right eye, look through the mirror that is to your right with your left eye, and repeat steps 8 and 9.

11. Remove the instrument and note the base reading.

12. If subsequent measurements are taken at a later date, the base is preset on the measurement previously used. This ensures that the measurements are made from the same reference point.

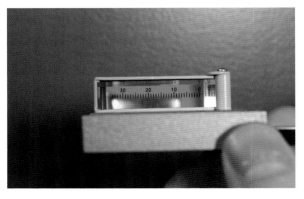

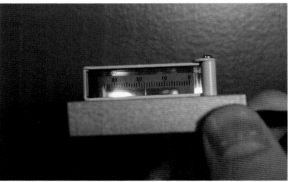

**FIGURE 5-44.** | (A) This is not the proper measuring position for Hertel exophthalmometry, because the two red lines are not overlapping. (B) When the examiner moves their head, the two red lines will appear to overlap at some point. The measurement of the corneal curvature intersection is taken from this position.

*Luedde Exophthalmometer*

1. Instruct the patient to open both eyes wide and to fixate on the distance target.
2. Position the exophthalmometer so that its concave end nests into the orbital rim of the patient's right eye at its outer canthus. Align the instrument so its long axis is parallel to the patient's line of sight both vertically and horizontally. Press the exophthalmometer gently but firmly into the outer canthus.
3. Using your sighting dominant eye, view the corneal apex by looking through the exophthalmometer perpendicular to its long axis to avoid parallax. Read off the position of the corneal apex in mm relative to the orbit.
4. Reposition the exophthalmometer at the lateral canthus of the patient's left eye. Attempt to press the instrument into position with the same force used for the right eye. Repeat step 3.

## Recording
- Hertel exophthalmometry readings are recorded as three numbers:
  - Measurement for the right eye
  - Measurement for the left eye
  - Base reading

- These numbers may be recorded separately, or as a fraction where the numerator is the proptosis measurements (OD–OS) and the denominator is the base measurement.
- Luedde exophthalmometer readings are recorded as single numbers for each eye.
- When recording exophthalmometry findings indicate which type of exophthalmometer was used.

### Examples
- Exophthalmometry: OD 21, OS 19, base 110—Hertel
- Exophthalmometry: OD 16, OS 21, base 105—Hertel
- Exophthalmometry: OD 17, OS 22—Luedde

### Expected Findings
- The average reading is 15–17 mm for all adults.
- The range of normal results is approximately 11–21 mm for White patients and 12–24 mm for African-American patients.
- A difference of 2 mm or more between the two eyes is considered significant.
- An increase in the reading of 2 mm or more over time is considered significant.

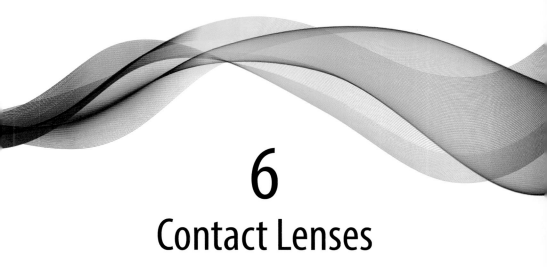

# 6

# Contact Lenses

Anita Gulmiri, OD, FAAO  /  Lance McNaughton, OD, PhD

## 6.1 INTRODUCTION TO THE CONTACT LENS EXAMINATION

The contact lens examination is an integral part of the core ocular examination. With over 45 million contact lens wearers in the United States alone, virtually all eye care providers will encounter contact lens wearers on a regular basis. Owing to the relentless growth of contact lens usage, it is essential to know the key components of a contact lens exam to ensure a maximum outcome for vision, comfort, and ocular health. This chapter describes basic procedures necessary for the fitting and evaluation of the most common contact lens types including soft and gas permeable (GP) designs. Due to their reduced prescribing frequency, some specialty lens types are beyond the scope of this chapter, though many of the basic procedures described in this chapter will apply to these lens types as well.

While a firm understanding of the overall structure of a contact lens exam creates a solid foundation, there will be instances when one or more side trips will be required to ensure a successful outcome. Indeed, contact lens patients have the same need for evaluation of refractive status, functional vision, and ocular health as all other patients. With this in mind, the procedures described in this chapter should be viewed as a regular part of your examination, just as your patient considers their contact lenses a regular part of their daily routine. Additionally, the procedures included in this chapter presume that the examiner is familiar with the prior procedures referenced in the text.

Because many providers choose to couple contact lens exams with routine comprehensive exams, this combined effort should flow seamlessly within the core ocular examination. For this to occur, you should be prepared to conduct tests that can be performed while the patient is wearing their lenses and others that should be done after the patient removes them. In general, tests requiring habitual correction, such as VA, entrance tests, and some functional tests, are more appropriately performed while the patient is wearing lenses. After the lenses are removed, keratometry, refraction, and ocular health assessment can be performed.

For the patient who presents for a comprehensive eye exam and is wearing contact lenses, **Figure 6-1** illustrates a proposed sequence of examination procedures. As stated above, certain circumstances may lead you to deviate from this sequence, though the overall components of the exam will still apply. For instance, if the patient habitually removes their contact lenses for prolonged periods of reading or other near work, you may want to delay near point testing until after the patient removes their lenses.

This chapter begins with a look at the contact lens case history, which is routinely incorporated into the general case history. The contact lens external examination includes procedures to help in the initial fitting of contact lenses. For both soft and GP lenses, inspection and verification, insertion and removal, and fit assessment are considered as part of the external exam. Next, to ensure maximum VA, a close look at contact lens over-refraction procedures will follow. Overall, the order in which these procedures are presented represents a logical sequence to be followed during a contact lens fitting examination.

When considered as a whole, all of the procedures in this chapter help the practitioner evaluate a patient's contact lens performance. By ensuring that a patient's lenses are fitting properly and not producing any adverse effects on the anterior segment, good quality vision and comfort can be assured.

Flow of Contact Lens Examination

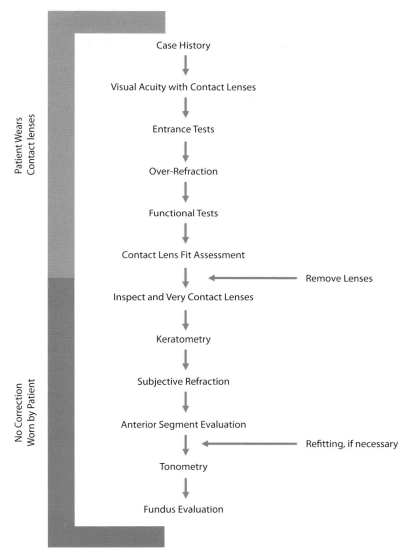

FIGURE 6-1 | Flowchart of the general eye examination incorporating the procedures for contact lens evaluation.

## 6.2 CONTACT LENS CASE HISTORY

### Purpose
Collecting a thorough contact lens history is one of the most important aspects of a contact lens examination. A patient's contact lens history should be thought of as a component of the patient's overall ocular and medical history, as each will influence clinical decision

making during the initial contact lens fitting process and future contact lens management. For a new contact lens wearer, the history questions will gather information that is useful in determining the patient's suitability for contact lens wear as well as in selecting the appropriate contact lens design and care regimen for the patient. For existing or past contact lens wearers, the case history questions will focus on previous contact lens wearing history, compliance and care practices, symptoms and comfort with current or previous lenses. When possible, the examiner should use open-ended inquiries to elicit the most comprehensive response.

## Procedure

*Note:* The questions below are examples of open-ended questions to guide the examiner in collecting a thorough contact lens history.

Gather information on the following:

1. Past and current ocular and medical history, including current medications (see Procedure 1.3)

2. For new contact lens wearers:

   a. "Why are you interested in wearing contact lenses?"

   b. "How often do you plan to wear your contact lenses?"

   c. Gather information regarding patient contact lens wearing demands based on the following:
      - Occupation
      - Hobbies
      - Driving history and demands
      - Social history, including smoking

3. For existing or past contact lens wearer:

   a. Reason for visit.

   b. "When was your last contact lens evaluation?"

   c. "What type of contact lenses do you wear now?"

      i. Based on the patient's answer, categorize the lens type between each of the following:
         - Soft, corneal rigid gas permeable (RGP), scleral RGP, or hybrid
         - Disposable or conventional
         - Spherical, toric, bifocal/multifocal, orthokeratology

   d. Wearing time:

      i. "What is your average wearing time per day?"

      ii. "How often do you wear your lenses (how many days per week)?"

      iii. "Do you wear your lenses as daily wear or extended wear?"
         "If extended wear, how many days in a row do you wear your lenses?"

      iv. "How often do you wear your lenses while sleeping or napping?"

      v. "How many hours have you worn your lenses today?"

   e. Vision and comfort:

      i. "Describe your vision with your contact lenses."

      ii. "Describe your comfort with your contact lenses."
         "Is your comfort consistent or does it decrease throughout the day?"

      iii. "Do you experience redness, irritation, itchiness, pain, discharge, tearing, dryness, or any other symptoms when wearing your lenses?"

 iv. "Do you use any rewetting drops or solutions while wearing your contact lenses?" "If so, which brand and product do you use?"

 v. "Do you have any other concerns regarding your contact lenses?"

f. Care and compliance:

 i. "Describe your current lens care regimen, including the solution brand used for cleaning, disinfection, and storage."

 ii. "Do you rub and rinse your lenses before storage?"

 iii. "Do you replace the cleaning solution in the lens case daily?"

 iv. "Have you used other types of care regimens in the past?"

 v. "Have you had problems using certain lens care products in the past?"

 vi. "How often do you replace your contact lens storage case?"

 vii. "How often do you replace your contact lenses?"

g. Past contact lens history:

 i. "How many years have you worn contact lenses?"

 ii. "Have you worn other types of lenses in the past?
 "Were you successful or unsuccessful with these types of lenses?"
 "Why did you discontinue that type of lens?"

 iii. "Have you had any contact lens–related problems in the past: dry eye, red eye, giant papillary conjunctivitis, infection, or ulcer?"

## Recording

- Record all collected information in the patient's record, including the pertinent negatives.

## 6.3 EXTERNAL EXAMINATION OF A CONTACT LENS PATIENT

### Purpose
The aim of this procedure is to obtain baseline measurements (lid position, palpebral aperture height, corneal diameter, pupil diameter, lid tension, and blink quality) that aid the examiner in selecting initial contact lens parameters, choosing a fitting technique, and assessing the appropriateness of currently prescribed contact lenses. *Note*: It is not necessary to perform the external examination for contact lens wearers as a separate sequence. Some measurements may be obtained in conjunction with other procedures. For example, pupil diameter is obtained during the pupil function assessment (see Procedure 2.15).

### Equipment
- Pupillary distance (PD) ruler with pupil gauge
- Penlight

### Setup
- No specific setup is required

### Procedure
*Lid Position*
1. Instruct the patient to view a distant target without squinting or wide-eyed staring (you may obtain a more reliable measurement if you do not tell the patient what you are measuring).
2. Observe the points at which the upper and lower lids cross the edge of the cornea for each eye.

*Note*: GP contact lens fits are most affected by variations in this measurement; an upper lid that covers part of the superior cornea is complementary to a superior lid attachment fit, whereas a lower lid that covers part of the inferior cornea may call for the use of a smaller lens diameter to minimize lens-lid interactions.

### Palpebral Aperture Height
1. Instruct the patient to view a distant target without squinting or wide-eyed staring.
2. For each eye, place a PD ruler vertically in front of the eye without touching the lashes or eyelids.
3. Measure the maximum vertical aperture (in millimeters) between upper and lower lid margins.

   *Note*: The ideal diameter of both GP and soft lenses depends on this measurement.

### Corneal Diameter or Horizontal Visible Iris Diameter (HVID)
1. Instruct the patient to view a distant target.
2. For each eye, place a PD ruler (or HVID ruler) horizontally in front of the eye as close to the cornea as is safe.  Be sure the ruler is aligned with the widest dimension of the cornea, i.e., the ruler should cover the inferior hemisphere of the cornea.
3. With a straight-on view, measure the corneal diameter from limbus to limbus to the nearest 0.5 mm.

   *Note:* A larger corneal diameter will often require a larger contact lens diameter. Some instruments such as certain corneal topographers can measure iris diameter and often do so diagonally, thereby providing an average measure of vertical and horizontal dimensions. When using such instruments, it may be wise to compare it to a manual measurement to ensure consistency of data.

### Pupil Diameter
1. Adjust the room lighting in preparation to measure pupil diameter under bright, dim, and average lighting conditions.
2. Instruct the patient to view a distant target.
3. For each eye, place a PD ruler horizontally (or a pupil gauge vertically) in front of the eye covering half the pupil.
4. Slide the gauge to match the pupil diameter or take your measurement directly from the PD ruler. In dim illumination, it may be necessary to hold a penlight obliquely from the temporal side to visualize the pupil.

   *Note:* Determining pupil size under dim illumination helps with the selection of an optic zone diameter (OZD) in GP lenses. Generally, the OZD should be 1–2 mm larger than the pupil to minimize nighttime glare. Pupil size is also important when fitting multifocal contact lenses.

### Lid Tension
1. During upper lid eversion of each eye, a subjective assessment of lid tension can be obtained.
2. Setup the patient in a slit lamp and instruct the patient to look down.
3. Grasp the lashes of the upper lid and pull outward.
4. The tension can be rated as tight, normal, or loose.

   *Note*: A tight lid is more likely to pull a contact lens upward or may squeeze it downward, and a loose lid may lead to an inferior position due to reduced pressure on the surface of the lens.

*Blink quality*
1. During a casual conversation with your patient, observe their eyes and note the completeness of the blink and the blink rate.

   *Note*: An incomplete blink can also promote a dry eye when contact lenses are worn.

## Recording
- For lid position, draw and/or describe the lid position.
- For palpebral aperture size, corneal diameter, and pupil diameter, record your measurements.
- For lid tension and blink quality, describe your observations.

## Example
- See **Figure 6-2**.

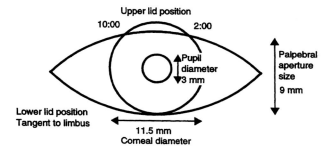

FIGURE 6-2 | Diagram of external measurements: lid position, palpebral aperture size, corneal diameter, and pupil diameter.

- Lid position: upper lid at 10:00 and 2:00; lower lid tangent to limbus
- Palpebral aperture size: 9 mm
- Corneal diameter: 11.5 mm
- Pupil diameter: 3 mm (bright), 4 mm (normal), 6 mm (dim)
- Lid tension: normal
- Blink quality: full, normal blink rate

## Expected Findings
- See **Table 6-1**.

| TABLE 6-1. Expected Findings on the External Examination of a Contact Lens Patient | |
|---|---|
| **MEASUREMENT** | **EXPECTED FINDINGS** |
| Lid position | Upper lid: Crosses superior limbus at 10:00 and 2:00<br>Lower lid: Less than 1 mm from the inferior limbus |
| Palpebral aperture height | 8–11 mm |
| Horizontal visible iris diameter | 10.5–12.5 mm |
| Pupil diameter | 2–8 mm, depending on lighting |
| Lid tension | Moderate with good elasticity |
| Blink quality | Full and complete 10–15 blinks per minute |

## 6.4 INSPECTION AND VERIFICATION OF SOFT CONTACT LENSES

### Purpose

The aim of this procedure is to inspect a soft contact lens for damage and contaminants, and to verify its power. *Note:* Hand hygiene using soap and water should be performed by the examiner before touching contact lenses.

### Equipment

- Lensometer
- Lint-free cloth or tissue
- Lens cleaner and saline
- Biomicroscope or a 10× head loupe
- Rubber-tipped tweezers

### Procedure

*Back Vertex Power*

1. Use a multipurpose contact lens solution to clean the contact lens and then rinse it thoroughly with saline solution.
2. Rotate the spring-loaded lens holder of the lensometer away from the lens stop and clean any ink or debris from the lens stop with a tissue. If available, install a disposable lens stop cover to minimize the risk of contact lens contamination.
3. Place the wet lens on a lint-free cloth or tissue and gently blot excess fluid from the lens surface without allowing the lens to become dehydrated since this will distort lens optics and potentially induce a change in lens power.
4. Center the lens on the lensometer with the concave surface against the stop. Drape the lens evenly so that there are no wrinkles or folds (**see Figure 6-3**).

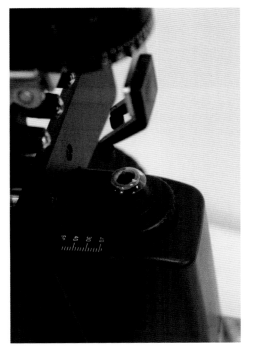

**FIGURE 6-3** | Positioning of a soft contact lens on the lensometer stop for back vertex power measurement.

5. Measure the lens power in the same way as spectacles (see Procedure 3.3). When reading the power, the mires may not be as clear as when measuring a GP lens. If a reasonably clear mire image is not obtained, rinse the lens with saline and repeat.

*Surface Inspection: Films and Spots*

1. Clean the lens surface with a multipurpose contact lens solution and rinse with sterile saline.
2. With the biomicroscope facing a dark background and set to low magnification, create a wide parallelepiped beam with the illumination arm swung out to a 90° angle.
3. While holding the lens with rubber-tipped tweezers, rinse it with sterile saline and shake off any excess fluid.
4. Hold the lens in the path of the light beam (**see Figure 6-4**).

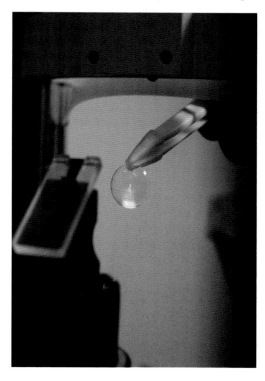

**FIGURE 6-4** | Surface inspection of a soft contact lens using the biomicroscope.

5. Move the lens back and forth until it comes into focus through the oculars of the biomicroscope.
6. Observe any film, hazy regions, or spots on the lens surface. Increase the magnification, if needed.
7. Look for milder deposits on the surface of the lens as it dries.

*Lens Inspection: Tears, Nicks, and Scratches*

1. The patient wears the lens of interest and is setup in the slit lamp so that it is comfortable for both you and the patient (see Procedure 5.2).
2. With the biomicroscope on low magnification, create a wide parallelepiped beam with the illumination arm at a 30° to 40° angle.

3. With the patient looking straight ahead, scan the lens surface for any physical defects.
4. With the patient looking up, inspect the inferior portion of the lens.
5. With the patient looking down, lift the upper lid and inspect the superior portion of the lens.

## Recording
- Document the appearance of any deposits.
- Document any tears, nicks, scratches, or other surface defects you observe.

## Types of Findings
- *Protein film:* Can range from a clear, transparent, thin film (mild deposition) to a semi-opaque, white, hazy film (severe deposition).
- *Lens calculi* (jelly bumps, mulberry spots): Raised, birefringent spots on the anterior lens surface that penetrate the lens matrix; growth rings may be seen under higher magnification.
- *Lipid deposits:* Greasy, shiny, smeary deposits that are displaced by rubbing, and often form a fingerprint pattern that is easily seen under low magnification.
- *Fungi:* Filamentary growths within the lens matrix appearing in a variety of colors: black, gray, brown, orange, pink, or white.
- *Hair spray:* Appears as a glistening, crystalized coating on the lens.

| INSPECTION AND VERIFICATION OF SOFT CONTACT LENSES at a glance | |
|---|---|
| **Parameter** | **Instrument** |
| Back vertex power | Lensometer |
| Lens surface | Biomicroscope |
| Films and spots | |
| Tears, nicks, and scratches | |

## 6.5 APPLICATION (INSERTION) AND REMOVAL OF SOFT CONTACT LENSES

### Purpose
The aim of this procedure is to apply and/or remove a patient's soft contact lenses.

### Indications
There are certain situations when the examiner must be able to apply and remove a patient's soft contact lenses. Since patients that are new contact lens wearers will be unable to perform these tasks independently, the examiner should apply and remove the trial lens during the initial lens fitting and assessment. Patients with poor manual dexterity or those new wearers who are still learning these skills will also have difficulty with these tasks and may need assistance in application and removal.

### Equipment
- Soft contact lens of interest (e.g., trial lens)
- Soft contact lens multipurpose solution
- Saline solution

### Setup
- Prior to handling lenses, the examiner must wash their hands with soap and water, using a soap that does not contain lotions or fragrances. The examiner should dry their hands with a lint-free towel. Do not use alcohol-based hand sanitizer before handling contact lenses.
- Inspect the lens orientation to ensure the lens is not inside out (**see Figure 6-5**).

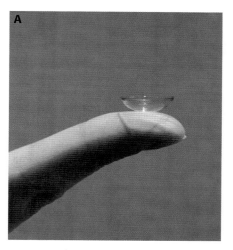

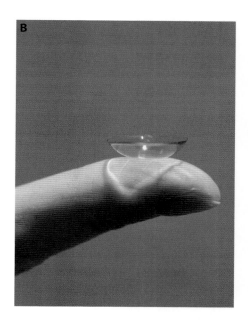

**FIGURE 6-5** | Assessment of lens orientation prior to insertion with lens (A) in proper orientation and (B) "inside out." Look at the very edge of the lens turned up or out.

- Inspect the lens for surface debris, tears, or other surface defects. The examiner may use a multipurpose soft contact lens solution or a saline solution to rinse and remove any debris. It is a good habit to rinse the lens with sterile saline solution even if it is a new lens and appears clean.
- Avoid touching the ocular (concave) surface of the lens once the lens is cleaned and rinsed.
- Dry the finger that will be used to apply the lens. A hydrophilic lens tends to stick to a wet finger more than to the patient's eye.
- For thin or low modulus lenses, it may help to allow the lens to air dry for several seconds on the finger before attempting to apply it.

## Procedure

*Application*

1. Place the lens on the tip of the index finger of your dominant hand.
2. Instruct the patient to look down. Place the index finger or thumb of your nondominant hand at the lid margin of the patient's upper lid. Retract the upper lid and hold it firmly against the upper brow.
3. Instruct the patient to look up. Place the middle or fourth finger of your dominant hand at the lower lid margin and retract the lower lid.
4. Gently apply the lens to the eye in one of three ways:
   a. While the patient is looking up, place the lens on the inferior sclera (**see Figure 6-6A**).
   b. Instruct the patient to look nasally and place the lens on the temporal sclera (**see Figure 6-6B**).
   c. Instruct the patient to look straight ahead and place the lens directly on the cornea (**see Figure 6-6C**).
5. If applying the lens to the inferior or temporal sclera, follow step 5a, otherwise skip to step 6.
   a. While maintaining control of the lids, instruct the patient to slowly look into the lens. This should allow the lens to center on the cornea. If the lens still has not centered, or

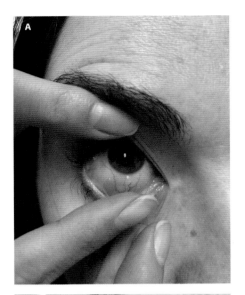

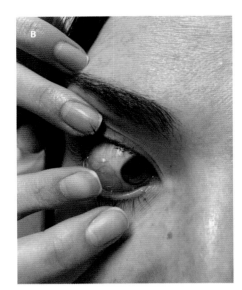

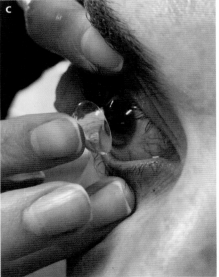

FIGURE 6-6 | Application of soft contact lens onto the (A) inferior sclera, (B) temporal sclera, and (C) straight onto the cornea.

if air bubbles are present under the lens, instruct the patient to look down, to the left, and then to the right. This will settle the lens onto the cornea.

6. Slowly release the lower lid, then the upper lid.

7. You can pat or massage the closed lid to help the lens further settle. You may also have the patient look left, right, up, and down while their eyes are closed.

*Removal*

1. Instruct the patient to look down. Hold the patient's upper lid against the upper brow with your nondominant hand.

2. Instruct the patient to look up. Retract the lower lid with your dominant hand's middle or fourth finger.

3. Place the index finger of your dominant hand on the inferior edge of the lens. Pull the lens down onto the sclera and in one continuous motion, place your thumb and index finger at the 5 and 7 o'clock position of the lens and gently pinch the lens off (**see Figure 6-7**).

4. Alternatively, instruct the patient to look nasally.

   a. Place the index finger of your dominant hand at the temporal edge of the lens and slide it temporally. Continue to slide it temporally until the lens comes out or is bunched up at the lateral canthus (**see Figure 6-8**). Gently pinch the lens off.

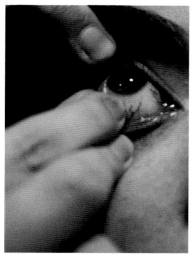

FIGURE 6-7 | Removal of soft contact lens from inferior sclera.

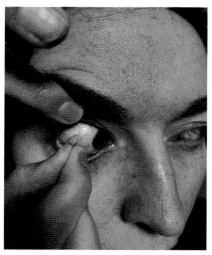

FIGURE 6-8 | Removal of soft contact lens by sliding it temporally, then pinching it off.

## 6.6 FIT ASSESSMENT OF SOFT CONTACT LENSES

### Purpose

The aim of this procedure is to determine whether a soft contact lens is fitting adequately so that vision and comfort are optimized, and contact lens-related anterior segment complications are minimized. A soft contact lens should be assessed for proper centration, full corneal and limbal coverage, and adequate movement. As the lens settles on the eye, it exhibits less and less lens movement. A push-up test is recommended in cases where limited lens movement is demonstrated by the soft lens. The examiner may use their judgment and only perform this test as necessary. In the event of a toric soft contact lens evaluation, rotational orientation and stability should also be assessed.

### Equipment

- Biomicroscope

### Setup

- Adjust the biomicroscope so that it is comfortable for both the patient and the examiner (see Procedure 5.2).
- Set the magnification to 10×.
- Set the illumination arm to approximately 30° from the straight-ahead position on the temporal side. Set the illumination level to medium to high. Open the slit beam to a wide parallelepiped or diffuse illumination.

## Procedure

1. After lens application, allow the lens to settle for 5–10 minutes or until initial reflex tearing has decreased.

2. Instruct the patient to look straight ahead, toward the back of the examination room. Alternatively, you can instruct the patient to look at your right ear.

3. Begin by focusing on the patient's right contact lens.

4. Assess lens centration: move the slit beam from temporal to the nasal lens edge and observe the lens position, both horizontally and vertically. If the vertical lens position is difficult to assess due to a small palpebral aperture, retract the patient's upper and lower eyelids away from the lens to evaluate the lens position. However, be aware that eyelid manipulation can alter lens position.

5. Assess corneal and limbal coverage: practice the same procedure as step 4, however this time observe the lens coverage.

6. Assess lens movement on blink: instruct the patient to blink once and observe the amount of lens movement induced in primary gaze. If you can see the lens edge at the inferior lens position, view the edge at this location. If not, view the lens edge adjacent to the lower lid on both nasal and temporal sides.

7. Assess lens movement on vertical lag: instruct the patient to look upward. Observe the amount of vertical lens movement demonstrated by the lens as the patient looks up. While the patient is looking up, instruct the patient to blink once. Observe the amount of lens movement induced.

8. Assess lens movement on lateral lag: instruct the patient to look straight ahead. Then instruct the patient to look to their right. Observe the amount of lateral lag movement demonstrated by the lens. Instruct the patient to look to their left. Again, observe the amount of lateral lag movement demonstrated by the lens.

9. Perform a push-up test (as needed): while the patient is looking straight ahead, use the patient's lower lid to push up on the inferior edge of the contact lens. Assess the ease or difficulty with which the lens moves upward.

   Steps 10 and 11 should be performed in the event the examiner is assessing a soft toric contact lens. For these assessments, the provider must make two additional observations: rotational orientation and stability. *Note:* Each lens manufacturer and brand will have unique and characteristic toric markings, the examiner should familiarize themselves with the markings of the brand of toric soft contact lens they are evaluating.

10. Assess toric rotational orientation: while the patient is looking in primary gaze, locate the toric lens marking(s) (**see Figure 6-9**).

    a. Grossly estimate the amount of rotation, using the clock hour method, where each clock hour is approximately equal to a 30° rotation.

    b. Alternatively, a more precise way to measure the amount of rotation, in degrees, is to use the slit lamp method. Ensure click stop position, narrow light beam and align with inferior toric marker (if toric marker is horizontally placed, set light beam perpendicular to the horizontal marker), then rotate the beam to align with the toric marker orientation. Read the rotation amount off the slit lamp, indicated in degrees (**see Figure 6-10**).

11. Note the direction of the lens rotation. This can be documented as either a clockwise or counterclockwise rotation. Alternatively, the direction of the lens rotation can be noted as either to the right or left from the examiner's perspective. If the lower lid is covering lens markings inferiorly, gently pull down the lower lid until you are just able to see the

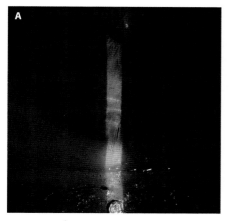 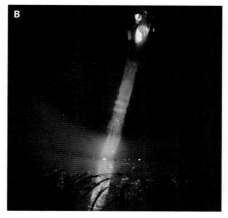

FIGURE 6-9 | (A) Localization of the soft contact lens toric marking. (B) Note the rotation of the slit lamp beam with the rotated marking.

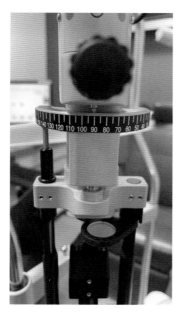

FIGURE 6-10 | Rotation of soft contact lens as measured with a biomicroscope.

markings. Be careful not to pull on the lid excessively because this can cause the lens to rotate. Do not have the patient look up because this can also cause the lens to rotate.

12. Assess rotational stability: instruct the patient to blink once. Observe whether the lens should return to the original position upon each blink.

13. Repeat steps 2 through 12 as needed for the left eye.

## Recording

- Record the lens position, corneal/limbal coverage, blink and lag movement, and push-up movement observed, if needed.
- If you are assessing a toric lens, also record the rotational orientation and stability observed.

## Examples

### Acceptable Soft Lens Fit

- Well-centered, full coverage, and optimal/adequate movement
  - Lens position: horizontally and vertically centered
  - Coverage: full corneal and limbal coverage
  - Blink movement: 0.5 mm in primary gaze, 1.0 mm in up-gaze
  - Lag movement: 1.0 mm in up-gaze and lateral gaze
  - Push-up movement: optimal

### Unacceptable Soft Lens Fit

- Tight-fitting lens:
  - Push-up movement: inadequate, difficult to move
  - Blink movement: less than 0.25 mm in primary and up-gaze
  - Lag movement: less than 0.5 mm in up-gaze and lateral gaze
- Decentration, inadequate coverage, and excessive movement:
  - Lens position and coverage: superior temporal, inadequate coverage inferior nasally
  - Blink movement: 2 mm in primary and up-gaze
  - Lag movement: 3 mm in up-gaze and lateral gaze
  - Push-up movement: easy
- Rotational orientation and stability:
  - Rotational orientation: 5° clockwise
  - Rotational orientation: 25° counterclockwise
  - Rotational orientation: 10° to the right
  - Rotation orientation: >30° to the left
  - Rotational stability: no rotation on blink
  - Rotational stability: rotates 10° on the blink, requires several seconds to return to original position

| SOFT CONTACT LENS FIT ASSESSMENT at a glance | |
|---|---|
| **Fit Characteristics** | **Expected Findings** |
| Lens position | The position of the contact lens relative to the cornea is assessed by observing the amount of lens overlap onto the sclera. The distance between the lens edge and the patient's limbus should be equidistant in all four quadrants (temporal, nasal, superior, and inferior). It is acceptable for the lens to sit slightly decentered, but it must maintain full coverage at all times. |
| Corneal coverage | The lens should extend 1–1.5 mm, overlap, and sit past the limbus in all four quadrants around the entire cornea (temporal, nasal, superior, and inferior). If you note any area of corneal exposure, there is inadequate corneal coverage. |
| Blink movement | The lens should exhibit 0.25–1.0 mm of vertical movement upon blink. |
| Lag movement | The amount by which the lens follows behind any eye excursion should be 0.5–2.0 mm. |
| Push-up movement | The ease with which the lens moves upward when pushed by the lower lid. The lens should move easily and freely when pushed by the lower lid. |
| Rotational orientation | The static position of the lens markings in primary gaze. Not more than 15–20° from intended. |
| Rotational stability | The amount of lens rotation demonstrated by the contact lens when the patient blinks. No rotation on the blink, or slight rotation with rapid return to original position. |

## 6.7 PHOROPTER-BASED OVER-REFRACTION OF SPHERICAL OR TORIC CONTACT LENSES

### Purpose

The aim of this procedure is to determine whether a patient's contact lenses are providing the optimal distance VA using a phoropter.

*Note*: This procedure assumes that the examiner is familiar with refraction procedures presented in Chapter 3. Before proceeding to over-refract your patient, ensure that a satisfactory lens fit is evident.

### Equipment

- Phoropter
- Distance VA chart
- Retinoscope

### Setup

- While the patient is wearing the contact lenses, position the patient behind the phoropter and use a starting point of plano in the phoropter or the net results of static retinoscopy over the contact lenses.

### Procedure

*Spherical Over-Refraction*

1. With the nontested eye occluded, assess the best-corrected VA (BCVA) provided by the current contact lens as it relates to the BCVA achieved in the subjective refraction.
2. Fog the eye with +0.75 D or to 20/40 and obtain monocular Maximum Plus to Maximum Visual Acuity (MPMVA) (see Procedure 3.6).
3. Repeat steps 1 and 2 for the fellow eye.
4. Unocclude both eyes and fog binocularly with +0.75 D or to 20/40.
5. Perform a binocular balance to obtain binocular MPMVA.

*Spherocylindrical Over-Refraction*

The spherocylindrical over-refraction can be performed when a spherical over-refraction alone does not provide adequate VA. This may occur in cases of moderate residual cylinder or with toric contact lenses. If the patient is wearing a toric lens, inspect the lens for rotation and be prepared to use a crossed-cylinder calculator if the resultant axis of the over-refraction is not aligned with the axis as seen on the eye.

1. With the nontested eye occluded, perform a monocular JCC test (see Procedure 3.9).
2. Fog with +0.75 D or to 20/40 and obtain monocular MPMVA.
3. Repeat steps 1 and 2 for the fellow eye.
4. Unocclude both eyes and fog binocularly with +0.75 D or to 20/40.
5. Perform a binocular balance to obtain binocular MPMVA.

### Recording

- Record the over-refraction results in the phoropter and the endpoint VA obtained for each eye and for both eyes.

### Examples

- Spherical over-refraction
  OD: −0.50 sphere, 20/20
  OS: −0.75 sphere, 20/25
  OU: 20/20

- Spherocylindrical over-refraction
  OD: +0.25 −0.75 ×165, 20/20
  OS: +0.50 −1.25 ×045, 20/20
  OU: 20/20

### Expected Findings
- Ideally, the BCVA in contacts will be at least as good as that achieved in the subjective refraction.
- If the contact lens power is appropriate for the patient, the over-refraction should yield a spherical equivalent of plano (with a cylinder component ≤0.50 D).

  *Note:* To ensure your patient is not over-minused, the vertexed spherical equivalent of the subjective refraction should be the same as the spherical equivalent of the final contact lens power, assuming the BCVA is the same.

## 6.8 LOOSE LENS OVER-REFRACTION OF SPHERICAL OR TORIC CONTACT LENSES

### Purpose
The aim of this procedure is to determine whether a patient's contact lenses are providing the optimal distance VA using spectacle trial lenses.

*Note*: This procedure assumes that the examiner is familiar with refraction procedures presented in Chapter 3. Before proceeding to over-refract your patient, ensure that a satisfactory lens fit is evident.

### Equipment
- Loose trial lenses
- Distance VA chart
- Occluder

### Setup
- With the patient in the examination chair, display several lines of a distance VA chart, ensuring the BCVA achieved in the subjective refraction occupies the bottom line.

### Procedure
*Spherical Over-Refraction*
1. With the nontested eye occluded, assess the best VA provided by the current contact lens as it relates to the BCVA achieved in the subjective refraction.
2. Move the lowest line the patient can clearly read to the top of the chart and have the patient focus on that line.
3. Place a +0.50 D trial lens in front of the eye.
    a. If the lens does not blur the top line, or if the line below it becomes clearer, continue to increase the plus power in +0.25 D steps until the patient reports blur. The last lens that did not cause blur is the over-refraction endpoint. At this point, determine the BCVA in contacts relative to that achieved in the subjective refraction.
4. If the +0.50 D trial lens produces blur, place a −0.25 D trial lens in front of the eye.
    a. If the lens causes blur, the letters become smaller or darker, or there is no improvement in VA, the spherical over-refraction endpoint is plano.
    b. If the −0.25 D lens improves clarity, continue to increase the minus power in −0.25 D steps as long as the VA improves by one line for each −0.25 D increase. This is the spherical over-refraction endpoint.

5. Repeat steps 1 through 4 for the fellow eye.

6. Place the respective endpoint lenses in front of the eyes binocularly. To ensure binocular MPMVA, obtain trial lenses with +0.25 D more plus for each eye and place in front of the eyes. If there is no loss in clarity, this is your binocular over-refraction endpoint.

*Spherocylindrical Over-Refraction*

If a spherical over-refraction fails to correct the patient to the same degree as the subjective refraction, a spherocylindrical over-refraction is indicated. In this case, the simplest approach would be to complete a phoropter-based over-refraction as outlined in Procedure 6.7.

### Recording
- Record the over-refraction and the endpoint VA obtained for each eye and for both eyes.

### Examples
- Spherical over-refraction:
  OD: plano, 20/20
  OS: +0.25, 20/20
  OU: 20/20
- Spherocylindrical over-refraction:
  OD: plano −0.50 × 090, 20/20
  OS: +0.25 −0.75 × 180, 20/20
  OU: 20/20

### Expected Findings
- Ideally, the BCVA in contacts will be at least as good as that achieved in the subjective refraction.
- If the contact lens power is appropriate for the patient, the over-refraction should yield a spherical equivalent of plano (with a cylinder component ≤ 0.50 D).
- **Table 6-2** provides tips on using loose lenses for contact lens over-refraction.

*Note:* To ensure your patient is not over-minused, the vertexed spherical equivalent of the subjective refraction should be the same as the spherical equivalent of the final contact lens power, assuming the BCVA is the same.

| TABLE 6-2. Loose Lens Over-Refraction Tips |
| --- |
| • If ±0.50 D does not improve visual acuity, the lens power is optimal. |
| • Binocular MPMVA often results in 0.25 D more plus than monocular MPMVA. |
| • Loose lens over-refraction is quicker and less constrained than with the phoropter. |
| • Loose lens over-refraction is more appropriate for monovision or bifocal contact lenses. |

## 6.9 EVALUATION OF THE MULTIFOCAL CONTACT LENS PATIENT

### Purpose
The aim of this procedure is to measure VA of patients with presbyopia wearing multifocal contact lenses. Multifocal contact lenses are available in a variety of optical designs, each with their own unique features that may affect VA differently. Most lens designs incorporate simultaneous vision optics, which place distance, near, and intermediate powers all within the optic zone. Therefore, optical quality may be somewhat compromised, and VA will not be as clear as with spectacles or single vision contact lenses. It is therefore important to recreate as realistic testing conditions as possible by controlling illumination and working distances.

Even when all testing conditions are optimal, VA at both distance and near may be worse than their BCVA as determined by refraction.

Another multifocal lens design uses translating vision optics, and at the time of this publication, it is available only as a corneal RGP lens. This type of design utilizes vertical movement of the lens to place a single zone in the visual axis, providing clear optics at each viewing distance. Translating lenses are available in bifocal, trifocal, and progressive lens designs. The evaluation of these corneal multifocal RGP lenses requires special considerations that are not covered in this text. Keep in mind, when measuring VA for multifocal contact lenses, VA will usually be better when measured binocularly as compared to monocularly.

## Equipment
- Distance acuity chart
- Near point card

## Setup
- Setup the patient in front of the distance VA chart to measure distance VA. It is best to measure distance VA in moderate room illumination to control pupil size for most daily visual tasks.
- Give the patient a near point card to measure near VA. An auxiliary lamp should be used to provide adequate lighting on the near point card.

## Procedure
*Distance and Near VA*
1. Measure the distance and near VA binocularly (both eyes together) first, then monocularly, using the procedure as outlined in Procedure 2.4.

## Recording
- Record VA at distance for each eye and both eyes together.
- Record VA at near for each eye and both eyes together.
- Specify that VA was assessed with the contact lens correction (cCL).

## Example
- Distance VA cCL: OD 20/25, OS 20/25, OU 20/20
- Near VA cCL: OD 20/30, OS 20/25, OU 20/25

## 6.10 LOOSE LENS OVER-REFRACTION OF MULTIFOCAL CONTACT LENSES

### Purpose
The aim of this procedure is to determine whether a patient's multifocal contact lenses are providing the optimal distance and near VA using spectacle trial lenses.

*Note*: When over-refracting multifocal contact lenses, each manufacturer has its own methods of optimizing VA based on clinical trial data and the specific lens design. Owing to their widespread popularity, this section deals with simultaneous vision multifocal lenses. To ensure the best outcome for your patients, please refer to manufacturer fitting guides for further assistance. Because the success of these lenses depends greatly on a well-centered fit, a thorough fit evaluation should be conducted before any attempt to over-refract the patient is made.

### Equipment
- Distance and near VA charts
- Occluder
- Loose trial lens set

*Note:* Because toric multifocal contact lenses are used much less often than their non-toric counterparts, this section omits the use of toric trial lenses that would be used for a sphero-cylindrical over-refraction.

## Procedure

*Spherical Distance Over-Refraction*

1. Complete a monocular over-refraction using loose spherical trial lenses as outlined in Procedure 6.8.
2. Recheck the over-refraction under binocular conditions. At times, additional plus power can be added to the over-refraction in the binocular state without adverse effects on distance vision.

*Spherical Near Over-Refraction*

1. With the patient in the examination chair, have them hold the near point card at an appropriate working distance.

   *Note:* It is important to be conservative when performing plus power over-refractions at near since patients will often accept increasingly high amounts of plus power to the detriment of distance VA.

2. With both eyes unoccluded, utilize loose trial lenses over the nondominant eye to determine the least plus power that provides an acceptable degree of near VA. See Procedure 3.10 for the ocular dominance check.
3. Have the patient view the distance VA chart with and without the over-refraction lens over the nondominant eye.

   a. If the over-refraction lens does not decrease distance VA, record the near over-refraction lens power and endpoint near VA.

4. If the over-refraction lens decreases distance VA, the patient should be asked if they would prefer to have better vision at distance or near. Record the final near over-refraction lens power and endpoint near VA according to their preferences.

## Recording

- Record the distance and/or near over-refraction and the endpoint VA obtained for each eye and for both eyes together.

## Examples

- Spherical distance over-refraction:
  OD: plano 20/25
  OS: −0.25 sph 20/25
  OU: 20/20
- Spherical near over-refraction:
  OD plano, 20/30
  OS +0.25 sph, 20/20
  OU 20/20

## Expected Findings

- If the contact lens power is appropriate for the patient, the distance and near spherical over-refractions should be plano to ±0.25 D.
- Owing to the simultaneous vision effect of multifocal contact lenses, endpoint VA may be slightly reduced to 20/25 or 20/30 in each eye, but binocular VA should be slightly better than monocular acuity.

## 6.11 EVALUATION OF THE MONOVISION PATIENT

### Purpose

The aim of this procedure is to measure VA and perform an over-refraction to improve vision for patients with presbyopia wearing one contact lens that is prescribed for distance vision and the other to optimize near vision. Thus, the monovision patient will have different acuities at distance and near for each eye.

The provider may use different methods to determine the "dominant eye," or the eye that will be corrected using the distance prescription. The ocular dominance check described in Procedure 3.10 is one method. Another method is the blur tolerance check and is described below. The eye corrected for near receives a lens prescription that is adjusted based on the amount of the patient's spectacle addition power.

The eye corrected with the distance contact lens should have good VA at distance, but comparatively worse VA at near. The eye corrected with the near contact lens should have good VA at near, but comparatively worse VA at distance. VA at both distance and near should be good with both eyes together, though the patient may notice that their vision is not as clear as when wearing spectacles.

### Equipment
- Phoropter or loose trial lens set
- VA chart
- Near point card

### Setup
- Position the patient in front of the distance VA chart to measure distance VA.
- Give the patient a near point card in good illumination to measure near VA.
- Use loose spectacle trial lenses to perform the over-refraction.

### Procedure

*Distance and Near VA*

1. Measure the distance and near VA binocularly (both eyes together) first, then monocularly, using the method as outlined in Procedure 2.4.

*Determining the Dominant Eye*

Ocular Dominance Check

See Procedure 3.10.

Blur Tolerance Check

1. With both eyes optimally corrected for distance, ask the patient to binocularly (both eyes together) view a target line that is one line larger than their BCVA on the VA chart.
2. Alternate holding a single loose trial lens of a power between +1.50 and +2.00 over each eye.
3. Ask the patient: "Which is blurrier: when the additional lens is held over your right eye or over your left eye?"
   a. The eye that the patient picks will be the dominant eye and thus will be corrected using the distance prescription.

*Distance Over-Refraction*

1. Using loose trial lenses, perform a spherical over-refraction at distance for each eye (see Procedure 6.8).
2. With both eyes unoccluded, perform a binocular balance.

3. Fog both eyes with +0.75 D or to 20/40 and obtain binocular MPMVA.
4. Record the spherical over-refraction and endpoint VA for each eye.

*Near Over-Refraction*
1. Have the patient hold the near point card at the appropriate working distance.
2. Keep both eyes open and unoccluded.
3. Using loose trial lenses, place lenses with powers ±0.25 and ±0.50 D over the eye corrected with the near contact lens.
4. Determine the least-plus lens power that provides the best near VA.
5. Have the patient view the distance VA chart with and without the over-refraction lens over the near eye. If the over-refraction lens does not decrease distance VA, record the near over-refraction lens power and endpoint near VA. If the over-refraction lens decreases distance VA, discuss with the patient if they would prefer better vision at distance or near. Record the final near over-refraction lens power and endpoint near VA based on the patient's preference.

## Recording
- Record VA at distance for each eye and both eyes together.
- Record VA at near for each eye and both eyes together.
- Specify that VA was assessed with the contact lens correction (cCL) and which eye is optimally corrected for distance and which is for near.
- Record the distance and/or near over-refraction and the endpoint VA obtained for each eye and for both eyes together.

## Example
- Distance VA cCL: OD 20/20, OS 20/100, OU 20/20 (monovision, OD: distance, OS: near)
  Near VA cCL: OD 20/100, OS 20/20, OU 20/20
  Distance over-refraction:
  OD plano, 20/20
  OS −1.50 sph, 20/20
  Near over-refraction:
  OS +0.25 sphere, OU 20/20

## Expected Findings
- The distance eye should have a distance over-refraction within +0.25 D of plano.
- The near eye should have a distance over-refraction that is equal to the amount of add power the lens is providing, but in minus power. For example, if the over-refraction is −1.50 D, the lens is giving the patient a +1.50 add.
- The near eye should have a near over-refraction that is within ±0.25 D of plano.

## 6.12 INSPECTION AND VERIFICATION OF CORNEAL AND SCLERAL GAS PERMEABLE CONTACT LENSES

### Purpose
The aim of this procedure is to determine the overall condition of a lens and to measure certain parameters of a patient's habitual lens(es), or to confirm that a new lens was made to specifications.

*Note:* Hand hygiene using soap and water should be performed by the examiner before touching contact lenses.

*Note*: Inspection and verification of GP contact lenses calls for the use of a variety of instruments designed to evaluate one or more parameters. Each instrument referred to herein is considered a representative option and is not implied to be the only device that can be used for the described purpose. This section is organized by each parameter of interest.

## Equipment
- Sterile saline solution
- Daily contact lens cleaner
- Lint-free cloth or tissues
- V-channel gauge
- Handheld magnifier (7× to 10×)
- Center thickness gauge or radiusgauge
- Biomicroscope
- Fluorescein strips (*optional*)

## Procedure

*Lens Diameter*

1. Use a multipurpose contact lens solution to clean the contact lens and then rinse it thoroughly with saline solution.
2. Blot the lens dry with a soft, lint-free cloth or tissue prior to measuring the lens diameter.
3. Place the lens concave side down into the wide end of the V-channel gauge.
4. With the narrow end of the gauge tilted downward, the lens will slide down the channel at which point a gentle tap on the gauge will cause it to firmly settle between the edges of the channel without the need to force it further down the channel.
5. Take the reading from the center of the lens, or at the point of touch with the edges of the channel (**see Figure 6-11**).

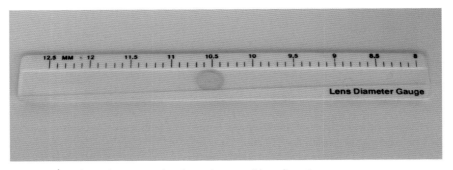

**FIGURE 6-11** │ V-channel gauge used to determine overall lens diameter.

*Optic Zone Diameter (OZD)*

1. Use a multipurpose contact lens solution to clean the contact lens and then rinse it thoroughly with saline solution.
2. Blot the lens dry with a soft, lint-free cloth or tissue prior to measuring the lens diameter and OZD.
3. Place the clean, dry lens with its concave side down on the distal end of the handheld magnifier.
4. Hold one edge of the lens gently against the magnifier with your index finger.

5. Hold the magnifier up to a light source and view the lens relative to the mires scale as seen through the magnifier (**see Figure 6-12**).

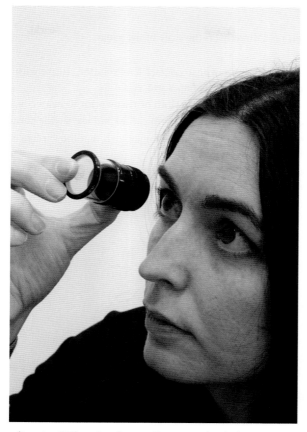

**FIGURE 6-12** | Lens diameter, OZD, and surface quality assessed with the measuring magnifier.

6. Move the lens with your index finger so that one edge is at the zero position and the lens is centered over the scale. While the lens is in this position, note the position of the opposite lens edge and read the overall lens diameter measurement directly off the scale.

7. Move the lens laterally so that one edge of the optic zone is aligned at the zero mark.

8. Note the position of the opposite edge of the optic zone and read the measurement directly off the scale.

   *Note*: If you find it difficult to see the edge of the optic zone, the magnifier can be rocked back and forth at the edge of a light source to obtain a better perspective. There is usually a change in the shadowing of the lens at the edge of each zone.

*Center Thickness*

1. If the center thickness gauge is not set to zero and requires a small adjustment, reset the gauge to zero by turning the dial face.

2. For a large adjustment, reset the gauge to zero by loosening the screw at the bottom of the center thickness gauge, resetting, and retightening.

3. Upon pressing the lever to open the center thickness gauge, hold the contact lens between the pins and then slowly release the lever so that the lens is gently braced between the pins.

4. The thickness is read directly off the scale of the gauge.

*Surface Quality*

1. Clean the lens with a multipurpose contact lens solution. Rinse with saline solution to remove any loose debris from the lens surface.

2. Blot the lens dry with a soft, lint-free cloth or tissue prior to inspecting the lens surface.

3. If using a biomicroscope, set to low magnification and use a wide parallelepiped beam.

4. Hold the lens between thumb and index finger such that the surface is facing the objective lens of the biomicroscope.

5. Bring the lens surface into focus by moving the lens back and forth, or by focusing the instrument (**see Figure 6-13**).

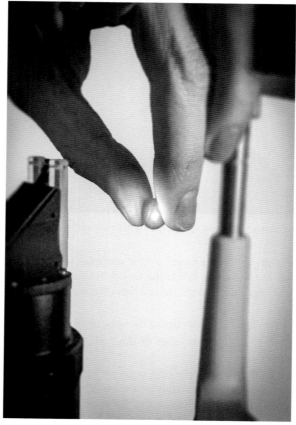

**FIGURE 6-13** | Gas permeable contact lens surface inspection using the biomicroscope.

6. Inspect the lens surface at low and medium magnification.

7. If using the measuring magnifier, place the lens on the end of the magnifier. Look through the ocular toward a light source.

8. Carefully look for films, spots, scratches, or chips.

*Surface Wettability*

1. Unlike the previous parameters, surface wettability is assessed with the contact lens on the eye. Fluorescein may be instilled to assess tear breakup time over the lens surface.

2. Adjust the biomicroscope so that it is comfortable for the examiner and the patient (see Procedure 5.2).

3. Set the magnification to the lowest setting (6× or 10×).

4. Set the illumination to a medium parallelepiped at low to moderate intensity.

5. If this assessment is to be performed immediately after lens insertion, wait 15 minutes to allow for lens stabilization.

6. Setup the slit lamp to create specular reflection off the anterior contact lens surface (see Procedure 5.4).

7. Instruct the patient to blink.

8. Observe the tear film on the front surface of the contact lens.

9. Assess the tear breakup time over the contact lens surface. This is the lens drying time.

## Recording

- Record the lens diameter and OZD to the nearest 0.1 mm.
- If the surface is clean with no deposits, cracks, or chips, record the surface as "clean."
- If deposits, cracks, or chips are present on the lens surface, draw and describe your findings.
- Draw and describe areas of rapid tear breakup or nonwetting.

## Examples

- *Protein film:* Can range from a clear, transparent, thin film (mild deposition) to a semi-opaque, white, hazy film (severe deposition).
- *Lipid deposits:* Greasy, shiny, smeary deposits that change by rubbing. Often seen in a fingerprint pattern, they are easily seen under low magnification.
- *Cracking and crazing:* Small lattice-type cracked appearance to lens surface. Can be cracks in a protein film or the lens surface itself.
- Areas of rapid tear disruption indicate poor wettability due to deposits, polish residues, or damaged lens surface.

| INSPECTION AND VERIFICATION OF GAS PERMEABLE CONTACT LENSES at a glance | |
|---|---|
| **Parameter** | **Instrument** |
| Lens diameter | V-channel gauge or hand-held magnifier (7× to 10×) |
| Optic zone diameter | Hand-held magnifier (7× to 10×) |
| Center thickness | Center thickness gauge or radiusgauge |
| Surface and edge quality | Biomicroscope or hand-held magnifier (7× to 10×) |
| Surface wettability | Biomicroscope or hand-held magnifier (7× to 10×) |
| Base curve radius | Radiuscope, radiusgauge, or Lensco-meter + keratometer |
| Back vertex power | Lensometer |
| Optical quality | Lensometer |

## 6.13 BASE CURVE (BC) RADIUS MEASUREMENT

### Purpose
The aim of this procedure is to determine or verify the BC radius of a GP contact lens with any one of several instruments.

### Equipment
- Radiuscope or radiusgauge (**see Figure 6-14**)
- Keratometer with Lensco-meter attachment

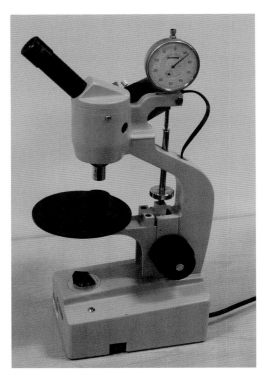

**FIGURE 6-14** | The radiuscope.

### Setup
- Use a multipurpose contact lens solution to clean the contact lens and then rinse it thoroughly with saline solution.
- Blot the lens dry with a soft, lint-free cloth or tissue prior to measuring the BC.

### Procedure
*Radiuscope or Radiusgauge*
The radiuscope has an internal measurement scale whereas the radiusgauge has an external dial where the measurement is read. Aside from this difference, the instruments are used in the same manner.
1. Place a drop of saline in the depression on the concave lens holder. Place the contact lens in the depression with the concave surface facing upward so that this surface remains dry.
2. Place the lens holder onto the support stage of the instrument and ensure that it is seated level in the stage.

3. Set the illumination control to 50%, or to a level that provides a reasonably bright image when you look into the oculars.

4. Check the aperture selector of the illuminator to be certain that the large aperture is in place.

5. Observe the green light coming from the objective and move the stage until the green beam appears to be centered on the contact lens.

6. Completely raise the objective of the instrument using the coarse adjustment knob.

7. For the radiuscope, look into the eye piece and bring the scale on the right side of the field of view into sharp focus using the scale focusing knob.

8. Lower the objective slowly using the coarse adjustment knob, until you see light come into focus on a spoked mire. Move the stage horizontally and vertically until the mires is centered in the field of view (**see Figure 6-15**).

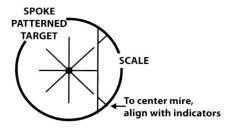

FIGURE 6-15 | Spoke-patterned target centered in the field of view of the radiuscope.

9. Continue to lower the objective. At one point, the filament of the lamp will come into focus. Disregard this image and continue lowering the objective with the coarse adjustment knob.

10. The spoke-patterned target will appear again. Bring the image of the target into sharp focus using the fine adjustment knob.

11. For the radiuscope, use the index adjustment knob to move the index line to zero. You may not be able to move the index line to zero. In this case, set the index line to the nearest whole number. For the radiusgauge, use the silver knob to adjust the dial until it reads zero.

12. Raise the objective until the original spoke pattern comes back into focus. Bring the image of the target into the sharpest focus possible using the fine adjustment knob.

*Lensco-meter*

1. Mount the Lensco-meter holder to the headrest of the keratometer in a manner that the end of the holder is roughly where a patient's eye would be during keratometry.

2. Select the steel ball with a depression on one end and a knob on the other. Add a small drop of a viscous gel or ointment into the depression followed by the lens.

3. Place the ball and lens assembly onto the end of the magnetized holder. Position the steel ball so that the concave surface of the contact lens is directly facing the center of the keratometer.

4. Use the keratometer to measure the horizontal and vertical curvatures as you would when doing conventional keratometry (see Procedure 3.16).

## Recording

*Radiuscope or Radiusgauge*

• For the radiuscope, if the original index line setting was zero, read the radius of curvature directly from the scale at the position of the index line. If the index line was set at +1, that must be added to the scale reading. For example, if the scale reads 6.54 mm and the index line was originally set at +1, the actual BC radius of the contact lens is 7.54 mm.

- Each number on the scale represents 1 mm. The scale is divided into 0.10-mm increments, indicated by the longer lines. The shortest lines represent 0.02-mm increments. Interpolation is required to read 0.01-mm increments (**see Figure 6-16**).

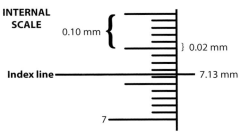

**FIGURE 6-16** │ Example of radiuscope reading. Interpolation is required to obtain the measurement of 7.13 mm.

- For the radiusgauge, read the millimeters from the small dial just inferior to the center of the gauge. If the needle is between two numbers, use the smaller of the two. Then, read the hundredths of a millimeter from the large dial. For example, if the small dial has the needle between 7 and 8, and the large dial has the needle at 40, the reading is 7.40 mm.
- Record the BC radius in millimeters to the nearest 0.01 mm.

*Lenscometer*
- Convert the dioptric readings to radius of curvature in millimeters using a conversion chart, or by dividing the dioptric value obtained into 337.5.
- Add a 0.03-mm correction factor for concave surfaces to your result to obtain the BC radius measurement, e.g., $7.54 + 0.03 = 7.57$.
- Record the BC radius in millimeters to the nearest 0.01 mm.

### Examples
- Base curve RGP BC OD 7.85, OS 8.10

## 6.14 BACK VERTEX POWER AND OPTICAL QUALITY

### Purpose
The aim of this procedure is to evaluate the optical quality of a GP contact lens and to verify its power.

### Equipment
- Lensometer

### Setup
- Use a multipurpose contact lens solution to clean the contact lens and then rinse it thoroughly with saline solution.
- Blot the lens dry with a soft, lint-free cloth or tissue prior to measuring the back-vertex power.

### Procedure
1. Rotate the spring-loaded lens holder of the lensometer away from the lens stop. Clean any ink or debris from the lens stop with a tissue. Turn on the lensometer.

2. Holding the contact lens by the edges, place the back (concave) surface of the lens against the lensometer stop. Make sure that the lens is centered (**see Figure 6-17**). Do not apply excessive pressure to the lens as it may warp and give you a falsely toric power.

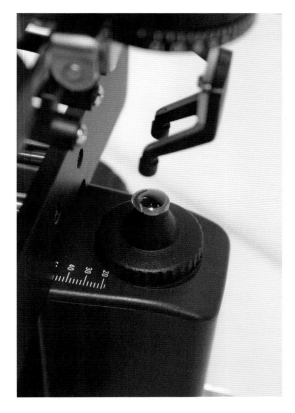

FIGURE 6-17 | Gas permeable contact lens positioned on the lensometer stop for back vertex power measurement.

3. Take a measurement as if you were measuring a pair of spectacles (see Procedure 3.3). Note the spherical power, amount of prism, and any toricity. Toricity in a presumed spherical lens can indicate warpage or distorted optics, or it can indicate that you are squeezing the lens too much while you are holding it in place.

4. Observe the sharpness of the mires. A cloudy, distorted, or double mire image indicates optical distortion.

### Recording
• Record the back-vertex power in diopters to the nearest 0.12 D.

### Examples
• RGP Power: OD + 2.50, OS + 3.00.

## 6.15 APPLICATION (INSERTION), REMOVAL, AND RECENTERING OF COR-NEAL GAS PERMEABLE CONTACT LENSES

### Purpose
The aim of this procedure is to apply and/or remove a patient's corneal RGP contact lens, and to recenter a lens onto the cornea when it has become dislodged.

## Indications

There are certain situations when the clinician must be able to apply and remove a patient's corneal RGP contact lens. Since patients that are new contact lens wearers will be unable to perform these tasks independently, the clinician should apply and remove the lens during the initial lens assessment. Patients with poor manual dexterity or those new wearers who are still learning these skills will also have difficulty with these tasks and may need assistance in application and removal.

## Equipment

- GP contact lens cleaning and wetting/conditioning solution
- Preservative-free artificial tears
- Small-suction RGP contact lens removal device *(optional)*

## Setup

- Prior to handling lenses, wash your hands with water and a soap that does not contain lotions or fragrances. Dry your hands with a lint-free towel. Do not use alcohol-based hand sanitizer before handling contact lenses.
- If using a trial lens from a diagnostic fitting set that was stored dry, clean the lens surface with a multipurpose GP contact lens solution. Rinse with saline solution to remove any surface debris. Condition the lens surface by rubbing a few drops of wetting solution onto the lens. This will promote on-eye wetting.

## Procedure

*Application*

1. Place the lens on the tip of your index or middle finger.
2. Put 1–2 drops of preservative-free cushioning solution, such as preservative-free artificial tears, into the lens bowl prior to application.
3. Direct the patient's gaze upward. Firmly grasp and retract the patient's lower eyelid with the middle or fourth finger of the hand holding the contact lens. Grasp the lid as close to the lid margin as possible.
4. Direct the patient's gaze downward. Retract the patient's upper lid with the thumb or index finger of the opposite hand.
5. Move the contact lens close to the patient's eye. Instruct the patient to look straight ahead, and at the same instant, gently but quickly apply the lens to the central cornea (**see Figure 6-18**).

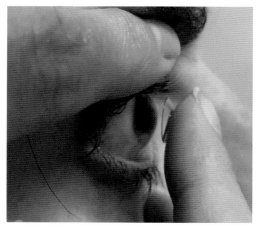

**FIGURE 6-18** | Insertion of a gas permeable contact lens.

6. When the lens appears stable on the central cornea, slowly release the lower lid and then slowly release the upper lid. The lens should maintain centration on the cornea.

   *Note:* An inexperienced wearer may be bothered by lens edge awareness. If so, have them close their eyes or look downward. This will temporarily relieve some of the discomfort.

### Removal

There are several methods to remove a corneal GP lens. Two of these methods are outlined below. The second method outlined requires the utilization of a suction removal device.

1. Direct the patient's fixation straight ahead toward the VA chart or some other distant target.

2. Place the tips of your index fingers or thumbs at the patient's lid margins at the 12:00 and 6:00 o'clock lens positions. Retract both upper and lower eyelids until the lid margins are just outside the lens edge. Be sure not to allow either lid to evert or the lens edge will slip under the lid.

3. Gently press the lids against the globe. Move the lids toward each other to scissor the lens until one edge pops up from the corneal surface. Continue to move the lids toward each other until the lens is removed (**see Figure 6-19**).

4. Instruct the patient to close their eyes. The lens will often stay on the eyelashes where it can be easily retrieved.

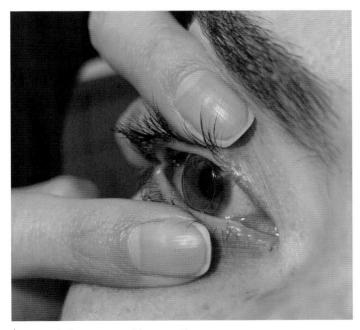

**FIGURE 6-19** | Removal of a gas permeable contact lens.

### Removal (With a Small Suction Removal Device):

1. Hold the removal device in your dominant hand using the thumb and index finger.

2. Place a drop of preservative-free fluid on the removal device.

3. Instruct the patient to look down. Place the index finger or thumb of your nondominant hand at the lid margin of the patient's upper lid. Retract the upper lid and hold it firmly against the upper brow.

4. Instruct the patient to look up. Place the middle or fourth finger of the dominant hand at the lower lid margin and retract the lower lid.

5. Place the removal tool on the lower one-third of the RGP lens.

6. Gently press up and pull the plunger away from the cornea and the lens should suction to the removal device (**see Figure 6-20**).

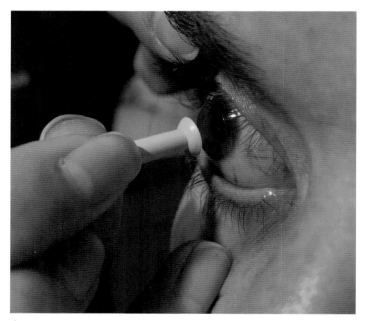

**FIGURE 6-20** | Removal of a gas permeable contact lens with suction device.

*Recentering*

1. Locate the lens on the eye. You may have to direct the patient's gaze and pull the lids away from the eye to do this.

2. Instruct the patient to look in the direction opposite to where the lens is located.

3. With two index fingers placed at the lid margins, use the lids to gently guide the lens toward the cornea (**see Figure 6-21**). Never directly touch the lens itself with your fingers.

4. When the lens is near the limbus and control of the lens is assumed, have the patient slowly look toward the lens. The lens should recenter onto the cornea.

   *Note:* If the lens has suctioned onto the eye, use the eyelid to break the suction by pressing on the sclera just outside the lens edge. Alternatively, the lens can be removed via the removal device, which can be placed on the decentered lens and then gently pulled off.

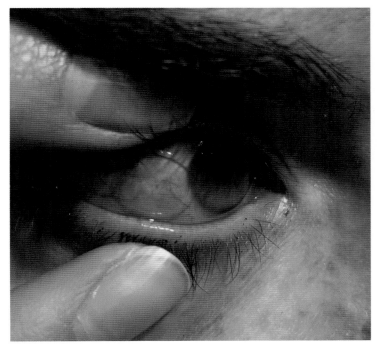

**FIGURE 6-21** | Recentering a gas permeable contact lens.

## 6.16 FIT ASSESSMENT OF CORNEAL GAS PERMEABLE CONTACT LENSES

### Purpose
The aim of this procedure is to determine whether a corneal RGP contact lens is fitting adequately so that vision and comfort are optimized, and contact lens-related anterior segment complications are minimized. A corneal RGP lens evaluation requires assessment of the fitting relationship between the lens and the cornea as well as the lens and the eyelids. A thorough lens evaluation will include assessment with the eyelids in normal position and with eyelids held apart. A fluorescein pattern evaluation is used to assess the cornea to lens relationship. Evaluating both types of fitting relationships will be crucial to the wearer's vision, comfort, and ocular surface health.

### Equipment
- Biomicroscope
- Yellow filter (Wratten #12 or #15); although not necessary, the yellow filter enhances the quality of the fluorescein pattern (**see Figure 6-22**)
- Fluorescein strips
- Sterile saline solution

### Setup
- Adjust the biomicroscope so that it is comfortable for both the patient and the examiner. The patient should be wearing the contact lens(es) to be assessed.
- Set the magnification to the lowest setting (6× or 10×).
- Set the light to the cobalt blue filter.

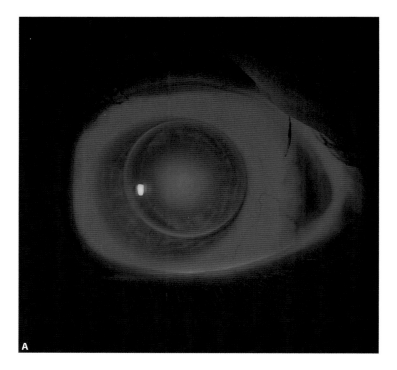

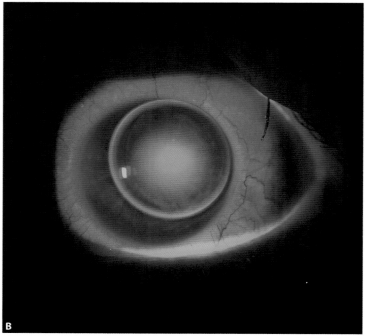

**FIGURE 6-22** | Gas permeable contact lens fit assessment using the biomicroscope: (A) without a Wratten filter and (B) with a Wratten filter to enhance fluorescence.

- Set the illumination arm to approximately 30° from the straight-ahead position on the temporal side.
- Set the illumination level to medium to high and open the slit beam fully.
- Place the yellow filter over the objective end of the biomicroscope. Do not place it over the cobalt blue light source.

## Procedure

1. Wet a fluorescein strip with a drop of sterile saline solution. Shake off the excess saline.
2. Instill a small amount of fluorescein into the inferior cul-de-sac or onto the superior bulbar conjunctiva of both eyes. Have the patient fully blink two to three times to pump the fluorescein underneath the contact lens. The patient should be instructed to blink normally thereafter.
3. Instruct the patient to look straight ahead or toward the back of the examination room. Alternatively, you can instruct the patient to look at your right ear.
4. Begin by focusing on the patient's right contact lens.
5. Observe the eyelid and lens interaction in between blinks.
6. Assess lens centration:  observe horizontal and vertical lens position on the cornea.
7. Assess lens movement: ask the patient to blink and observe dynamic aspects of the fit.
   a. Assess movement on blink
   b. Assess stability on blink
8. Assess and note the fluorescein pattern. This should be viewed first with the eyelids positioned normally. If the lens is decentered, the examiner should manually center the lens on the cornea to assess the central fitting relationship. The patient's eyelids may be used to manipulate the lens position or to pump fluorescein under the lens, as needed.
9. Fluorescein pattern should be evaluated systematically by assessing the amount of fluorescein present in three regions or zones of the lens: apical, midperipheral, and peripheral.
10. Repeat steps 5 through 9 for the left eye.

## Recording

- Record the lens position, blink movement, stability, and fluorescein pattern observed for each eye.

## Examples

- Acceptable fit (**see Figure 6-23**)
  - Eyelid and lens interaction: lid attachment
  - Lens position: central
  - Blink movement: good—approximately 2 mm
  - Stability: good—remains central
  - Fluorescein pattern: central alignment, midperipheral touch, moderate peripheral clearance
- Unacceptably steep fit (**see Figure 6-24**)
  - Lens position: inferior-nasal
  - Blink movement: poor—approximately 1 mm
  - Stability: poor—drops between blinks
  - Fluorescein pattern: excessive central clearance, midperipheral bearing, and minimal peripheral clearance

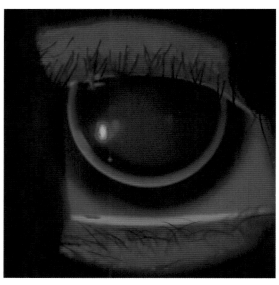

**FIGURE 6-23** | Acceptable gas permeable contact lens fit with superior central position.

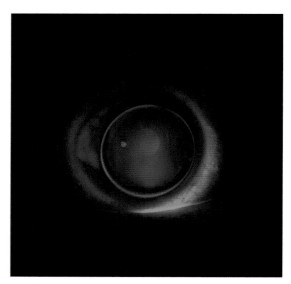

**FIGURE 6-24** | Unacceptably steep gas permeable contact lens fit.

- Unacceptably flat fit (**see Figure 6-25**)
  - Lens position: inferior-temporal, crossing the limbus
  - Blink movement: excessive—traverses past limbus
  - Stability: poor—drops between blinks
  - Fluorescein pattern: central touch, midperipheral clearance, and wide band of peripheral clearance

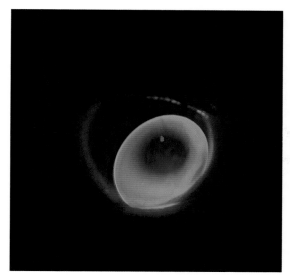

**FIGURE 6-25** │ Unacceptably flat gas permeable contact lens fit.

| GAS PERMEABLE CONTACT LENS FIT ASSESSMENT at a glance | |
|---|---|
| **Fit Characteristics** | **Expected Findings** |
| Eyelid and lens interaction | The eyelid-lens interaction is observed during each blink. The lens may interact with the eyelids in one of following ways:<br>• Lid attachment: The superior edge of the lens is tucked underneath the upper eyelid.<br>• Interpalpebral: The lens is centered over the pupil and the lens is fully resting on the cornea. It is sitting between the upper and lower eyelids.<br>• Lower lid: The lens is resting on the lower lid margin. |
| Lens position | Corneal location where the lens settles after the blink is expected to be central to superior-central |
| Movement on blink | The amount of vertical excursion the lens makes across the cornea after the blink is expected to be between 1.5 and 2 mm (vertically). |
| Stability | The lens is expected to remain stable upon each blink and promptly return to the same position upon blink |
| Fluorescein pattern | The amount of fluorescein, and therefore tears, underneath the lens should be evaluated in the apical/central, midperipheral, and peripheral zones of the lens. Darker areas indicate touch or bearing, while greenish-yellow areas indicate clearance or pooling of tears. Areas of alignment between the contact lens back surface and the cornea appear an even greenish-black. The expected fluorescein pattern is central alignment to minimal clearance, midperipheral alignment, and moderate peripheral clearance. |

## 6.17 FIT AND ASSESSMENT OF ORTHOKERATOLOGY LENSES

### Purpose

The aim of this procedure is to determine whether an orthokeratology contact lens is fitting adequately so that vision and comfort are optimized, and contact lens-related anterior segment complications are minimized. Orthokeratology lenses are corneal RGP lenses with a reverse geometry lens design. Modern orthokeratology lenses are worn overnight to reshape the corneal curvature for refractive correction upon lens removal. Contrary to corneal GP fit assessments where eyelids play a major role in lens function, orthokeratology lenses are best assessed without eyelid interaction. A fluorescein pattern evaluation is used to assess the cornea to lens relationship. Since the lenses are primarily worn in a closed-eye state, assessment of an orthokeratology lens in an open-eye state should always be accompanied by a corneal topography scan for a comprehensive performance evaluation of an orthokeratology lens (see Procedure 9.3).

### Equipment

- Biomicroscope
- Yellow filter (Wratten #12 or #15); although not necessary, the yellow filter enhances the quality of the fluorescein pattern
- Fluorescein strips and sterile saline solution

### Setup

- Adjust the biomicroscope so that it is comfortable for the patient and examiner.
- Set the magnification to 10×, the illumination level to medium to high, and the slit beam to diffuse illumination.
- Set the light to the cobalt blue filter.
- Set the illumination arm to approximately 30° from the straight-ahead position on the temporal side.

  *Note:* For application and removal instructions, see Procedure 6.15.

### Procedure

1. Wet a fluorescein strip with a drop of sterile saline solution. Shake off the excess saline.
2. Instill a small amount of fluorescein into the inferior cul-de-sac or onto the superior bulbar conjunctiva of both eyes. Have the patient fully blink two to three times to pump the fluorescein underneath the contact lens. The patient should be instructed to blink normally thereafter.
3. Instruct the patient to look straight ahead or toward the back of the examination room. Alternatively, you can instruct the patient to look at your right ear.
4. Begin by focusing on the patient's right contact lens.
5. Assess centration, observe horizontal and vertical lens position on the cornea. Observe centration with eyelids held apart to predict lens position in a closed-eye state without the influence of eyelid interaction.
6. Assess lens movement: ask the patient to blink and observe lens movement upon blink.

   a. Assess movement on blink.

   b. Assess stability on each blink.

7. Observe and note the fluorescein pattern. This should be observed without eyelid interaction, therefore carefully hold the eyelids apart to observe the fluorescein pattern. If the lens is decentered, the examiner should manually center the lens on the cornea to assess the central fitting relationship. The patient's eyelids may also be used to manipulate the lens position or to pump fluorescein under the lens, as needed.

a. The fluorescein pattern should be evaluated systematically by assessing the amount of fluorescein present in three regions or zones of the lens: apical, midperipheral, and peripheral. For fluorescein pattern descriptions, see Procedure 6.16.

**8.** Repeat steps 5 through 7 for the left eye.

### Recording

- Record the lens position, blink movement, stability, and fluorescein pattern observed for each eye.

### Examples

- Acceptable fit (**see Figure 6-26**)

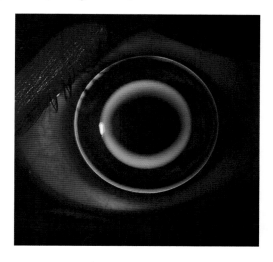

**FIGURE 6-26** | Acceptable orthokeratology fit.

- Lens position: central
- Blink movement: good—approximately 1 mm
- Stability: good—remains central and returns to position upon blink
- Fluorescein pattern: bull's eye pattern, central touch, paracentral pooling, midperipheral touch, low peripheral clearance

| ORTHOKERATOLOGY CONTACT LENS FIT ASSESSMENT at a glance ||
| --- | --- |
| **Fit Characteristics** | **Expected Findings** |
| Lens position | Corneal location where the lens settles after the blink is expected to be central. |
| Movement on blink | The amount of vertical excursion the lens makes across the cornea after the blink is expected to be approximately 1.0 mm (vertically). |
| Stability | The lens is expected to remain stable upon each blink and promptly return to the same position upon blink. |
| Fluorescein pattern | The amount of fluorescein, and therefore tears, underneath the lens should be evaluated in the central, midperipheral, and peripheral zones of the lens. Darker areas indicate touch or bearing, while greenish-yellow areas indicate clearance or pooling of tears. Areas of alignment between the contact lens back surface and the cornea appear an even greenish black.<br>The expected fluorescein pattern should be a characteristic "bulls-eye" pattern with apical touch or light alignment, paracentral ring of fluorescein pooling, wide band of midperipheral touch/bearing, and low peripheral clearance. |

## 6.18 APPLICATION (INSERTION) AND REMOVAL OF SCLERAL CONTACT LENSES

### Purpose
The aim of this procedure is to apply and/or remove a patient's scleral GP contact lenses.

### Indications
There are certain situations when the examiner must be able to apply and remove a patient's scleral contact lenses. Since patients that are new scleral contact lens wearers will be unable to perform these tasks independently, the examiner should apply and remove the trial lens during the initial lens assessment. Patients with poor manual dexterity or new wearers who are still learning these skills will also have difficulty with these tasks and may need assistance in application and removal.

### Equipment
- GP contact lens daily cleaner
- Preservative-free saline solution
- Large suction cup device for contact lens application
- Small suction cup device for contact lens removal

### Setup
- Prior to handling lenses, wash hands with water and a soap that does not contain lotions or fragrances. Dry hands with a lint-free towel. Do not use alcohol-based hand sanitizer before handling contact lenses.
- Inspect the lens for surface debris, cracks, or other surface defects.
- If using a trial lens from a diagnostic fitting set that was stored dry, clean the lens surface with a multipurpose GP contact lens solution. Rinse with saline solution to remove any surface debris. Condition the lens surface by rubbing a few drops of wetting solution onto the lens. This will promote on-eye wetting.
- Avoid touching the ocular (concave) surface of the lens once it has been cleaned and rinsed.
- Give the patient a towel or several paper towels to place on the counter or on their lap to catch the saline solution that will spill out from the lens upon scleral lens application.

### Procedure
*Application*
1. Hold the suction cup device with your dominant hand.
2. Place the convex surface of the lens on the large suction device. Center the lens on the device. The examiner may choose to suction the lens on the device for better stability during the application process. If suction will be used, a gentle squeeze of the device will suction the scleral lens to the device.
3. Fill the scleral lens with sterile preservative-free saline solution until the lens is completely full.
4. If desired, a fluorescein strip can be dipped into the fluid of the scleral lens bowl. This technique will instill fluorescein dye into the lens to allow the examiner to more easily visualize the post-lens tear layer (**see Figure 6-27**).
5. Instruct the patient to bring their head down so that their face is parallel to the floor. Instruct the patient to tuck their chin against their chest and give them a target on the floor to view.

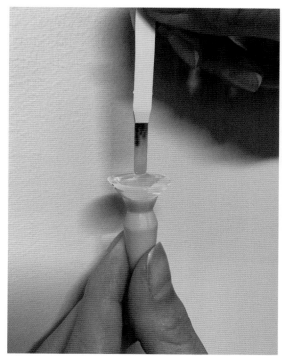

**FIGURE 6-27** | Scleral lens with fluorescein for fit assessment.

6. Instruct the patient to retract their lower lid away from the globe and hold it pressed against the inferior orbital bone. If the patient is unable to do so, use your middle or ring finger of the hand holding the suction device to hold the lower lid.

7. Instruct the patient to look down. Place the index finger or thumb of your nondominant hand at the lid margin of the patient's upper lid. Retract the upper lid and hold it firmly against the upper brow.

8. While the patient is looking down, place the lens directly on the center of the cornea (**see Figure 6-28**). Slightly push the lens upward until the lens is against the eye, but do not apply excessive force.

9. If suctioned to stabilize the lens, gently squeeze the plunger to relieve the suction and remove the suction device. Excess saline solution will spill out from the lens as it settles on the eye.

10. Instruct the patient to blink. They can then lift their head to an upright position and look straight ahead.

*Removal*

1. Place the patient's head in an upright position with their chin pointed slightly upwards. Instruct the patient to look down. Hold the patient's upper lid against the upper brow with your nondominant hand.

2. Place the small suction device (without the air hole) toward the top edge of the scleral lens (**see Figure 6-29**). Place it as close to the edge as possible while still maintaining good suction on the lens. Do not place the device in the center of the lens.

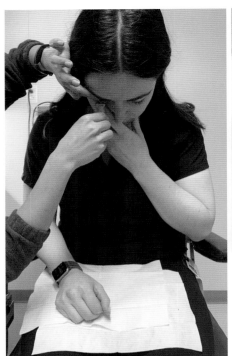

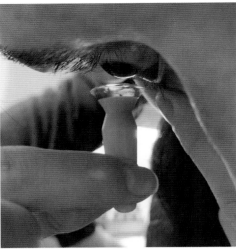

FIGURE 6-28 | Insertion of scleral contact lens.

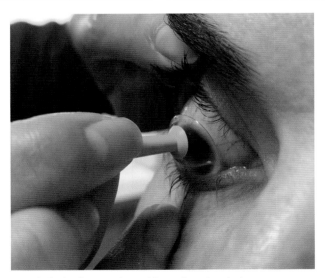

FIGURE 6-29 | Removal of scleral contact lens with small suction device.

3. With your nondominant hand, apply mild pressure to the superior bulbar conjunctiva through the upper eyelid to relieve the seal between the lens and the eye. Gently rocking the suction device can help relieve the seal.

4. Once the seal has been relieved, gently rotate the suction device downward to lift the lens off the eye.

## 6.19 FIT ASSESSMENT OF SCLERAL CONTACT LENSES

### Purpose

The aim of this procedure is to determine whether a scleral contact lens is fitting adequately so that vision and comfort are optimized, and contact lens-related anterior segment complications are minimized. A scleral contact lens is a large-diameter RGP contact lens that extends out to the sclera and is intended to rest on the conjunctiva. Prior to application on the eye, a scleral lens is filled with preservative-free saline solution. During the first hours of lens settling, there is a gradual decrease in the fluid clearance between the cornea and the lens, however an important goal in fitting a scleral lens is to avoid contact with the posterior contact lens surface and the anterior cornea and limbus. For the duration that the scleral lens sits on the eye, it should maintain fluid clearance across the cornea and the limbus, and land evenly 360° around the sclera. A scleral lens evaluation will begin at the optic zone (central cornea) and then extend limbus to limbus, before an assessment of the scleral lens landing zones.

### Equipment

- Biomicroscope

### Setup

- Biomicroscope setup will vary throughout a scleral lens assessment, depending on the aspect of the scleral lens being evaluated. Therefore, any evaluation technique that requires a different setup than below will preclude a biomicroscope setup under the procedure section below.
- Adjust the biomicroscope so that it is comfortable for the patient and examiner.
- Set the magnification to 10×, the illumination level to medium to high, and the slit beam to a wide parallelepiped or diffuse illumination.
- Set the illumination arm to approximately 30° from the straight-ahead position on the temporal side. The patient should be wearing the scleral lens(es) of interest.

### Procedure

1. Instruct the patient to look straight ahead, toward the back of the examination room. Alternatively, you can instruct the patient to look at your right ear.
2. Begin by focusing on the patient's right contact lens.
3. Assess lens centration: move the slit beam from temporal to the nasal lens edge and observe the lens position, both horizontally and vertically. If the vertical lens position is difficult to assess due to a small palpebral aperture or larger scleral lens, retract the patient's upper and lower lids away from the lens to evaluate the lens position. However, be aware that lid manipulation can alter lens position.
4. Assess lens movement: ask the patient to blink and observe the lens edge for any signs of lens movement.
5. Assess the optic zone of the lens: increase the magnification to 16×. Set the illumination arm to approximately 45° from the straight-ahead position on the temporal side. Narrow the beam to an optic section with white light beam and set the illumination level to high.
   a. Start at the corneal apex and then scan across the lens from limbus to limbus, horizontally and vertically.
   b. Estimate the amount of fluid clearance between the lens and corneal optic zone (centrally), midperipherally, and at the limbal zones. If fluorescein was used during lens application, the fluid clearance between the lens and the cornea will highlight green.

The amount of clearance under the lens is estimated by comparing the known center thickness of the lens to the fluid layer behind the posterior lens surface to the anterior surface of the cornea. Take note of the clearance values at the corneal apex, remarkable areas of high or low clearance, and the limbus.

6. Assess the scleral landing zones: change the magnification to 10×. Set the illumination arm to approximately 30° from the straight-ahead position on the temporal side. Set the illumination level to low to medium. Open the slit beam to a wide parallelepiped or diffuse illumination.

   a. Inspect the conjunctiva and sclera under the peripheral (haptic) portion of the scleral lens landing zone. Assess the haptic areas superiorly, inferiorly, nasally, and temporally. Note areas of vessel blanching (whitened areas), conjunctival impingement, and edge lift.

7. Repeat steps 3 through 6 for the left eye.

## Recording
- Record the lens position.
- Record the lens clearance centrally, any remarkable areas in the midperipheral cornea and over the limbus, particularly nasally and temporally.
- Record the peripheral (haptic) fitting relationship in all four quadrants.

## Examples
- Lens position: central
  - Optic zone assessment: adequate clearance centrally without fluorescein (**see Figure 6-30**)
  - Adequate clearance limbus to limbus
  - Peripheral fit: even alignment on sclera 360°
- Apical/central touch (**see Figure 6-31**)
  - <100 microns of clearance in the midperiphery, clearance at the limbus
  - Scleral lending zone: edge lift at 12:00 and 6:00, alignment at 3:00 and 9:00
- Peripheral fit: blanching 360° with impingement (**see Figure 6-32**)
- Excessive clearance centrally (**see Figure 6-33**)
  - >500 microns of clearance centrally, touch inside nasal limbus, clearance at limbus temporally, superiorly, and inferiorly

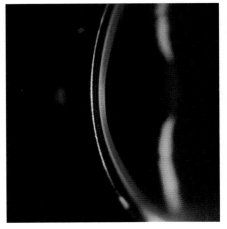

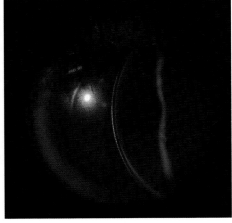

**FIGURE 6-30** | Acceptable scleral lens fit with adequate central clearance.

**FIGURE 6-31** | Unacceptable scleral lens fit with <100 microns of clearance.

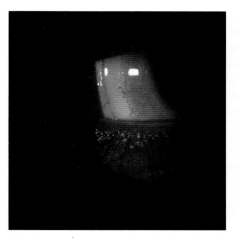

FIGURE 6-32 | Unacceptable scleral lens fit with 360-degree impingement and blanching.

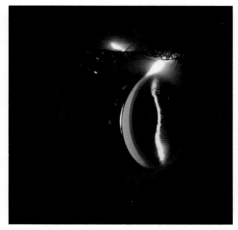

FIGURE 6-33 | Unacceptable scleral lens fit with excessive central clearance.

| SCLERAL CONTACT LENS FIT ASSESSMENT at a glance | |
|---|---|
| **Fit Characteristics** | **Expected Findings** |
| Lens position | Lens position relative to the cornea is assessed by observing the amount of lens overlap onto the sclera. The distance between the lens edge and the patient's limbus should be equidistant in all four quadrants (temporal, nasal, superior, and inferior). |
| Lens movement | There should be very minimal to absence of lens movement. |
| Optic zone assessment | The estimated amount, in microns, of tear fluid between the posterior surface of the scleral lens and the anterior surface of the cornea. The ideal initial post-lens fluid layer should be between 250 and 350 microns of central clearance. As the lens settles, the post-lens fluid layer will decrease by approximately 100 microns. A settled lens should exhibit 150–250 microns of central clearance. |
| Limbal zone assessment | The estimated amount, in microns, of tear fluid between the posterior surface of the scleral lens and the anterior surface of the cornea. There should be a gradual tapering of post-lens fluid from the central aspect of the scleral lens to the limbal aspect. |
| Scleral lens landing zone assessment | The scleral lens should land evenly on the conjunctival vessels 360° around the sclera. There should be an absence of whitening of blood vessels (blanching), an absence of lens digging into the conjunctiva/sclera (impingement), and an absence of edge lift. |

## 6.20 WRITING A CONTACT LENS PRESCRIPTION

### Purpose

The aim of this procedure is to write a clear and comprehensive prescription for contact lenses that will be recognized, understood, honored, and filled by any optician or optical lab. In contrast to eyeglass prescriptions, contact lens prescriptions are often much more complex owing to an array of additional details that are needed. A complete prescription will avoid errors or delays in contact lens orders submitted by the patient or those submitted by you on behalf of the patient. Dispensing complete and accurate contact lens prescriptions is an essential part of a successful practice. In this section, basic components of a contact lens prescription are outlined for soft and GP lenses.

*Note*: Prescriptions for GP lenses and scleral lenses can be overly complex and incomplete due to proprietary details that are not routinely released by the manufacturer. Under these circumstances, prescriptions are often collected by patients for record purposes since replacement lens orders are normally made through the prescribing doctor's office without the need for a physical prescription.

### Equipment
- Computer for electronically generated or printed prescription

### Procedure
1. There are several key elements which must be included on every contact lens prescription. **Table 6-3** contains a list of essential components required for all contact lens prescriptions.

| TABLE 6-3. Essential Components for All Contact Lens Prescriptions | |
| --- | --- |
| **Predesignated** | **Custom details** |
| • Clinic name<br>• Clinic address, phone, and fax<br>• Prescribing doctor's name, professional degree(s), license number | • Patient name and date of birth<br>• Date of prescription issue and expiration |

a. **Table 6-4** lists essential and optional details required for a disposable soft contact lens prescription.

| TABLE 6-4. Components of Soft Contact Lens Prescription | |
| --- | --- |
| **Required** | **Optional** |
| • Lens series name<br>• Lens base curve and diameter<br>• Lens power<br>• Lens replacement frequency<br>• Lens quantity corresponding to one full Rx cycle<br>• Prescribing doctor's signature | • Manufacturer |

b. **Table 6-5** lists essential and optional details required for a GP contact lens prescription.

| TABLE 6-5. Components of Gas Permeable Contact Lens Prescription | |
| --- | --- |
| **Required** | **Optional** |
| • Manufacturer<br>• Lens series name<br>• Lens material<br>• Lens base curve and diameter<br>• Lens power<br>• Distinct lens colors or dot on OD lens<br>• Prescribing doctor's signature | • Center thickness<br>• Optic zone diameter<br>• Secondary and tertiary base curves and zone widths |

c. **Table 6-6** lists essential and optional details required for a scleral contact lens prescription.

| TABLE 6-6. Components of Scleral Contact Lens Prescription | |
|---|---|
| **Required** | **Optional** |
| • Manufacturer<br>• Lens series name<br>• Lens base curve and diameter<br>• Lens power<br>• Sagittal depth<br>• Distinct lens colors or dot on OD lens<br>• Prescribing doctor's signature | • Center thickness<br>• Optic zone diameter<br>• Lens material<br>• Secondary and tertiary base curves |

2. Once you have filled out the prescription with the necessary details outlined above, review it for accuracy and provide your patient a copy for their records. In preparation for the possibility that an electronic facsimile of the prescription is required, ensure that the font of the document and your signature appear in black ink for the best resolution and greatest contrast.

## Examples
• An example of a contact lens prescription is seen in **Figure 6-34**.

## Notes
• A copy of every prescription should be maintained on file in the patient's chart.

**ABC Vision**
**Center for Eye Care**
**930 Commonwealth Ave**
**Boston, MA 02215**
**Office Ph:  (617)262-2020**

**ABC Vision**

**Patient Name: James Test**
**Address:** 930 Commonwealth Avenue   Boston, MA  02215
**Exam Date:**05/03/2022

**Date of Birth:** 07/01/1989
**Print Date:** 5/3/2022
**Expires:**05/03/2023

| | Manufacturer | Brand | BC1 | BC2 | DIA | Sph | Cyl | Axis |
|---|---|---|---|---|---|---|---|---|
| OD | Best | Daily Lens | 8.6 | | 14.2 | -3.00 | | |
| OS | Best | Daily Lens | 8.6 | | 14.2 | -3.50 | | |

| | Add | Seg | Prism | Tint | Series | Type | | QTY |
|---|---|---|---|---|---|---|---|---|
| OD | | | | | | Final Rx | | 4 x 90 Unit Boxes |
| OS | | | | | | Final Rx | | 4 x 90 Unit Boxes |

Benjamin Young, OD

LIC#:  99X9

**FIGURE 6-34** | An example of an electronic or printed soft contact lens prescription.

# 7

# Systemic Health Screening

Maureen Hanley, OD / Bina Patel, OD, FAAO

## 7.1 INTRODUCTION TO SYSTEMIC HEALTH SCREENING

Primary eye care practitioners frequently encounter manifestations of systemic disease. A number of systemic diseases, particularly those of infectious or inflammatory nature, affect the eyes as well as other organs or tissues within the body. Ocular related findings such as headaches or blurred vision are often the first symptom of a variety of systemic conditions, and the primary eye care provider may be the first healthcare professional sought by the patient for their concerns.

Occasionally, ocular signs present that may suggest the presence of a potentially life-threatening condition such as a space-occupying lesion in the brain, severe hypertension, or carotid artery disease. Many of these conditions can be detected by carefully listening to the patient's symptoms and the use of the problem-specific procedures described in this chapter. The patient is then referred to the appropriate provider in a timely manner.

The procedures included in this chapter are generally not considered part of the core ocular examination. Rather they are problem-specific tests that are employed when indicated by the patient's symptoms, case history, or abnormal test results noted during other procedures. Most of the techniques in this chapter will be used more frequently in examining elderly patients because they are at higher risk for many systemic diseases. Practitioners with a predominantly elderly patient population may choose to include some of these techniques in their core routine examination. Blood pressure measurement is sometimes performed routinely as an initial screening procedure, especially in offices that utilize ancillary personnel. All of these techniques may be used with any age group, when indicated.

Throughout this chapter, reference is made to the *standard precautions* whenever the examiner touches the patient (see Procedure 2.2). These standards are essential in the prevention of the spread of infection. Vigorous hand washing with soap and water or an alcohol-based hand sanitizer is recommended by the Centers for Disease Control and Prevention (CDC) before and after every patient encounter. Disposable surgical gloves may also be used but should not substitute for hand washing.

## 7.2 BLOOD PRESSURE EVALUATION (SPHYGMOMANOMETRY)

### Purpose

Sphygmomanometry with the use of a stethoscope is used to determine blood pressure. This method determines the pressure in the arteries at the height of ventricular contraction (systolic pressure) and ventricular relaxation (diastolic pressure). Measurement readings are recorded in millimeters of mercury (mmHg).

### Equipment

- Stethoscope with a two-sided head (bell and diaphragm).
- Blood pressure cuff is commonly used with an aneroid manometer. Other types are available, such as automated, hybrid or mercury, the latter, less commonly used due to its safety profile. Use appropriate cuff size (pediatric, adult, and large adult size)

### Setup

- The patient is seated in a quiet setting/room for at least 5 minutes.
- The patient should not have consumed any caffeine-containing products, exercised, or smoked within 30–60 minutes before the reading is taken.
- The patient is relaxed and seated with a back support, feet resting on the ground and uncrossed. Their arm should be flexed and resting with the palm facing upward, supported on either a table or arm of a chair, at the level of the left atrium. Perform the procedure on bare skin and avoid rolled up sleeves as it may excessively constrict the upper arm.
- The examiner uses standard health precautions before touching the patient.
- The examiner is seated in front of or to the side of the arm being tested.

### Procedure

1. Inform the patient that you will be checking their blood pressure by wrapping a cuff around their arm and inflating the cuff with air. Advise the patient that they will feel pressure around their arm as you inflate the cuff, but that they should not experience any pain.
2. Palpate the patient's radial artery by placing your index and middle finger on the patient's wrist in between the bone and tendon of the thumb. Press firmly feeling for the arterial pulsation (**see Figure 7-1**). Ensure the patient's elbow or brachial artery and is at heart level (left atrium).
3. Center the bladder length of the cuff (indicated by an arrow or circular symbol or other marking on the cuff) on the patient's upper arm overlying the brachial artery. Use the appropriate cuff size. Ensure the bladder of the cuff is encircling the arm approximately 75–100%.
4. Adjust the cuff so that its lower edge is approximately 2–3 cm (~1 inch) above the antecubital crease/fossa.
5. Secure the cuff at this location and determine that it is wrapped snug along the upper arm. The examiner should be able to slip one finger between the patient's arm and the cuff edge and with two fingers it should feel snug (**see Figure 7-2**). If more of a gap is present, the cuff is too loose. If less of a gap is present, the cuff is too tight.

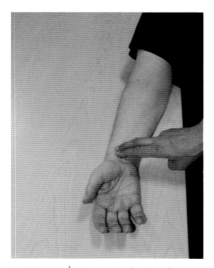

FIGURE 7-1 | Examiner palpating the patient's radial arterial pulse.

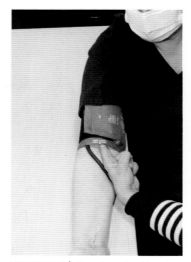

FIGURE 7-2 | Examiner checking the fit of the blood pressure cuff.

6. Determine the palpable systolic pressure to avoid discrepancies produced by an auscultatory gap:

   a. Use the index and middle finger on one of your hands to gently palpate the radial pulse on the patient's wrist. This is the side closest to the side of their thumb.

   b. Lock the air valve and inflate the cuff to 30 mmHg above the level at which the radial pulse disappears.

   c. Unlock the air valve, then smoothly and slowly release the air from the cuff at a rate of 2 to 3 mmHg per second (mmHg/s), until the radial pulse is felt again. Make a mental note of the manometer reading when the pulse reappears. Deflate the cuff completely. For subsequent inflations, and to prevent patient discomfort from higher than necessary cuff pressures, use the summation of the 30 mmHg and your tentative systolic reading as a target pressure.

7. Use standard precautions for disinfection of the stethoscope. Position the earpieces of the stethoscope so they are facing forward in your ears and make the necessary adjustments with the headset.

8. The stethoscope has a chest piece that has a diaphragm (flat side) and a bell (**see Figure 7-3**). Click the diaphragm side in place so it is transmitting sound through the stethoscope. Gently place the diaphragm over the brachial artery between the antecubital crease/fossa and the lower edge of the cuff (**see Figure 7-4**).

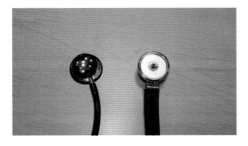

FIGURE 7-3 | Bell (left side of image) and diaphragm (right side of image) of the stethoscope.

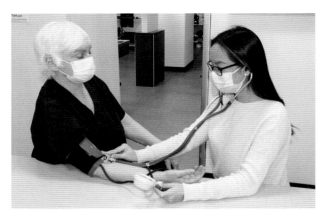

**FIGURE 7-4** | Proper positioning of the cuff and stethoscope head.

9. Lock the air valve and inflate the cuff 20–30 mmHg above the palpated systolic pressure value determined in step 6c.

10. Unlock the air valve. Smoothly and slowly at a rate of 2–3 mmHg/s, release the air from the cuff, listening for the Korotkoff sounds (**see Table 7-1**). Note the first audible sound and the manometer reading (Korotkoff phase I sounds are classified as tapping sounds). This is considered the systolic blood pressure reading. Continue to slowly release air from the cuff and note the manometer reading when the Korotkoff phase V sound occurs (loss of all sounds). This is considered the diastolic blood pressure.

| TABLE 7-1. The Korotkoff Sounds |
|---|
| • Phase I: The sudden appearance of regular tapping sounds—indicates the systolic pressure reading |
| • Phase II: A swishing, softening of sounds |
| • Phase III: Crisper sounds, increasing in intensity |
| • Phase IV: An abrupt muffling of sounds (diastolic pressure I) |
| • Phase V: The complete cessation of sounds (diastolic pressure II)—indicates the diastolic pressure reading |

11. Continue to reduce the air valve for 10 to 20 mmHg to confirm that all sounds have disappeared. Then rapidly deflate the cuff completely.

12. It is recommended that the blood pressure readings are taken twice at one sitting. Take the second reading 1–2 minutes after the first. *Note:* It has been recommended to take blood pressure on both arms the first time establishing a reading on a patient, or if peripheral vascular disease is expected.

## Recording
- Systolic pressure/diastolic pressure: recorded to the nearest whole number
- Right arm or left arm
- Posture: sitting, standing, or lying down
- Time of the day
- Cuff size—if other than regular size

## Examples

- 120/80, right arm, sitting, @ 1:30 PM, large adult cuff
- 110/70, left arm, sitting, @ 10:00 AM, pediatric cuff
- 160/95, right arm, sitting, @ 2:00 PM, 120/80, left arm, sitting, @ 2:00 PM
- 150/95, left arm, supine position @ 9:00 AM

## Expected Findings

Various organizations have guidelines for interpreting sphygmomanometer values and guidelines for diagnosing hypertension, **see Table 7-2**. These include:

**TABLE 7-2. Interpreting Sphygmomanometry Values**

| Blood Pressure Category | Systolic mmHg (upper number) | And/Or | Diastolic mmHg (lower number) |
|---|---|---|---|
| Normal | Less than 120 | and | Less than 80 |
| Elevated | 120–129 | and | Less than 80 |
| High Blood Pressure (Hypertension) Stage 1 | 130–139 | or | 80–90 |
| High Blood Pressure (Hypertension) Stage 2 | 140 or higher | or | 90 or higher |
| Hypertensive Crisis (consult your doctor immediately) | Higher than 180 | and/or | Higher than 120 |

*Source: Data from the American Heart Association. Healthy and unhealthy blood pressure ranges. American Heart Association website. https://www.heart.org/en/health-topics/high-blood-pressure/understanding-blood-pressure-readings. Accessed April 28, 2022.*

- Diurnal variations in blood pressure are normal. Blood pressure is usually highest in the mid-morning and lowest during sleep.
- A 5–10 mmHg discrepancy between the two arms is considered normal. Differences of greater than 10–15 mmHg are abnormal and could be indicative of atherosclerotic narrowing of the subclavian or brachiocephalic arteries or part of subclavian steal syndrome.
- False low blood pressure readings may occur as the result of:
  - the blood pressure cuff being too wide;
  - the patient's arm being above heart level;
  - deflating the cuff too rapidly (affects the systolic reading); and
  - an auscultatory gap, which underestimates the systolic pressure and overestimates the diastolic pressure.
- False high blood pressure readings may occur as the result of:
  - patient anxiety or fear ("white coat syndrome"); automated sphygmomanometry has been shown to produce more precise in-office measurements in these patients;
  - the blood pressure cuff being too small or narrow;
  - deflating the cuff too slowly (affects the diastolic reading);
  - the patient's arm being below heart level;
  - the patient's legs are crossed; and
  - constrictive clothing on the upper arm.

## 7.3 CAROTID ARTERY EVALUATION

### Purpose
The aim of this procedure is to assess the carotid arterial system for occlusive vascular disease. These in office techniques maybe helpful in referring for appropriate care and workup; the standard of care for evaluating the carotids is a noninvasive carotid Doppler.

### Indications
This evaluation is indicated for any patient who presents with signs and/or symptoms of atherosclerotic plaque formation within the cerebrovascular arterial system.

### Equipment
- Double headed stethoscope which has a chest piece with a two-sided head. One side is the diaphragm (flat side), and other side is the bell.

### Setup
- The patient sits comfortably in a chair with a back-support in front of the examiner.
- The patient should be relaxed, and the room should be quiet.

### Procedure
*Palpation of the Carotid Pulses*
1. Perform a gross inspection of the patient's neck looking for any significant prominent pulsations.
2. Inform the patient that you will be placing your fingers on their neck to check their pulse.
3. To palpate the patient's right carotid pulse:
   a. Stand to the right of the patient and instruct the patient to tilt their head to the left and tilt their chin slightly upward.
   b. Using the tips of the index and middle finger of your left hand, gently place your fingers near the upper neck. Palpate the patient's neck in the groove located lateral to the trachea and medial to the sternocleidomastoid muscle (at the level of the cricoid cartilage), feeling for the pulse of the right common carotid artery.
   c. Feel the pulse for 10 to 15 seconds. Note the pulse rhythm, pulse rate, and pulse force.
4. To palpate the patient's left carotid pulse, repeat step 3, and stand to the left of the patient. Instruct the patient to turn their head to the right and tilt their chin slightly upward. Use the tips of the index and middle finger of your right hand to gently palpate for the pulse of the left common carotid artery (**see Figure 7-5**). Make a note of pulse equality between right and left side.

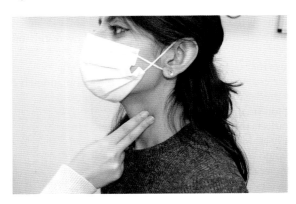

**FIGURE 7-5** | Examiner palpating the left carotid pulse.

*Note: Do* not apply excess pressure on the carotid artery during palpation. **Never** palpate both the right and left carotid arteries at the same time. Excessive carotid massage (avoid stimulating the Vagus nerve) can cause slowing of the pulse or a drop in blood pressure.

### Auscultation of the Carotid Arteries

1. Inform the patient that you will be placing a stethoscope on their neck to check the circulation through the blood vessels.
2. Be sure the room is quiet.
3. To auscultate the patient's right carotid artery, stand to the right of the patient. Instruct the patient to turn their head to the left and tilt their chin slightly upward.
4. Use standard precautions for disinfection of the stethoscope. Position the earpieces of the stethoscope so they are facing forward in your ears and make the necessary adjustments with the headset.
5. Turn the head of the stethoscope so that the bell is "clicked" into position so it is transmitting sound through the stethoscope. The bell transmits low frequency sounds and its size fits within the contour of the neck. The diaphragm can also be used, which transmits higher frequency sounds.
6. Place the bell of the stethoscope at the base of the patient's neck approximately 2.5 cm or 1 inch above the clavicle. This position allows you to listen to the common carotid.
7. Instruct the patient to hold their breath and listen for the presence of a bruit. This is an abnormal systolic sound with turbulent blood flow (vascular turbulence) through an area of stenosis, described as a "whooshing" or "swishing" or "blowing" sound. The artery is stenosed approximately 50% for a bruit to be heard.
8. Instruct the patient to exhale. Reposition the bell of the stethoscope further up the neck. This position allows you to listen to the carotid bifurcation area. Repeat step 7.
9. Instruct the patient to exhale. Reposition the bell of the stethoscope further up the neck at the angle of the jaw. This position allows you to listen to the internal carotid artery. Repeat step 7.
10. To auscultate the patient's left carotid artery, stand to the left of the patient. Instruct the patient to turn their head to the right and tilt their chin slightly upward.
11. Repeat steps 6 through 9 on the left carotid artery. **See Figure 7-6**.

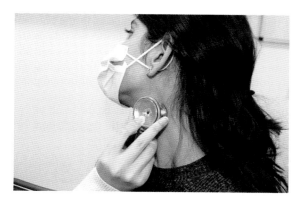

**FIGURE 7-6** | Examiner auscultating the left carotid artery bifurcation.

## Recording
- Palpation of the carotid pulses:
  - Grade the pulse amplitude:
    - 0 = no palpable pulse
    - 1+ = detectable but faint pulse
    - 2+ = stronger pulse, but slightly decreased intensity
    - 3+ = normal pulse
    - 4+ = bounding pulse
  - Evaluate the symmetry between the right and left sides.
- Auscultation of the carotid arteries:
  - Note the presence or absence of a bruit on the right and left side.

## Examples
- Palpation of carotid pulses: R: 3+ L: 3+
  Auscultation of carotid arteries: R: no bruits L: no bruits
- Palpation of carotid pulses: R: 2+ L: 1+
  Auscultation of carotid arteries: R: no bruits L: bruit

## Expected Findings
- Normal
  Palpation of carotid pulses: 2+ to 3+ pulses without asymmetry
  Auscultation of carotid arteries: no bruits on the right or left sides
- Abnormal
  Palpation of carotid pulses: decreased pulse amplitudes or asymmetry
  Auscultation of carotid arteries: presence of a bruit on right and/or left side

## Notes
- Checking the carotid pulse and performing carotid auscultation for bruit could be considered on patients presenting with symptoms and or signs related to carotid artery stenosis. These may include symptoms such as transient ischemic attacks and presence of Hollenhorst plaque(s), or signs of ocular ischemic syndrome on ocular examination.
- If the stenosis is significant, the bruit may be more audible.
- If the stenosis is greater than approximately 85% of the cross-sectional diameter of the artery, it is likely associated with low blood flow in the carotid artery resulting in an inaudible bruit. Thus, an *absence* of a bruit does not rule out atherosclerotic plaque formation.
- It is recommended that individuals that do *not* present with signs and/or symptoms of atherosclerotic disease should not be screened for bruit. The evidence on the outcomes of management and treatment, outweighs the benefits for asymptomatic individuals. This continues to be debated.
- Common methods used for assessing the carotid artery include cerebral angiography, magnetic resonance angiography, carotid Doppler ultrasound, duplex ultrasonography, and computerized tomography angiography.
- Not all carotid bruits are due to atherosclerotic occlusion. Some may be the result of:
  - transmitted murmurs from valvular aortic stenosis, severe aortic regurgitation, or a damaged mitral valve;
  - vigorous left ventricular ejection (more common in children); and
  - venous hums (heart murmur) (more common in younger patients).

## 7.4 LYMPH NODE EVALUATION

### Purpose

The aim of this procedure is to determine the presence of lymphadenopathy, which may provide information about the differential diagnosis of a red eye.

### Equipment

- No specific equipment is required.

### Setup

- The patient sits comfortably in a chair with their chin slightly elevated, facing the examiner.
- The examiner sits or stands in front of the patient.
- The examiner uses standard health precautions before and after touching the patient.

### Procedure

*Palpating the Preauricular Lymph Nodes*

1. Place your hands on the patient's face so that the index and middle finger or the middle and ring finger of each hand are positioned in front of the patient's external ear. Usually both the right and left preauricular region are tested at the same time.

2. Locate the bony structures of the temporomandibular joint, applying minimal pressure.

3. Slowly move your fingers in a circular motion to slide the patient's skin over the underlying bony structures. Search for a depression of the joint (normal) or an elevated nodular lesion (swollen lymph node indicating lymphadenopathy), **see Figure 7-7**. A tender swollen preauricular node will feel like a pebble or bean under the patient's skin.

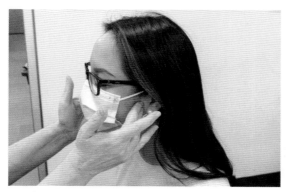

**FIGURE 7-7** | Examiner palpating the preauricular nodes.

4. Compare the right and left sides noting the presence or absence of palpable nodes. If a swollen node is present, note its size, whether or not it is mobile, and if there is warmth overlying or surrounding the node. Ask the patient if the area is tender when touched.

*Palpating the Cervical, Submandibular, and Submental Lymph Nodes*

1. Place the fleshy tips of your index, middle, and ring fingers of each hand on the patient's neck.

2. To palpate the cervical nodes, begin at the angle of the jaw. Gently rotate the patient's skin between your fingers and the underlying sternocleidomastoid muscle. Slowly move your fingers down, continuing to palpate, following the sternocleidomastoid muscle to the base of the neck (**see Figure 7-8**).

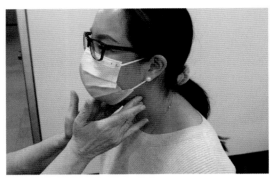

FIGURE 7-8 | Examiner palpating the cervical nodes.

3. Compare the right and left sides, noting the presence or absence of palpable nodes. If a swollen node is present, note its size, whether or not it is mobile, and if there is warmth overlying or surrounding the node. Ask the patient if the area is tender when touched.

4. To palpate the submandibular nodes, place your fingertips along (but under) the edge of the jawbone, and massage the patient's skin between your fingers and the underlying tissue (**see Figure 7-9**).

5. To palpate the submental lymph nodes, place your fingertips under the tip of the chin and massage the patient's skin between the fingers and the underlying tissue.

6. If a swollen node is present, note its size, whether or not it is mobile, and if there is warmth overlying or surrounding the node. Ask the patient if the area is tender when touched.

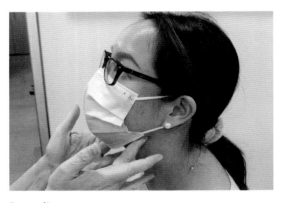

FIGURE 7-9 | Examiner palpating the submandibular nodes.

### Recording
- Record if nodes are palpable (positive finding) or not (negative finding).
- If nodes are palpable characterize them by:
  - laterality: unilateral or bilateral;
  - tenderness: tender or nontender; usually if tender, one thinks of viral etiology; if hard, classically malignancy & granulomatous infection, and if rubbery one thinks of lymphoma;
  - mobility: mobile or immobile;
  - size: small or large; and
  - *warmth:* presence or absence.

### Examples
- No palpable preauricular, cervical, submandibular, or submental lymph nodes.
- Positive right preauricular node. Approximately 1 cm in size, mobile, tender, with no overlying warmth. No palpable cervical, submandibular, or submental lymph nodes.

### Expected Findings

- *Normal:* No palpable lymph nodes.
- *Abnormal:* Palpable lymph nodes (lymphadenopathy) are commonly seen in the following conditions:
  - viral conjunctivitis: preauricular lymphadenopathy often greater on the side of the more involved eye;
  - severe bacterial lid conditions such as preseptal cellulitis or infection in the medial canthal region: preauricular or submental lymphadenopathy;
  - Parinaud's oculoglandular conjunctivitis: preauricular lymphadenopathy;
  - upper respiratory infection: cervical and submandibular lymphadenopathy; and
  - non-Hodgkin's and Hodgkin's lymphoma.

## 7.5 GLUCOMETRY

### Purpose

The aim of this procedure is to determine the blood glucose level of a patient who may present with signs or symptoms of hypo- or hyperglycemia. This procedure is also helpful in the differential diagnosis of the patient with a significant shift in refractive error.

### Equipment

- Glucose monitor (glucometer)
- Test strips
- Disposable lancets
- Lancing device
- Alcohol swabs
- Disposable latex-free examination gloves
- Sharps container
- Biohazard container

### Setup

- The patient sits comfortably in front of the examiner.
- The patient should be relaxed.
- The glucose monitor and test strips should be kept at room temperature.

### Procedure

1. Prepare the patient:

    a. Instruct the patient to wash their hands with soap and water or use an alcohol swab to clean their fingertip.

    b. Explain the purpose and procedure of the test to the patient to decrease any anxiety they may have.

2. Wash your hands with soap and water, thoroughly dry them, and then put on a pair of sterile examination gloves.
3. Turn the glucometer on and insert a fresh test strip.
4. Wait for the monitor to prompt you to apply a sample of blood to the test strip.
5. Insert a sterile lancet into the lancing device and activate the spring-loaded tension device.
6. Place the lancing device firmly along the side of the patient's finger.
7. Press the lancing device's release button, which will cause the lancet to penetrate the patient's skin surface.
8. You may massage the patient's fingertip to create a well-formed drop of blood.
9. Touch the drop of blood to the target area of the test strip.

10. Once the target area is adequately covered with blood, the monitor will begin a count-down and then display a number.
11. Record the number in milligrams per deciliter (mg/dL) (**see Figure 7-10**).
12. Dispose of used lancets in a sharps container.
13. Dispose of used alcohol swabs, used test strips, and used rubber gloves in a biohazard container for appropriate removal. Perform hand hygiene following glove removal.
14. Turn off the glucometer.

**A**

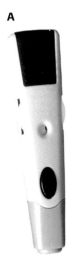

**B**

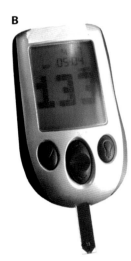

**FIGURE 7-10** | (A) Lancing device and (B) digital readout showing results of glucometry, recorded in milligrams per deciliter (mg/dL).

### Recording
- Glucometry (list brand of instrument)
- Record the number displayed in mg/dL
- Date and time of sample
- Time of last meal (if known)
- Any other comments

### Examples
- Glucometry (brand): 100 mg/dL; 12/27/21 @ 4 pm
- Glucometry (brand): 40 mg/dL; 12/28/21 @ 10 am, 2 hours postprandial; patient light-headed

### Expected Findings
- According to the CDC, a fasting blood sugar level (no food for 8 hours) of 99 mg/dL or lower is normal, 100 to 125 mg/dL indicates you have prediabetes, and 126 mg/dL or higher indicates you have diabetes. A random blood sugar of greater than 200 is suggestive of diabetes.
- Findings vary depending on the time since last meal. Findings may also vary depending on medications used, the presence of blood dyscrasias, and grossly elevated triglycerides or cholesterol.
- Refer to the owner's manual of the instrument you are using for the normal ranges of that given instrument.
- Notify the patient's primary care physician or endocrinologist with any abnormal results.

# 8

# Cranial Nerve Screening

Benjamin Young, OD, FAAO

## 8.1 INTRODUCTION TO CRANIAL NERVE SCREENING

Cranial nerves (CN) 2, 3, 4, and 6 are all either directly or indirectly assessed during routine eye examination. However, patients will often present to their eye care provider with neurologic dysfunction involving one or more of the other eight CNs because many of the diseases that affect these nerves present with visual or ocular symptoms such as diplopia, blurry vision, or reduced peripheral vision. For example, a patient with a new-onset Bell's palsy may present to their optometrist because they are experiencing ocular dryness or observed a new onset ptosis in the mirror. In situations such as this, optometrists need to be able to determine if their patient's condition warrants monitoring, treatment, or referral. If monitoring is called for, the optometrist must be confident that no harm will come to the patient while they wait and watch the patient's condition over an extended period of time.

If treatment of neurologic dysfunction is required and falls within the optometrist's scope of practice, appropriate testing is necessary to accurately diagnose the condition and prescribe appropriate therapy. If the treatment falls outside the optometrist's scope of practice, they need to decide the type of specialist the patient will be referred to and within what time frame. In order to make these decisions, the optometrist uses data about the neurological status of the patient through problem-specific tests such as the chair-side procedures described in this chapter.

A thorough exposition of the entire general neurological examination is beyond the scope of this text and can be found in other sources (see References for Chapter 8). This chapter is limited to problem-specific procedures for assessing the functions of the CNs, because ocular or visual symptoms that are likely to motivate a patient to see an eye care specialist are likely to affect the functions of the CNs. The reader should remember that many of the routinely performed entrance tests also assess the function of certain CNs. For example, tests of visual acuity, color vision, visual fields, and ophthalmoscopy assess the structure and function of the optic nerve, while extraocular muscle movement testing and cover test assess the oculomotor, trochlear, and/or abducens nerves.

The techniques described in this chapter require no unusual or special instrumentation. They are easy to perform and use equipment and supplies that are readily available in most optometric settings.

## 8.2 LID AND PTOSIS MEASUREMENTS

### Purpose
The aim of this procedure is to measure the placement of the lids in relation to the pupillary reflex and each other.

### Indications
This test is indicated when the difference in pupil sizes is not equal in bright and dim illumination, or when a patient presents with a new onset ptosis.

### Equipment
- Penlight or transilluminator
- Small ruler marked in millimeters (e.g., PD ruler)

### Setup
- Position yourself directly in front of the patient.

### Procedure
Three separate measurements are typically made when evaluating upper and lower lid positioning: interpalpebral fissure (IPF), margin to reflex distance 1 (MRD-1), and margin to reflex distance 2 (MRD-2). These measurements allow the examiner to distinguish between different conditions such as CN 3 palsy, lid laxity, and Horner's syndrome.

*IPF*
1. Hold the light source between your eyes pointing directly at the patient and tell them to look at the light.
2. Begin with the right eye. While holding the light in one hand, use the other hand to measure the distance between the upper lid margin and lower lid margin using the ruler as in **Figure 8-1**.
3. Repeat step 2 on the left eye.

*MRD-1*
1. While holding the light in one hand, use the other hand to measure the distance between the upper lid margin and the corneal light reflex.
2. Repeat step 1 on the left eye.

*MRD-2*
1. While holding the light in one hand, use the other hand to measure the distance between the corneal light reflex and the lower lid margin as in **Figure 8-2**.
2. Repeat step 1 on the left eye.

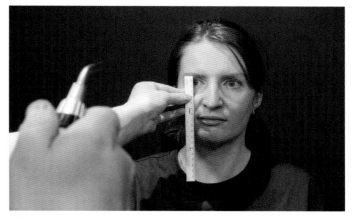

**FIGURE 8-1.** | Measurement of the IPF using a transilluminator as a fixation target.

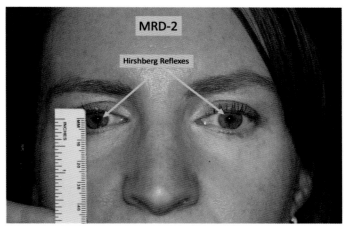

**FIGURE 8-2.** | Measurement of MRD-2.

## Recording
- Record each measurement separately.
- Indicate which measurement was performed.
- The reading for the right eye is recorded first and the reading for the left eye is recorded after.

## Examples
- IPF: 11 mm/8 mm
- MRD-1: 3 mm/1 mm
- MRD-2: 8 mm/7 mm

## Notes
- The MRD-1 and MRD-2 values should generally add up the IPF value of the same eye.
- Expected IPF norms: 10 mm ± 2 mm. >1 mm difference between eyes is also significant.
- IPF distances greater than norms may indicate lid retraction, as in Graves' ophthalmopathy.
- Symmetry between eyes is expected for all three measurements. Asymmetry >1mm between eyes may indicate the presence of ptosis, reverse ptosis, or lid retraction.

## 8.3 LEVATOR FUNCTION TEST

### Purpose
The aim of this procedure is to provide additional diagnostic information about the levator palpebrae superioris muscle.

### Indications
This test is indicated when external observation reveals a ptosis or the pupils appear to be unequal in size during routine pupillary entrance testing.

### Equipment
- Bright light source (e.g., exam-lane lamp, transilluminator, or direct ophthalmoscope)
- Distance fixation target (projected 20/400 optotype)
- Small ruler marked in millimeters (PD ruler) or pupil gauge

### Setup
- Position yourself directly in front of the patient and slightly below their line of sight.

### Procedure
1. With the patient looking straight ahead at the distance fixation target, use the PD ruler to measure the size of the IPF, MRD-1, and MRD-2 in millimeters (see Procedure 8.2).
2. Instruct the patient to look all the way down. Bracing your hand against the side of the patient's face, hold the ruler with the 0 mm marking intersecting the upper eyelid margin.
3. Carefully keeping your hand and ruler in place without moving, instruct the patient to look all the way up. Record in mm where the upper eyelid margin intersects with the ruler.
4. Repeat steps 1 and 2 at least three times followed by a repeat measurement of the IPF in primary gaze. Look for any significant change in levator function or IPF that occurs upon repeated testing in either eye.

### Recording
- Record the size of each palpebral aperture in millimeters for straight ahead gaze (i.e., the IPF) and in upgaze (i.e., the levator function) for each of the 3 total measurements. If both apertures are equal and intersect the normal position (approximately 2 mm below the superior limbus in upgaze), record "no ptosis of the upper lid."
- If the lower lids clear the lower limbus at the same time when the patient looks upward, record "no ptosis of lower lid" or "no reverse ptosis." If one lid clears the limbus sooner than the other, record "ptosis of the lower lid" and indicate which lid cleared second.

### Examples
- No ptosis of upper or lower lid. IPF: 9 mm OD and OS.
- (+)Ptosis of upper and lower lids OS. IPF 12 mm OD and 9 mm OS.

### Notes
- As an alternative, the examiner may have the patient sustain up-gaze for 30–60 seconds and observe.
- A fatigable ptosis should raise concern for myasthenia gravis, and an icepack test should be performed in this case.

> Note: An icepack test is a quick and simple procedure in office that has a relatively high sensitivity and specificity for myasthenia gravis. The examiner first measures the IPF and MRD-1 in both eyes before applying an ice pack to the suspected eye (or eyes) for 2 min. IPF and MRD-1 measurements are then repeated. An increase of 2 mm is considered positive and suspicious for myasthenia gravis.

## 8.4 NEAR (ACCOMMODATIVE) PUPIL TESTING

### Purpose
The aim of this procedure is to test the responsiveness of the pupil to a near target.

### Equipment
- Non-accommodative distance fixation target (e.g., 20/400 optotype)
- Near accommodative target with a line or isolated letter one to two lines above the patient's near visual acuity

### Procedure
1. Instruct the patient to maintain fixation on the distance optotype while you hold up a near accommodative target at 10–40 cm from their eyes. *Note*: If the patient is myopic, it is necessary to hold the target closer to their eyes, preferably well within their far point, in order to stimulate accommodation.
2. Instruct the patient to direct their gaze toward the near target. Look for pupillary constriction. *Note*: This is known as the "near" or "accommodative" response of the pupil.
3. Instruct the patient to return their gaze to the distance target. Look for dilation of the pupil to confirm that it had constricted during near viewing.
4. Compare the accommodative reaction of the pupil to the light reaction (see Procedure 2.15).

### Recording
- If all pupillary functions are within normal limits, add the letter "A" after the "PERRL" (pupils equal round reactive to light) when recording the results of pupillary testing (see Procedure 2.15).
- If the abbreviation "PERRL" does not apply to your patient, write "pupils constrict to near" or "pupils unresponsive to near," or "near response more brisk than light response," depending on the result.

### Examples
- PERRLA, (-)RAPD
- OD unresponsive to light direct or consensual; both pupils constrict to near; OS responds to direct and consensual light

## 8.5 PHARMACOLOGICAL PUPIL TESTING

### Purpose
The aim of this procedure is to distinguish pathological from nonpathological causes of anisocoria. In cases of pathological etiologies, pharmacological testing can help localize the pathology within the postganglionic, preganglionic, or central components of the neurological circuitry for pupillary reaction.

### Equipment
- Slit lamp
- Penlight or transilluminator
- Pupil gauge
- Stopwatch, clock, or watch accurate to the min
- The particular pharmaceutical test agent to be used (**see Table 8-1**)
- Camera equipped to take close-up photographs of the face showing both eyes

**TABLE 8-1. Summary of Pharmacologic Tests of the Pupil**

| Indication: Primary Purpose of the Test | Drug and Concentration | Check In (min) | Nonpatho-logical Response | Response of Compromised Pupil | Mode of Action (Basis of Test) |
|---|---|---|---|---|---|
| To confirm or rule out oculosympathetic paresis | Apraclonidine 0.5%* | 40 | No dilation | Dramatic dilation and reversal of anisocoria | Denervation supersensitivity |
| To distinguish postganglionic from preganglionic or central locations of pathology in oculosympathetic paresis | Hydroxyam-phetamine (Paredrine) 1.0% | 40–60 | Dilation | Reduced dilation if the lesion is postganglionic; Normal dilation if the lesion is preganglionic or central | Directly stimulates the release of norepinephrine from nerve endings |
| To distinguish postganglionic from preganglionic or central locations of pathology in oculosympathetic paresis | Phenylephrine 1.0% | 30 | Slight dilation | Dramatic dilation if the lesion is postganglionic; Slight dilation if the lesion is preganglionic or central | Denervation supersensitivity |
| To confirm or rule out Adie's tonic pupil | Pilocarpine 0.125% or 0.063% | 30 | No miosis | Miosis only if there is a postganglionic parasympathetic lesion, such as in Adie's pupil | Denervation supersensitivity |
| To confirm or rule out pharmacologic block of the sphincter of the pupil | Pilocarpine 2.0% or 4.0% | 30–40 | Miosis | No miosis if the cholinergic receptors of the sphincter are pharmacologically blocked | Direct acting cholinergic agonist |

*Cocaine has been historically used to confirm or rule out oculosympathetic paresis. However, its extremely limited availability as a controlled substance makes it impractical in most clinical settings. Apraclonidine is much more readily available and has been shown to be an acceptable replacement for cocaine.

## Setup

- Prior to instilling the test agent, perform and record a complete assessment of pupillary measurements in dim and bright light (see Procedure 2.15). Check for the presence of a ptosis and measure and record the widths of the palpebral apertures in primary gaze and up-gaze (see Procedures 8.2 and 8.3).
- Perform a thorough slit lamp examination of both eyes and ensure that neither eye is at risk for angle closure should the agent have the potential to cause pupillary dilation. See Procedure 5.7 for other precautions before drop instillation including assessment of allergies.
- Take a pretest baseline picture of the face showing the pupils of both eyes.

## Procedure

1. Instill one drop of the test agent in each eye with as little interval as possible between medicating the two eyes. Record the time of instillation (see "Notes" section below).

2. Monitor the state of the pupils at the earliest interval indicated on **Table 8-1**, comparing the sizes of the pupils in the two eyes. Repeat close-up photography of the pupils at this time.

3. Continue comparing the responses and sizes of the pupils in the two eyes until a definitive difference in pupillary behavior is observed or until the longest time indicated in **Table 8-1** has elapsed (if a time interval is provided). Repeat photography of the pupils as needed.

4. Use **Table 8-1** to assist in interpretation of the findings.

### Recording
- Record the agent used and the time of its instillation.
- Record the final response of each pupil (e.g., full dilation, minimal dilation, miosis, depending on the agent used) and the time of observation.

### Examples
- 1 gtt phenylephrine 1% at 3:30 pm OD & OS; Slight dilation OD, large dilation OS at 4:05 pm
- 1 gtt Paredrine 1% at 11:10 am OD & OS; OD pupil = 7 mm, OS pupil = ~4 mm at 11:40 am

### Expected Findings
- See **Table 8-1** for the response of a nonpathological pupil and the response of a compromised pupil for each pharmaceutical test agent.

### Notes
- Alexander, Skorin, and Bartlett recommend instillation of two drops of each test agent separated by a few min.
- Instillation of test agent in both eyes is indicated except in cases of suspected bilateral pharmacological block; in such cases, place the test agent in only one eye and make a comparison between the pupils 30–40 min later.

## 8.6 PARK'S THREE-STEP METHOD FOR A PARETIC VERTICAL MUSCLE

### Purpose
The aim of this procedure is to detect a paretic muscle in a non-comitant deviation with a vertical component.

### Equipment
- Occluder
- Distance acuity chart (for fixation target)
- Penlight (*optional*)

### Procedure
1. Perform cover test in all positions of gaze by following the procedure for alternating cover test outlined in Chapter 2. Identify which eye is the hyperdeviated eye and measure the deviation with prism bars (see Procedure 2.9).

   a. Pay careful attention to the relative magnitude of the hyperdeviation in primary gaze, right gaze, and left gaze as those assessments are pertinent to the three-step method.

2. Instruct the patient to tilt their head slightly to the right and repeat alternating cover test. Repeat with the patient's head tilted to the left. Again, pay careful attention to the relative magnitude of the hyperdeviation.

3. Trace through the flowchart in **Figure 8-3** to identify the paretic muscle.

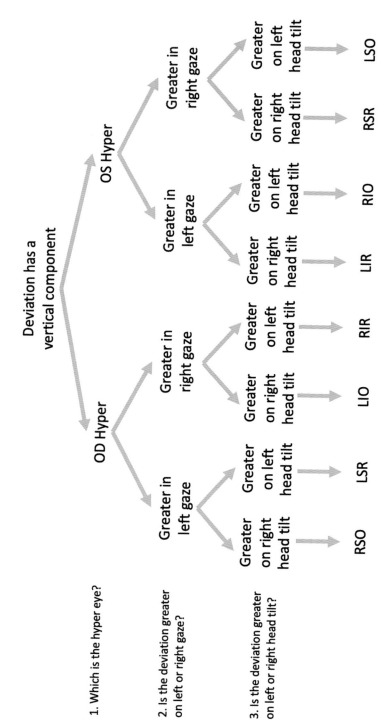

**FIGURE 8-3.** | Flowchart to interpret the findings when identifying a paretic muscle by the Park's three-step method.

### Recording
- Write "Park's three-step" followed by the identity of any paretic muscle or muscles.

### Examples
- Park's three-step: paretic LIO
- Park's three-step: paretic RSO

### Notes
- If no significant difference is found in the vertical deviation in multiple positions of gaze, the patient may have a vertical tropia or decompensated vertical phoria instead of a muscle paresis.

## 8.7 RED LENS TEST FOR A PARETIC HORIZONTAL MUSCLE

### Purpose
The aim of this procedure is to identify a subtle non-comitant muscle paresis in a deviation that is purely horizontal.

### Equipment
- Transilluminator (or penlight)
- Red lens

### Setup
- The patient removes their spectacles and holds the red lens over their right eye.
- The examiner holds the transilluminator.

### Procedure
1. Perform the Hirschberg procedure as described in Chapter 2 (see Procedure 2.12).
2. Give instructions to the patient:

   "Follow the light with your eyes without moving your head. You may see two lights instead of one, and if so, one will be white and the other will be red. Please tell me if they get closer together or further apart while I move the light."

3. Start with the light on and pointed directly at the patient while holding the transilluminator 40–50 cm away. This is called the "primary position of gaze."
4. Move the light all the way to the right and all the way left before returning to the primary position of gaze. *Note:* the order in which the positions are tested is not important. It is critical, however, to test gaze in all three positions and maintain a sooth movement of the light across the patient's midpoint.
5. Determine if a horizontal deviation is present, and if so, whether it is an exo or eso deviation. *Note:* If the patient reports that the red light is to the left of the white light, they have an exo deviation, and if they report that red light is to the right of the white light, they have an eso deviation. If the patient only sees one light throughout testing, they are either fusing normally or suppressing one eye and the procedure should be discontinued.
6. Determine if the deviation is greater in the patient's left or right gaze by asking the patient when the separation between the two lights is greatest.
7. Trace through the flowchart in **Figure 8-4** to identify the paretic muscle.

### Recording
- Record the type of deviation (eso or exo) and the direction of gaze in which the deviation is greater.
- Record the identity of the paretic muscle.

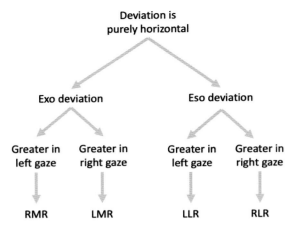

**Deviation is purely horizontal**

- Exo deviation
  - Greater in left gaze → RMR
  - Greater in right gaze → LMR
- Eso deviation
  - Greater in left gaze → LLR
  - Greater in right gaze → RLR

**FIGURE 8-4.** | Flowchart to interpret the findings when identifying a paretic horizontal muscle.

## Example
- Eso deviation > on left gaze: paretic LLR.

## Notes
- A red lens is not necessary if the patient has an externally observable and obvious eso or exo deviation. In this situation, it is appropriate to simply confirm that the patient sees two white lights next to each other and determine if the horizontal diplopia is greater in right or left gaze.

## 8.8 TRIGEMINAL NERVE FUNCTION TEST

### Purpose
The aim of this procedure is to test the functional integrity of the trigeminal CN, CN-V (or CN-5).

### Equipment
- Two sterile cotton tipped applicators with a small amount of cotton pulled out to form a point
- Piece of lint-free tissue (or cotton tipped applicators)

### Setup
- Have the patient seated and looking straight ahead. No other setup is needed.

### Procedure
*V1-V3—Ophthalmic, Maxillary, and Mandibular Branch (Sensory)*
1. Show the patient the cotton tip applicator and say that this is what you will be using for the test. Then ask them to close their eyes.
2. Instruct the patient to tell you when they feel you touch their face and to compare the strength of the touch on the left and right sides of their face.
3. Test the patient's touch sensation by lightly dragging the tip of the cotton tip applicator 5 cm from left to right or right to left at each of the six locations diagrammed in **Figure 8-5**: the left and right forehead, the left and right cheek near the upper lip, and the left and right chin or lower lip.

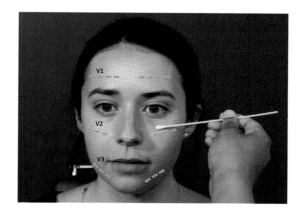

**FIGURE 8-5.** | Photo illustrating where to stimulate the patient's face using a cotton tip applicator when performing the trigeminal nerve (CN-V) sensory function test.

*Note*: These locations allow sampling of areas innervated by each of the branches of the trigeminal nerve. The points of touch should be symmetrical with respect to the midline of the patient's face.

An alternative to step 3 is to simultaneously touch the face with equal pressure in two mirror image locations. Have the patient report if the touches are equal or if one is stronger than the other.

### V1—Ophthalmic Branch, Corneal Sensitivity

1. With cleaned hands, pull apart the tip of two cotton tip applicators to make a small wisp of cotton. Hold one in each hand.

2. Have the patient open their eyes and look up and to the left. Approach the patient in such a way that they cannot see your hand. Touch their right cornea near the limbus with the wisp of cotton at the end of the cotton tipped applicator. Observe the strength of the reflex blink response in this eye (**see Figure 8-6**).

3. Have the patient look up and to the right. Using the second cotton tipped applicator, approach the patient in such a way that they cannot see your hand. Touch the left cornea near the limbus with the wisp of cotton at the end. Observe the strength of the reflex blink response in this eye.

*Note*: During steps 2 and 3 be sure to avoid touching the eyelashes of either eye.

4. Compare the strength of the blink responses elicited by touching the right and the left corneas.

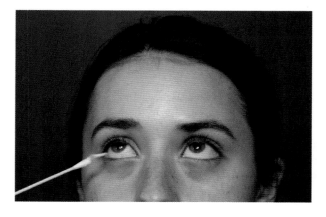

**FIGURE 8-6.** | Photo illustrating the corneal sensitivity test using a wisp of the cotton tip applicator. Notice the examiners inferior approach as the patient looks up.

*V3—Mandibular Branch (Motor)*

1. Ask the patient to open their mouth as wide as they can while you apply gentle but firm resistance by pushing up on the jaw upwards with one hand. Observe carefully for a deviation of the jaw toward the left or right.
2. Ask the patient to close their mouth and clench their jaw.
3. Palpate the masseter and temporal muscles, feeling for a difference in muscle tone between the right and left side.

## Recording

- If all functions of the trigeminal nerve are normal and both sides of the face are equally sensitive and equally strong, record "trigeminal nerves intact" or "trigeminal nerves symmetrical."
- If the patient has reduced sensitivity, record "fine touch reduced" and indicate the part of the face that is affected.

## Examples

- CN-V: sensory divisions intact and symmetrical.
- Trigeminal nerve: reduced light touch sensitivity upper left forehead. Other sensory divisions intact. Motor divisions symmetrical.
- Trigeminal nerve (CN-5): reduced light touch and pain sensation in lower left jaw. Muscles weaker on left. Other divisions intact.

## 8.9 FACIAL NERVE FUNCTION TEST

### Purpose

The aim of this procedure is to assess the functional integrity of the somatic motor, taste, and parasympathetic divisions of the facial nerve, CN-VII (or CN-7), and its supranuclear control pathways.

### Equipment

- Table salt
- Glass of water
- Two sterile cotton tipped applicators with a small amount of cotton pulled out to form a point
- Equipment for a Schirmer #1 test (see Procedure 5.10)
- Small ruler marked in millimeters

### Setup

- The patient should be seated upright in normal room illumination.

### Procedure

1. Carefully examine the patient's face, comparing the left and right sides, looking for asymmetries such as loss of facial wrinkles or the nasolabial fold on one side of the face when the patient relaxes their facial muscles. Look for asymmetries in the upper and the lower face separately.
2. Place all four fingers of both your hands over the patient's eyebrows. As you pull down gently, instruct the patient to attempt to raise both eyebrows together. Compare the strength with which they can pull their right and left eyebrows against the resistance of your fingers. Look for left versus right asymmetries in the amount of wrinkling of the forehead skin.

3. Instruct the patient to "furrow" or pull their eyebrows together. Look for asymmetry in their ability to pull the left and right brow together.

4. Instruct the patient to close their eyes tightly and look at the lids and lashes of both eyes. The base of the lashes should be hidden by lid tissue. Compare the left and right eyes.

5. Instruct the patient to close their eyes tightly while you attempt to pull their eyes open. Compare the ability of the right and left orbicularis oculi muscles to resist the forced opening of the eyes. *Note*: Look for a Bell's phenomenon (an upward and sometimes outward rolling of the eyes on attempted eyelid closure).

6. Instruct the patient to inflate or "puff out" both cheeks simultaneously. Instruct them to attempt to smile, then to frown. Then, have the patient purse their lips or attempt to whistle. Look for asymmetries in the size and tightness of the left and right cheek.

7. Measure the distance between each outer canthus and the ipsilateral corner of the mouth.

8. Instruct the patient to rinse out their mouth with clean water and stick out their tongue. Sprinkle a small quantity of salt on one side near the front of the tongue and have the patient report what they taste. Have them rinse out their mouth again and sprinkle salt on the other side of the tongue. Instruct the patient to compare their taste sensation on the two presentations to the best of their ability.

   *Note*: As an alternative, sprinkle salt and sugar on their tongue and ask them to identify what they are tasting.

9. Perform a Schirmer #1 test (see Procedure 5.10) to assess lacrimal gland function.

### Recording
- If all CN-VII functions are within normal limits, record "all facial muscles symmetrical, taste WNL," and record the results of the Schirmer #1 test per the instructions for that test.
- Describe any facial asymmetry or functional abnormality observed.

### Examples
- CN-VII: All facial muscles symmetrical, taste WNL, Schirmer #1: 20 mm OD and OS in 5 min.
- Facial Nerve: Weakness of upper and lower muscles on left face; taste intact; Schirmer #1: 22 mm OD and 7 mm OS / 5 min.

## 8.10 SCREENING TESTS FOR CN I, VIII, IX, X, XI, AND XII

### Purpose
The aim of this procedure is to rapidly and superficially test the functions of the CNs not closely associated with ocular functions.

### Equipment
- Two or three vials containing different aromatic substances, such as coffee, vanilla, chocolate powder, soap, or oil of wintergreen

   *Note*: Avoid noxious chemicals
- Penlight (*optional*)

### Setup
- The patient should be seated comfortably in the examination chair under bright illumination.
- The patient closes their eyes.

## Procedure

*Olfactory Nerve (CN-I):*

1. Have the patient occlude their left nostril. Hold one of the vials containing an aromatic substance beneath their right nostril and have them inhale. Ask them if they smell anything, and if so, what the substance is.

2. Have the patient occlude their right nostril. Hold another vial containing a different aromatic substance beneath their left nostril and have them inhale. Ask them if they smell anything, and if so, what the substance is.

3. Ask the patient to report any differences they may have noticed in their sense of smell in the right and left nostril.

*Vestibulocochlear Nerve (CN-VIII):*

1. Tell the patient that you will be making a sound on either side of their head near their ears. Instruct them to tell you when they first hear the sound and to point to the ear in which they hear it.

2. Hold your hand approximately 50 cm away from the patient's right ear and rub your index finger and thumb together gently to produce a soft sound. Slowly move your hand toward the patient's right ear until they report that they hear the sound. Note the distance at which this takes place.

3. Repeat step 2 for the patient's left ear and compare the distance at which each ear first heard the fingers rubbing together.

4. Instruct the patient to hum. Ask them if their voice sounds louder in one ear or the other or if it sounds equally loud.

   *Note:* A ticking watch can be used as an alternative to rubbing fingers.

*Glossopharyngeal Nerve (CN-IX) and Vagus Nerve (CN-X):*

1. Instruct the patient to swallow and observe for any difficulty or delayed response. Ask the patient if they experienced any difficulty when swallowing. Alternatively, the patient can be given a cup of water and asked to take a small sip and swallow.

2. Instruct the patient to open their mouth wide and say "ah." Observe the elevation of the soft palate on each side of the back of the throat or deviation of the uvula. A penlight may aid in observation.

*Accessory Nerve (CN-XI):*

1. Observe the relative height of the patient's shoulders.

2. Have the patient shrug both shoulders simultaneously. Compare the elevation of the left and right shoulders during the shrug.

3. Place both hands on the patient's shoulders and push down gently.

4. Have the patient shrug both shoulders and compare the force with which the left and right shoulders push against the resistance of your hands holding them down.

*Hypoglossal Nerve (CN-XII)*

1. Instruct the patient to stick their tongue straight out.

2. Note whether the tongue lies straight along the patient's midline or if it deviates to one side or the other.

## Recording

- Record the CN tested.
- Describe the patient's response to the test.

## Examples

- CN-I: correctly identified coffee and chocolate in left and right nostril

  CN-VIII: heard fingers at 35 cm right ear/at 5 cm left ear. Hum sounded louder in right ear

  CN-IX and X: uvula deviates to the right, poor left sided soft palate elevation. Reports difficulty when swallowing

  CN-XI: left shoulder lower than right/right shoulder elevates more during shrug

  CN-XII: tongue deviates to the right

- CN-I: correctly identified coffee and chocolate in left nostril, barely able to smell in right nostril/failed to ID coffee or chocolate

  CN-VIII: heard fingers @ 35 cm right ear/@ 35 cm left ear. Hum sounded equal in both ears

  CN-IX and X: symmetrical elevation of uvula. Able to swallow without difficulty

  CN-XI: shoulders at equal height during rest and during shrug

  CN-XII: tongue protrudes to the left

For a quick guide to other CNs not addressed in this procedure, **see Table 8-2.**

| TABLE 8-2. Summary of Cranial Nerve Assessment Tests | | |
| --- | --- | --- |
| **Cranial Nerve** | | |
| **Number** | **Name** | **Procedures That Assess the Functions of This Nerve** |
| I | Olfactory | Screening test included above* |
| II | Optic | Visual Acuity<br>Color vision<br>Pupils<br>Screening visual fields<br>Finger counting visual fields<br>Tangent screen |
| III | Oculomotor | Extraocular motilities<br>Pupils<br>Red lens test for a paretic horizontal muscle<br>Pharmacological tests of the pupil<br>Cover test |
| IV | Trochlear | Extraocular motilities<br>Park's three -step method for a paretic vertical muscle |
| V | Trigeminal | Trigeminal nerve function test |
| VI | Abducens | Extraocular motilities<br>Red lens test for a paretic horizontal muscle |
| VII | Facial | Facial nerve function test<br>Schirmer tests |
| VIII, IX, X XI, and XII | Vestibulocochlear, glossopharyngeal, vagus, accessory, hypoglossal | Screening tests included above* |
| *Screening tests for CNs I, VIII, IX, X, XI, and XII are outlined above in Procedure 8.10.<br>CN, cranial nerves | | |

# 9
# Ocular Imaging

Elena Biffi, OD, MSc, FAAO / Anita Gulmiri, OD, FAAO / Maureen Hanley, OD

## 9.1 INTRODUCTION TO OCULAR IMAGING

Ocular imaging technology has become an integral part of eye care and revolutionized our approach to disease identification, diagnosis, and management. The high sensitivity of various ocular instruments with their superior imaging capabilities can provide detailed information on ocular structures, aiding in deeper understanding of disease pathophysiology and progression, thus laying the groundwork for a more objective, image-driven diagnostic approach to common and rare ocular diseases. This chapter provides the foundation for a procedural approach when using these tools in clinical care.

As technology continues to evolve, newer and more specialized instruments are introduced to increase the quality of patient care. The focus in this chapter will be on the most common ocular imaging technologies used by primary eye care providers today for a variety of ocular conditions ranging from corneal dystrophies to optic nerve abnormalities. While ocular imaging has become an integral part of managing certain ocular conditions such as in diabetic retinopathy, it is important to note that imaging does not replace the dilated exam and is meant to be supplemental. The provider is responsible for carefully and critically reviewing all ocular imaging acquired for their patient in addition to providing the standard of care for each condition they manage.

While proper analysis of the image acquired for any of the procedures listed in this chapter is essential for proper patient care, it is beyond the scope of this text to provide a comprehensive review of every possible anomalous result that may manifest on each of these instruments. Instead, proper recording is outlined in order to provide the examiner with the framework to apply the information when clinically relevant according to their expertise.

Many of the devices used for ocular imaging store patient information for proper review and therefore must be secure and password protected (see Procedure 1.2). Furthermore, all acquired images should be securely stored and archived as part of the patient record or file to safeguard protected health information.

## 9.2 OCULAR PHOTOGRAPHY

### Purpose
The aim of this procedure is to image anterior and posterior segment ocular structures for the purpose of photo-documentation and diagnosis and management of ocular disease. A variety of filters and imaging modalities can be used for fundus photography highlighting structures and pathologies otherwise not visible on ophthalmoscopy alone.

### Equipment
- Slit lamp camera (anterior segment imaging)
- Fundus camera (posterior segment imaging)
  *Note:* The examiner should review the instructions provided by the manufacturer for the specific model and fundus camera configuration. Various posterior segment cameras offer a variable angle of view ranging from 30° to ultra-widefield (up to 200°) and can be mydriatic or non-mydriatic. In standard color fundus photography, retina is illuminated by white light and examined in full color. In contrast to the traditional monochromatic photography scanning confocal laser is another type that uses lasers of different wavelengths scanning across the retina in a raster pattern and allowing for a wider angle of view even without the need of dilation to acquire the image. In addition, fundus cameras can have different filters and various imaging modalities, including red-green-blue channel split, multicolor photography, fluorescein angiography, indocyanine green angiography and fundus autofluorescence. Some cameras have multiple modifiable settings, while other cameras are fully automatic. Some fundus cameras are contraindicated for patients with epilepsy and seizure disorder due to the bright flash and medical history should be confirmed prior to imaging.
The following components are common to all fundus cameras:
- Adjustable chin rest and forehead rest to support the patient's head comfortably during testing and to align the instrument with the patient's eye or outer canthus
- A button to raise and lower the instrument table to a comfortable height for the patient
- Focus control button or a joystick to move the instrument toward the patient until focus of desired structures is achieved
- A focusing target (internal within the device or external that is attached to device exterior) for the patient to fixate
- Device-dependent internal focus and position controls (can be automated or manual)

### Setup
- The patient may need to be dilated prior to the start of the procedure for posterior segment imaging (see Procedure 5.7 and eyedrop/dilating precautions). In addition, lubricating eyedrops may need to be used to prevent dry eye related reduction in image quality.
- The patient removes their glasses. Contact lenses should be removed for anterior segment imaging unless the lenses are the subject of the image. Contact lenses may remain in place for certain fundus cameras but may contribute to ocular dryness while images are being acquired.
- Instrument setup:
  - Turn on the instrument's power.
  - Remove the lens cap from the front lens, if applicable.

- Disinfect the chin rest and forehead rest by wiping it with alcohol and drying it with a tissue.
- Open imaging software if applicable and enter new patient's information or find the existing patient.
• Adjust the height of the patient's chair and the instrument to a comfortable position for both the patient and the examiner.
• Instruct the patient to position their chin on the chinrest and forehead against the headrest. *Note:* Some instruments have a single chinrest while others have one to position the patient for right eye image acquisition and another for the left eye.
• Raise or lower the chin rest until the patient's outer canthus is aligned with the hash mark on the upright support of the instrument or with the pointer on the side of the instrument.

## Procedure

*Slit Lamp Camera*

1. Position the patient in the slit lamp so that it is comfortable for both the patient and the examiner (see Procedure 5.2).
2. Use desired illumination, magnification, and beam width and height to focus on the particular structure to be imaged. Slit lamp cameras often have a separate screen to preview the tentative image before the photo is captured.

   *Note:* Many slit lamp cameras have a diffuser which cuts down on harsh concentrated light and prevents the structures from being "washed out" in the image.

3. When desired focus and centration are achieved, click the joystick, button, or touchscreen to take the image.
4. Repeat steps 2-3 on the patient's other eye and/or for each structure or finding to be imaged, as necessary.
5. Review acquired images for quality and repeat imaging as necessary.

*Fundus Camera*

1. Use the joystick, relevant knobs, or buttons, to position the device so that the pupil is in the center of the alignment image.

   *Note:* Some ultra-wide field instruments require the patient to move their head to one side and/or move closer or further from the camera for image acquisition, and the examiner may have to help guide the patient.

2. Adjust the height, focus, and centration according to the specification of the particular fundus camera used. Most instruments display the tentative image on a screen and these controls may be adjusted to maximize image quality.
3. When desired focus and centration are achieved, click the joystick, button, or touchscreen to take the image. On some devices, images would be taken automatically when desired positioning and focus are accomplished.

   *Note:* Posterior pole imaging often has an internal target for the patient to fixate. If another region of the retina is desired for imaging, the internal fixation target (or external fixation target) can be moved to image other retinal areas.

4. Repeat steps 1–3 on the patient's other eye and/or for each imaging modality, as necessary.
5. Review acquired images for quality and repeat imaging as necessary.

## Recording

Write down the following:
• Type of procedure performed and image modality
• Location: right/left eye

- Quality of the image
- Pertinent findings
- Comparison to the previous images, if applicable
- Summary or impression of the image(s)
- Plan of action including when patient should return to clinic (RTC)

*Examples*

- Fundus photography performed today for baseline on both eyes with good reliability OU. Color images showed oval greenish-gray lesion of ~1–1.25 DD in size with no obvious elevation and with distinct borders; location: along inferior temporal arcade OD; (–)drusen and (–)lipofuscin (**see Figure 9-1**). The lesion disappeared with the red-free filter and became more prominent with green-free filter. Left eye was normal. Impression: choroidal nevus OD, Plan: RTC 4–6 months for follow-up to ensure stability.

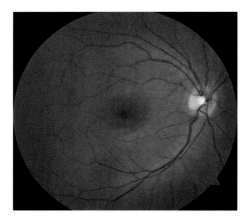

**FIGURE 9-1.** | Fundus photography example of the right eye. For documentation of this image, see the recording under section "Examples."

## 9.3 CORNEAL TOPOGRAPHY

### Purpose

The aim of this procedure is to obtain information on the corneal profile and curvature, including the power, and shape of the cornea. It is also valuable in the diagnosis of corneal conditions, initial fitting and monitoring of contact lens fits, such as for orthokeratology (see Procedure 6.17), and for selecting eligible candidates for refractive surgery and monitoring these patients postoperatively. Corneal topography may also be used to assess the integrity of the ocular surface, including the tear film.

The traditional method of collecting information on the cornea has been with a manual keratometer (see Procedure 3.16), however this method only provides information on approximately the central 3 mm of the corneal surface. When more information on the cornea is needed, a corneal topographer can be used to provide up to 10 mm of data points (depending on scan quality).

### Equipment

- Corneal topographer

  *Note:* There are several different types of corneal topographers available on the market. These modalities include:

  - *Placido disc technology:* Uses reflection for curvature analysis. Concentric white rings of light are displayed on a black background and the reflection from the tear film and the anterior cornea is projected on a corneal map. Quantitative and qualitative information on the corneal curvature is recorded. The drawback to placido disc technology is the lack of information provided on the posterior corneal surface. **See Figure 9-2.**

- *Scanning-slit technology:* Uses multiple projected scanning slit beams to capture the reflected beams to create data points on both the anterior and posterior corneal surface, and corneal pachymetry.
- *Scheimpflug technology:* Uses a rotating camera to capture cross-sectional images of the cornea and anterior chamber. This method provides superior accuracy and resolution and corrects for any image distortion that comes with capturing the non-planar corneal shape. It also provides information on the anterior and posterior corneal surface, as well as global corneal pachymetry and information on the anterior chamber angle.

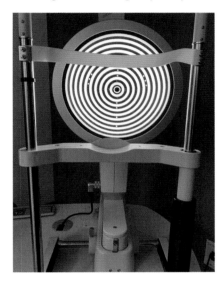

FIGURE 9-2. | Concentric rings (mires) of the corneal topographer utilizing placido disc technology.

Depending on the specific model and type of corneal topographer, the examiner should review the specific instructions provided by the manufacturer. The following components are common to most corneal topographers:

- An automatic method to raise and lower the instrument table to a comfortable height for the patient
- Adjustable chin rest and forehead rest to support the patient's head comfortably during testing
- A knob to raise or lower the chin rest to align the patient's outer canthus with the dash marker on the instrument
- A joystick for focusing and alignment
- A fixation target (typically internal within the device)
- A computer system housing the corneal topography software and patient database
- Device-dependent internal focus and position controls

## Setup
- Disinfect the chin rest and forehead rest of the corneal topographer by wiping it with alcohol and drying it with a tissue.
- Ask the patient to remove their glasses and/or contact lenses.
- Turn on the instrument's power.

- Turn on the computer system connected to the corneal topographer then open up the corneal topographer software application.
  - The corneal topography software houses a database of patient information. Enter the new patient's demographic information and medical record number as prompted by the software or find the existing patient from the database.
- Adjust the height of the patient's chair and the instrument to a comfortable position for both the patient and the examiner.
- Unlock the instrument controls. This is necessary on some corneal topographers.

## Procedure

1. Explain the procedure and the reason for conducting the procedure to the patient.
2. On the corneal topography software, select the option to acquire a new image. *Note: Another option will allow the examiner to review or analyze a previously acquired image.*
3. Instruct the patient to place their chin in the chin rest and their forehead against the headrest.
4. Raise or lower the chin rest until the patient's outer canthus is aligned with the hash mark on the upright support of the instrument or with the pointer on the side of the instrument.

   *Note:* Lubricating eye drops may be used to prevent dry eye related reduction in image quality.
5. Slide the topography instrument head to the examiner's left to capture the patient's right eye.
6. Push the joystick forward toward the patient's right cornea.
7. Instruct the patient to maintain fixation on the target (typically a colored light).
8. Depending on the device, the computer/corneal topography software will display focusing and positioning prompts such as:

   a. Rings of corneal mires: Focus the mires such that each ring is clear in quality, even in size, and uniform in spacing compared to other rings.

   b. Prompts for centration (**see Figure 9-3**): Use the joystick to adjust the positioning to best align the eye for image acquisition. Follow prompts given by the software. Often only very fine adjustments are required for optimal centration and alignment.

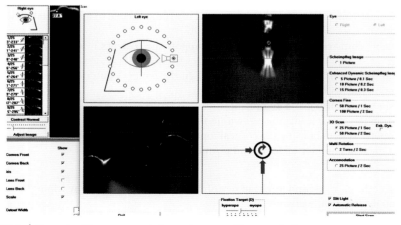

**FIGURE 9-3.** | Example of image prompts for center corneal topography image.

9. Once focused, the image will capture automatically. Most corneal topography software applications also have a manual image acquisition mode, in which case, the examiner will click the joystick or press "capture image" on the computer to acquire the image.

10. Repeat steps 5–9 but now moving the instrument to the examiner's right side to capture images for the patient's left eye.

11. Ask the patient to sit back.

12. On the corneal topography software, select the option that allows the examiner to analyze the acquired images. Ensure appropriate image scan quality. Repeat image acquisition as necessary.

## Recording

After image acquisition, corneal topography color maps are generated by the software system for analysis. Corneal topography image maps are analyzed, and image interpretations are recorded. These maps will provide both qualitative and quantitative data points in a variety of ways:

- Simulated keratometry readings provide an average keratometry reading across the steep and flat meridians of the anterior cornea.
- Axial display maps provide a color-coded map of the absolute corneal power across the anterior corneal surface.
- Tangential display maps are more sensitive than axial maps and they provide information on the shape of the anterior corneal surface.
- Elevation maps are displayed based on a theoretical "best-fit sphere" reference. Areas of relative elevation and depression are mapped compared to this reference. Elevation maps are more accurate for scanning slit and Scheimpflug technology compared to placido disc technology.
- Astigmatism is represented on the map as a bow-tie pattern. Symmetrical astigmatism is displayed as an even bow on either side, whereas asymmetrical astigmatism is displayed with irregularity and unevenness in the colors and size of the bow-tie patterns.
- Steep areas of the cornea are color-coded as red, or warmer colors and flat areas of the cornea are color-coded as blue, or cooler colors.
- Record for each eye separately.
- Record the quality of the scan.
- Record the power and the meridian for the flat meridian first, then the steep meridian.
- Record the amount of corneal astigmatism in diopters and the type of astigmatism as displayed by bow-tie pattern:
  - WTR or WR—with the rule (more corneal power in the vertical meridian, corneal map will display red bowtie vertically;
  - ATR or AR—against the rule (more corneal power in the horizontal meridian, corneal map will display red bowtie horizontally;
  - OBL or Obl.—oblique (major meridians within ±15° of 45° and 135°); and
  - Irregular—the two principal meridians are not 90° apart.
- Record the condition of the mires: mires clear and regular or mires irregular and distorted.
- If previous corneal topography maps are available, state whether the current map is stable, or a significant change is noted. Comment on any progression of an irregularity.

## 9.4 OPTICAL COHERENCE TOMOGRAPHY (OCT)

### Purpose

The aim of this procedure is to obtain cross-sectional images of the cornea, anterior chamber (cornea-to-iris) angle, retina, macula, optic nerve, and ocular vasculature for the purpose of diagnosis and management of ocular pathologies, otherwise not visible with ophthalmoscopy or ocular photography.

### Indications

OCT is used as a diagnostic device to aid in the detection and management of patients with narrow angles, corneal pathologies, retinal diseases, macular conditions, optic nerve abnormalities, and vascular/systemic ocular conditions. It is indicated for in-vivo, cross-sectional, and three-dimensional images of anterior and posterior ocular structures, including cornea, retina, retinal nerve fiber layer, ganglion cell layer, macula thickness, and optic nerve head. OCT is particularly useful for monitoring condition progression as small changes in the order of microns can be observed. Each manufacturer uses their own normative database and segmentation analysis to provide qualitative and quantitative information, thickness of retinal layers, optic nerve parameters and vascular flow.

### Equipment

- OCT instrument

  *Note:* Depending on the specific model and OCT configuration, the examiner should review the specific instructions provided by the manufacturer. There are many OCT imaging modalities, that include:

  - *OCT-Anterior Segment (OCT-AS):* Used to obtain cross-sectional images of cornea to detect layers of the cornea in detail and assess for corneal pathology. This mode can aid in the assessment of corneal thickness or to assess the fit of a scleral contact lens. This mode also offers imaging of anterior chamber angle evaluation and may include software for cornea-to-iris angle analysis.
  - *OCT-Retina:* Used to obtain cross-sectional detailed images of various retinal layers in the macular area, as well as other fundus locations. Detailed line scans can provide in depth information about the integrity and pathology within the retina. Quantitative (based on the normative database) analysis can provide information of macular thickness in fovea and peri-foveal areas.
  - *OCT-Optic Nerve:* Used to obtain analysis of the optic nerve head, retinal nerve fiber layer, and macular ganglion cell layers. Both qualitative and quantitative information about the optic nerve can assist greatly in diagnosis and management of optic nerve abnormalities.
  - *OCT-Angiography (OCT-A):* Used to obtain three-dimensional information about retinal and choroidal vascular structure and flow to facilitate comprehensive clinical assessment.
  - Some OCT instruments have multiple modifiable settings, and some are fully automatic.

The following components are common to all OCT instruments:

- Adjustable chin rest and forehead rest to support the patient's head comfortably during testing and align the instrument with the patient's eye or outer canthus
- A button to raise and lower the instrument table to a comfortable height for the patient
- Focus control button or a joystick to move the instrument toward the patient until focus of desired structures is achieved

- A focusing target (internal within the device or external that is attached to device exterior) for the patient to fixate
- Device-dependent internal focus and position controls (can be automated or manual)

## Setup
- The patient may need to be dilated prior to the start of the procedure for posterior segment imaging (see Procedure 5.7 and eyedrop/dilating precautions). Dilation is associated with better image quality for posterior segment images. In addition, lubricating eyedrops may need to be used to prevent dry eye related reduction in image quality.
- The patient removes their glasses. Contact lenses should be removed for anterior segment imaging unless the lenses are the subject of the image.
- Instrument setup:
  - Turn on the instrument's power.
  - Remove the lens cap from the front lens, if applicable.
  - Disinfect the chin rest and forehead rest by wiping it with alcohol and drying it with a tissue.
  - Open imaging software if applicable and enter new patient's information or find the existing patient.
- Adjust the height of the patient's chair and the instrument to a comfortable position for both the patient and the examiner.
- Instruct the patient to position their chin on the chinrest and forehead against the head-rest. *Note:* Some instruments have a single chinrest while others have one to position the patient for right eye image acquisition and another for the left eye.
- Raise or lower the chin rest until the patient's outer canthus is aligned with the hash mark on the upright support of the instrument or with the pointer on the side of the instrument.

## Procedure
1. Chose the desired imaging mode: anterior segment, retina, optic nerve, or angiography.

   *Note:* Some instruments with an anterior segment imaging modality require that a different lens be attached to the instrument, or a new headrest bar is put in place to allow the device to focus on anterior segment structures.
2. Use the joystick, relevant knobs, or buttons to position reticle (target) in the middle of the patient's pupil.
3. Adjust the height, focus, and centration according to the specification of the OCT instrument. In most instruments, a preview of the image will appear on the screen showing both the en face image of the ocular structures and the cross section. The examiner may assess the image quality, brightness, and centration using this preview and adjust as needed.
4. When desired focus and centration are achieved, click the joystick, button, or touchscreen to take the image. On some devices, images would be taken automatically when desired positioning and focus are accomplished.
5. Repeat steps 1–4 on the patient's other eye and/or for each ocular structure, region, or imaging modality, as necessary.
6. Review acquired images for quality and repeat imaging as necessary.

## Recording
Write down the following:
- Type of procedure performed and image modality
- Location: right/left eye

- Quality of the image
- Pertinent findings
- Comparison to the previous images, if applicable
- Summary or impression of the image(s)
- Plan of action including when patient should RTC

## Examples

- OCT-Macula Thickness performed today for baseline on both eyes with good reliability (Signal Strength 6/10 OD and 6/10 OS). In the right eye, macular thickness was increased in the fovea (517 μm) and in all other sectors 360° surrounding the fovea. In the left eye, macular thickness was normal in the fovea (238 μm), but borderline thickening was seen superiorly. Right eye shows (+)intra-retinal fluid with (+)pseudohole and (+)pseudocyst foveally. The contour of the photoreceptor layer and retinal pigment epithelium layers appears normal in both eyes. **See Figure 9-4.** Impression: Severe epiretinal membrane OD with (+)pseudohole and intra-retinal fluid. Mild epiretinal membrane OS. Consider referral for surgical treatment of epiretinal membrane.

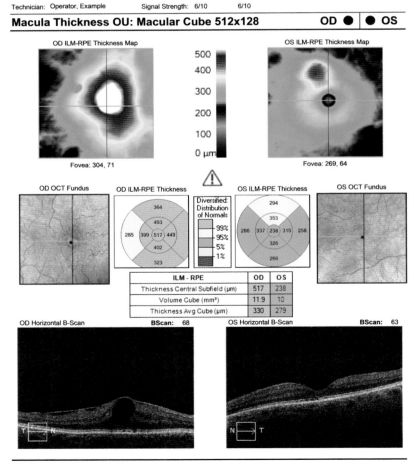

**FIGURE 9-4.** | Macular OCT scan example. For documentation of this image, see the recording under section "Examples."

## 9.5 OCULAR BIOMETRY

### Purpose
Ocular biometry is an important technology used to assess the length of the various structures within the eye. The past and current primary use of ocular biometry is to determine eye length for the purposes of calculating appropriate intraocular lens power. Ocular biometry is being used more commonly to measure axial length (AXL) during myopia management. Excessive AXL is an important contributor to variety of ocular diseases, and it is important to assess posterior pole pathology.

### Indications
- To obtain biometric measurements of ocular structures inside the eye:
  - Corneal curvature and thickness
  - Anterior chamber depth (ACD)
  - Lens thickness
  - AXL
  - The size and ultrasound characteristics of masses inside the eye
- To determine the power of the intraocular lens needed at the time of cataract extraction surgery, using a formula that includes the AXL of the eye, lens thickness, and the corneal curvature (keratometry)
- To manage the progression of myopia by tracking the rate of change of AXL during treatment. Depending on the treatment modality, it may also be indicated to obtain measurements of the central corneal thickness and ACD to account for changes in those measurements when monitoring progression of myopia.

### Contraindications
Ocular biometry has traditionally been obtained using amplitude scan (A-scan) ultrasound (e.g., A-2500 Sonomed, Echoscan US-800), which required topical anesthesia. The contraindications of using an A-scan are those of using topical anesthetics. Nowadays, optical biometers are more commonly used. There are three main types of optical biometers: (1) based on partial coherence interferometry (PCI) (e.g., IOLMaster 500, AL-Scan, Pentacam AXL), (2) based on A-scan optical low-coherence interferometry (e.g., Lenstar LS 900, Aladdin), and (3) based on B-scan swept-source optical coherence tomography (SS-OCT) (e.g., IOLMaster 700, Galilei G6 ColorZ, OA-2000, ARGOS). No contraindications are expected from optical biometers as the light exposure is brief and well under the permissible limits.

Even though not considered a contraindication, the following ocular pathologies may lead to inaccurate AXL measurements: corneal diseases, corneal distortions from diseases or from contact lens wear, and significant ocular lens opacities.

### Equipment
- Ocular biometry unit/instrument (this procedure will describe the use of optical biometers)

*Basic Components of the Optical Biometry Unit*
The examiner shall review the specific instructions provided by the manufacturer and become familiar with the use of the instrument before using it on patients. Manufacturers offer training sessions to learn the use of the devices. The following components are common to all optical biometers:
- Adjustable chin rest and forehead rest to support the patient's head comfortably at the correct position during testing

- A focusing target (internal within the device or external that is attached to device exterior) for the patient to fixate during the measurements
- Device-dependent internal focus and position controls (can be automated or manual) to focus the mires on the patient's ocular surface

## Setup

- Patient removes their glasses or contact lenses prior to the procedure.
- Device setup, before the patient arrives:
  - Turn on the instrument's power.
  - Calibrate the instrument (as necessary) following manufacturer's instructions. Typically, the instrument needs to be calibrated daily or weekly.
  - Enter new patient's information or find the existing patient, if applicable.
  - Disinfect the chin rest and forehead rest of the instrument by wiping it with alcohol and drying it with a tissue.
- Adjust the height of the patient's chair and the instrument to a comfortable position for the patient. Ensure the patient has their feet on the floor for stability (**see Figure 9-5**). For young children, standing may be a better option.
- Instruct the patient to position their chin on the chin rest and forehead against the headrest.
- Raise or lower the chin rest until the patient's outer canthus is aligned with the hash mark on the upright support of the instrument or with the pointer on the side of the instrument.

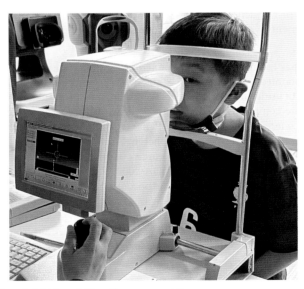

FIGURE 9-5. | Setup of child for axial length measurement.

## Procedure

*Note:* The procedure described below references the Zeiss IOLMaster 700 user manual, but the authors make no specific recommendation on instrument selection.

1. Pull the instrument base toward the examiner and move it in front of the patient's eye to be examined.
2. Using the joystick or relevant knobs, position the device so that the pupil is in the center of the aligned image.

3. Adjust the height, focus, and centration according to the specification of the manufacturer.

4. When desired focus and centration are achieved, click the joystick or press "capture image" on the instrument screen to take the measurements. On some devices, measurements would be taken automatically when desired position is accomplished.

5. Repeat steps 1-4 on the patient's other eye and/or for each imaging modality, as necessary.

### Recording
- Record each eye separately.
- Record the AXL of the eye. If the device provides other measurements, such as ACD or lens thickness, these may also be recorded, as needed.
- Record keratometry measurements: the power and the meridian for the horizontal meridian first (the primary meridian, K1) and the power and meridian for the vertical meridian (secondary meridian, K2).
- If indicated, calculate and record the power of IOL. *Note:* There are numerous equations that may be considered for IOL calculation, the discussion of which is outside the scope of the text.

### Examples
- Ocular biometry:

| OD | AXL 24.35 | ACD 3.46 | K1 41.55 at 172, K2 42.75 at 082 |
| OS | AXL 24.25 | ACD 3.41 | K1 41.75 at 004, K2 42.98 at 094 |

## 9.6 B-SCAN ULTRASOUND

### Purpose
B-scan ultrasonography is an important adjunct ocular imaging technology used to assess a variety of ocular diseases, providing a dynamic real-time evaluation of the retina and choroid. In comparison to light-based ocular imaging technologies, sound waves can bypass various pathology; thus, making B-scan an invaluable test for assessing posterior pole disorders in the presence of media opacity.

### Indications
B-scan ultrasonography can be safely done in both adult and pediatric populations, as well as in inpatient and outpatient settings. Below are the conditions for which B-scan ultrasound can be indicated:
- Evaluation of ocular structures when visualization is obscured by media opacity:
  - Eyelid pathology (lid edema, tarsorrhaphy, etc.)
  - Corneal opacity (corneal scar, edema, etc.)
  - Anterior chamber opacity (hyphema, hypopyon, severe uveitis, etc.)
  - Miosis
  - Dense cataracts
  - Vitreous opacity (vitreal hemorrhage, vitritis, etc.)
- Evaluation of posterior segment disorders:
  - Ciliary body lesions (ciliary body cyst, etc.)
  - Ocular tumors (choroidal melanoma, etc.)
  - Vitreous pathology (asteroid hyalosis, persistent hyperplastic primary vitreous, etc.)
  - Retinal detachment (serous, rhegmatogenous, exudative, etc.)
  - Differentiation of posterior vitreous detachment from retinal or choroidal detachment
  - Differentiation of optic disc edema from optic disc drusen
- Detection, localization, and characterization of intraocular foreign body

## Contraindications

B-scan ocular ultrasonography is a non-invasive procedure, and contraindications are rare. Below is the list of potential contraindications and risk factors:

- If examination is performed on an eye with an open lid, improper probe positioning can lead to corneal abrasions
- Scleral laceration
- Rupture or suspected rupture of the globe after trauma

## Equipment

- B-Scan ultrasound instrument is a portable device that consists of the following:
  - A probe that sends acoustic waves into the globe.
  - A marker which acts as a reference point that indicates the top of an echogram.
  - Display video screen that displays echogram image.
    Some newer models have the probe connected directly to any computer/laptop for image display.
- Coupling gel (e.g., ophthalmic methylcellulose solution): Used for better transmission of acoustic waves to minimize reflection and refraction.
- Anesthetic eyedrops (e.g., 0.5% proparacaine): Used if technique is performed on an eye with open lid. Due to the absorption of acoustic waves by ocular structures, B-scan ultrasonography would have the best resolution when done on an eye with an open lid.
- Foot pedal (*optional*): Used to start/stop dynamic scanning to obtain photographic image.

## Setup

- Turn on the B-scan ultrasound device.
- Adjust settings to the desired frequency and length of signal penetration. B-scan ultrasonography uses acoustic waves with high frequencies between 7 million oscillations per second (MHz) to 15 MHz. This is the ideal frequency needed for sound to travel to the posterior portion of the average-size globe. The longer the wavelength (shorter frequency), the deeper the penetration. Some models operate with even higher frequencies of 20-40 MHz range.
- Adjust gain, if indicated, to make sure that it's on the "high" setting. Always start on high gain.
- Position the patient comfortably in a chair with the patient's head comfortably against the headrest.
- Apply a small amount of coupling gel to the tip of the probe.
- Hold the probe in your dominant hand.
- Use your nondominant hand to stabilize patient's head, if needed.
- Position your foot comfortably on the foot pedal (if used).
- When the probe is applied to the patient's testing eye, use one or two fingers for stabilization.

## Procedure

*Probe Positions*

B-scan ultrasonography can be performed in three different orientations (**Table 9-1**):

- *Transverse Scan:* Determines lateral extent of a lesion, imaging mid-periphery or periphery circumferentially between 4 and 6 o'clock hours of the globe.
- *Longitudinal Scan:* Determines radial extent of a lesion extending from anterior (periphery) to posterior (posterior pole) at a specific clock hour.
- *Axial Scan:* Locates lesions in the posterior pole in either vertical or horizontal directions. This is the scan of choice to image optic nerve related abnormalities.

Positioning of the probe, the marker, and the patient's fixation determine where in the globe acoustic waves are traveling to and what part of retina is being imaged on the echogram.

The position of the marker is always displayed at the top of the echogram; whereas patient's fixation is always displayed in the middle axis of the echogram (**see Figures 9-6** and **9-7** for examples).

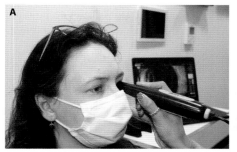
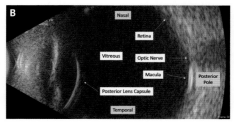

FIGURE 9-6. | (A) Setup of the B-scan probe for an axial scan. Note the marker is beneath the examiner's thumb, and aligned nasally here. (B) This is the corresponding echogram. Note the location of the labeled parts of the globe, nasal, posterior pole, and temporal for this axial scan.

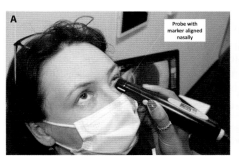
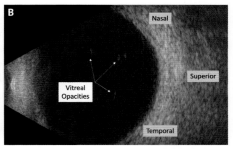

FIGURE 9-7. | (A) Setup of the B-scan probe for a superior transverse scan. (B) Note the locations on the nasal, superior, and temporal aspects of the globe here in the corresponding echogram.

*Basic Screening Procedure*

1. Performed when media opacity obscures the view of the posterior portion of the globe.
2. Perform transverse scan in the 12:00 o'clock position: patient looks superiorly, probe is positioned on inferior conjunctiva with marker orientation nasally (**see Table 9-1** and **Figure 9-6**).
3. Use limbus-to-fornix approach to scan for lesions dynamically. Start at the limbus (less peripheral) and slowly move probe to the fornix (more peripheral).
4. Perform transverse scan in the 3:00 o'clock position: patient looks left, probe is positioned on right conjunctiva with marker orientation superiorly (**see Table 9-1**). Start at limbus and slowly move probe to fornix.
5. Perform transverse scan in the 6:00 o'clock position: patient looks inferiorly, probe is positioned on superior conjunctiva with marker orientation nasally (**see Table 9-1**). Start at limbus and slowly move probe to fornix.
6. Perform transverse scan in the 9:00 o'clock position: patient looks right, probe is positioned on left conjunctiva with marker orientation superiorly (**see Table 9-1**). Start at limbus and slowly move probe to fornix.

7. If a lesion is seen on the transverse scan, then the examiner should proceed to perform "Topographical Evaluation Procedure," see below.

8. After transverse scan was performed at the 12:00, 3:00, 6:00, and 9:00 o'clock orientations, then the posterior pole should be assessed by doing a horizontal axial scan to view the posterior lens surface, optic nerve, and macula simultaneously. The patient looks straight ahead, and the probe is placed on the lid directly over the cornea with the marker oriented nasally (**see Table 9-1**).

9. If indicated, vertical axial scan can be performed to get a vertical cross-section of either macula or optic nerve. The patient looks straight ahead, and the probe is placed on the lid, directly over the cornea with the marker oriented superiorly (**see Table 9-1**).

*Topographical Evaluation of the Lesion Procedure*

1. Performed for diagnostic purposes of orbital lesions and for lesions diagnosed via Basic Screening Procedure.

2. Once the clock hour of a lesion was determined, then transverse scan is performed to obtain lateral extent of the lesion (**see Table 9-1**). The patient looks toward the lesion and the probe is positioned on the opposite side of the globe with the marker being perpendicular to the patient's fixation.

3. Limbus-to-fornix technique should be used when assessing lesions with transverse scan.

4. To determine the radial extent of the lesion, longitudinal scan should be performed next. The patient continues to look toward the lesion, probe is oriented perpendicular to the limbus and continues being positioned on the opposite side of the globe. The marker should be rotated in the way that it would be pointing to the cornea.

5. Limbus-to-fornix technique should be used when assessing lesions with longitudinal scan.

6. Axial scans can be performed, if indicated.

| **TABLE 9-1. Summary of Three Scan Orientations and Corresponding Location of the Retina Being Imaged for Different Directions of Probed Position, Marker Orientation, and Patient's Fixation** | | | | |
|---|---|---|---|---|
| **Scan Orientation** | **Imaged Location of the Globe** | **Patient Fixation** | **Probe** | **Marker** |
| **Transverse:** Lateral extent of a lesion mid-peripherally and peripherally | Superior 9:00 → 3:00 | Up | Inferior conjunctiva | Nasally at 9:00 |
| | Nasal 12:00 → 6:00 | Nasally | Temporal conjunctiva | Superiorly at 12:00 |
| | Inferior 9:00 → 3:00 | Down | Superior conjunctiva | Nasally at 9:00 |
| | Temporal 12:00 → 6:00 | Temporally | Nasal conjunctiva | Superiorly at 12:00 |
| **Longitudinal:** Radial extent of a lesion | Specific clock hour | Toward the direction of the lesion | Opposite side to patient's fixation | Toward the cornea |
| **Axial:** Posterior pole, macula and optic nerve | Horizontal 9:00 → 3:00 | Straight | Center of the cornea | Nasally at 9:00 |
| | Vertical 12:00 → 6:00 | Straight | Center of the cornea | Superiorly at 12:00 |

### Recording

- B-scan ultrasonography images can be recorded as a video or saved as digital or printed images in a patient's chart. It is important to label the type of scan used, as well as to specify retinal location at the top of the echogram, in the middle axis of the echogram, and the bottom of the echogram.

### Examples

- No pathology seen OU with the Basic Screening Procedure.
- Basic Screening Procedure revealed retinal detachment OD superiorly. Superior Transverse scan showed the extent of the lesion from 11 to 2 o'clock. Superior Longitudinal scan showed the radial extent to mid-periphery, not involving posterior pole or macula.

## 9.7 AUTOMATED VISUAL FIELD

### Purpose

The aim of this procedure is to map the patient's visual field whether peripheral or central.

### Indication

This procedure is indicated if the patient is a glaucoma suspect, has glaucoma, or has unexplained or suspected visual field loss. Also indicated if you suspect that the patient may have a neurological visual field defect, or a known or suspected pituitary adenoma. If the patient is taking a medication that needs to be monitored for small changes in visual field sensitivities, this test may be warranted.

### Equipment

- Perimetry instrument
- Eyepatch (if using bowl-style perimeter)

### Setup

Be sure to read the owner's manual for the individual perimeter that you are using. Different makes and models within a brand can vary greatly.

- Dim the lights in the room (so most perimeters will calibrate correctly).
- Turn on standard bowl perimeter or virtual reality (VR) device.
- Find the existing patient or enter the new patient's name, date of birth (DOB), ID or medical record number (MRN), and enter the Rx you will be using to do the test. *Note*: Some instruments offer an Rx calculation feature.
- Disinfect the chin rest and forehead rest with an alcohol wipe and dry with a tissue.
- Choose the appropriate visual field you wish to test:
  - This may include testing the central 10°, 24°, 30°, G and M programs (Octopus), 180°, or a binocular visual field. Some models of perimeters can do custom as well as kinetic visual fields. *Note*: A 30° visual field means the radius of the visual field is 30°.
  - Choose what mode of testing you wish, screening or threshold:
    - Choose which mode of screening, e.g., Humphrey 3 zone or Fast Screening by Octopus. There are many different options in all instruments.
    - Choose which mode of threshold testing, e.g., SITA Fast (Humphrey) or TOP (Tendency Oriented Perimetry by Octopus). Each perimeter has many different modes to choose.
  - The examiner should be familiar with the perimeter they are using, e.g., in some perimeters, the patient needs to be corrected for a 30 cm working distance and therefore you must calculate the appropriate add for that working distance. The working distance

also needs to be considered if the patient is dilated. In other perimeters, the instrument requires you to use the patient's distance Rx either because the add is built into the instrument or the lights are theoretically projected from infinity.

## Procedure

*Note:* The following assumes a bowl-style perimeter.

1. Explain to the patient why they are having this particular test done.

2. Patch the non-tested eye.

3. Position the patient near the perimeter on a safe (sturdy and stable) chair or stool.

4. Place the buzzer in the patient's right hand and explain how to depress the buzzer.

5. Show the patient the fixation target, or on models where you cannot see the fixation target from outside the bowl, explain the concept of the fixation target to the patient.

6. Position the patient so that their chin sits comfortably in the instrument and raise or lower the patient's chin so their pupil can be aligned with the center of the fixation target. Some instruments have optical monitoring devices (screens) which will help you align the patient and help you monitor fixation as the field progresses. Some test for gaze initialization and monitor with gaze tracking.

7. Explain to the patient that they will see lights in their side vision. Some will be bright, and some will be dim. They should always remain looking forward but when they see a light, they should depress the buzzer. They should be instructed to only look at the fixation target.

8. Begin the demo. If the demo is successful (they are responding to the lights and maintaining fixation) then start the real test, if the demo is not successful remove the patient's head from the bowl and re-explain the test to the patient. Some instruments have prepared scripts that a *new* operator can follow to instruct the patient.

9. As the test is progressing, the examiner should be monitoring the patient's fixation by manually watching the patient's eye in the optical monitoring device, monitoring the Heijl Krakau fixation losses, or in some devices also watching the gaze tracker. If fixation is poor, then you should stop the test, reexplain and restart the test again.

10. The examiner should also monitor false positive and false negative results if your mode of testing has these options engaged.

11. When the right eye is done you can give the patient a brief break and then patch the other eye. The patient may have to switch sides on the chinrest for some instruments to align the other eye. Once the other eye is aligned, initiate the test and repeat steps 9 and 10.

12. When the test is done, save and then either print or show on the computer display. The interpretation of the test should be included in the patient's exam record as well as the digital or paper printout for each eye tested.

13. As with all imaging studies, the doctor should explain the testing results to the patient. If this is the first field, explain that the physiological blind spot is normal. The grayscale is very helpful to explain the results to most lay people. If this is not the patient's first field, then show them how this present field compares to past fields.

## Recording

- In many offices, visual fields will be scanned right into the patient's electronic medical record or viewed in an imaging software, but an interpretation still must be written.
- Record the results for each eye separately.
- The quality of the test should be recorded by including parameters such as fixation loses, false negatives, and false positives to ensure you have a valid field. In some testing modes

the only variable the examiner may have available to record is the quality of the gaze track-er and false positives.

- It should be indicated if the test was the baseline exam, or a follow up, and if a follow up, a comparison to previous exams should be included.
- It should be indicated if the patient was dilated or not.
- The general metrics for each eye should be recorded including the Mean Deviation (MD) and Pattern Standard Deviation (PSD) or square root of Loss Variance (sLV).

## Examples

- Humphrey 24-2 Sita Fast, First Field
  OD: (undilated) Fixation Losses 0/12, False Positives 0%, False Negatives 9 %, GHT out-side normal limits, MD −2.44 dB, PSD 8.82. Dense scotoma in inferior Bjerrum area. Find-ings correlate with optic nerve appearance of significant notching of the superior-temporal rim. **See Figure 9-8**.
- Octopus G standard White on White TOPS catch trial 1/8
  OS: undilated, MS 25.0 dB, MD 4.0 dB, sLV 3.2. Moderately dense nasal step inferior with scattered inferior scotomas in Bjerrum area, but stable from last two visual fields and con-sistent with long-standing superior temporal notch from primary open angle glaucoma.

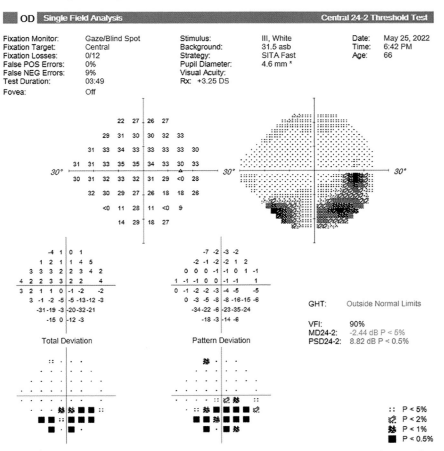

**FIGURE 9-8.** | Visual field example of the right eye. For documentation of this image, see the recording under section "Examples."

**Notes**

- Compare your patient's decibel value at each point with the age acceptable norms at each point. This is called total deviation or comparison.
- Compare your patient's decibel value compared to themselves, pattern deviation or corrected comparison which "filters out" the overall depression to theoretically compensate for overall depressions and help point out deeper defects.
- Evaluate the MD. *Note:* On some instruments a positive (+) MD means the average (or weighted average) of all the dB values for each point was "x-number" of dB better than the average for a person their age (Humphrey style), and in other brands of perimeters a (+) MD means worse than average (Octopus style).
- Evaluate the pattern standard deviation or sLV to evaluate how the slope of your patient's hill of vision deviates from the normal hill of vision.

# 10

# Advanced Ocular Procedures

Elena Biffi, OD, MSc, FAAO / Anita Gulmiri, OD, FAAO / Bina Patel, OD, FAAO

## 10.1 INTRODUCTION TO ADVANCED OCULAR PROCEDURES

Advanced ocular procedures are techniques that go beyond the standard or routine ophthalmic examination. These techniques are usually problem specific and performed by eyecare practitioners when clinically indicated. Many advanced procedures include manipulating ocular structures directly, performing minimally invasive surgical procedures (such as intralesional steroid injection and suturing), removing ocular foreign body (FB), and using anterior segment lasers. The following procedures in this chapter presume that the examiner is intimately familiar with and has mastered the prior procedures mentioned in the text. The goal of this chapter is to provide procedural knowledge on various advanced techniques, ophthalmic lasers, and microsurgical procedures used for treatment and management of ocular diseases.

A number of techniques described in this section involve instruments that are placed in direct contact with ocular surfaces or fluids. It is critical that these instruments be sterile or disinfected following the guidelines set forth by the Centers for Disease Control and Prevention (CDC) (or other local legal requirements if outside the United States), see Procedure 2.2, "Infection Control." The examiner should also observe Standard Precautions whenever a procedure involves touching a patient, e.g., vigorous hand washing with soap and water before and after every patient encounter to prevent the spread of infection. Clear instructions given to the patient are also crucial in maximizing safety and accuracy.

*Note:* Procedures outlined in this chapter may require additional advanced training, privileges, and certification in order to perform them in the patient care setting; restrictions may be in place in certain states and jurisdictions. This text is not intended for any practitioner to use this book alone without the proper hands-on training of the techniques and post-procedural care and management training. Injection training, certification, and/or licensure is a prerequisite for all advanced procedures that require injections. The examiner should consult with regional authorities to ensure the proper training and credentials are obtained before performing these procedures in patient care.

## 10.2 PUNCTAL PLUG INSERTION (TEMPORARY SHORT DURATION IN-TRACANALICULAR COLLAGEN IMPLANT)

### Purpose
The aim of this procedure is to determine if permanent punctal occlusion to treat ocular surface disease or increase drug retention time using temporary short duration intracanalicular collagen implants is effective for diagnostic purposes.

### Indications
Some indications include moderate to severe dry eye disease, to increase drug retention time for ocular lubricants or other ophthalmic drugs, refractive surgery, contact lens wearers, and other ocular surface disease.

### Contraindications
Contraindications to this procedure include allergy to bovine short duration temporary intracanalicular collagen plugs, nasolacrimal infections such as darcryocystitis (acute or chronic), canaliculitis, nasolacrimal obstruction, long term inflammation to the ocular surface, lid changes such as ectropion, and/or conjunctivitis or significant blepharitis.

### Equipment
- Slit lamp (biomicroscope)
- Sterilized or disposable surgical forceps, e.g., Jeweler's forceps
- Topical anesthetic, e.g., 0.5% proparacaine
- Temporary short duration intracanalicular collagen plugs—variety of sizes with diameter of 0.20 mm, 0.30 mm, and 0.40 mm, and 1.60 mm and 2.00 mm in length.
- Cotton tip applicator (*optional*)
- Punctal gauge (*optional*)
- Magnifying loop (*optional*)

### Setup
Slit lamp setup is the same as Procedure 5.2 with the following specifications:
- Adjust the slit beam to a medium width parallelepiped, low to moderate intensity, and set the illumination arm of the biomicroscope centered at 0° or angled between 30 and 45°. Use low magnification of 6× to 10×.
- Disinfect the forceps according to manufacturer and CDC guidelines (or other local legal requirements if outside the United States)
- Instill a drop of a topical anesthetic into the eye to be examined (*optional*) or apply the topical anesthetic to a cotton tip applicator (see Procedure 5.7). Hold the moistened applicator over the puncta (lower or upper) for approximately 30–60 seconds.

## Procedure

*Slit Lamp Technique*

1. Ensure the patient is comfortably seated, and properly position the patient in the slit lamp with their forehead and chin positioned appropriately against the rests.

2. Instruct the patient to look upwards and direct their gaze temporally. Gently and slightly pull down the lower lid to locate the lower puncta.

3. Determine the size of the punctal plug to be used by either using a sterilized punctal size gauge or visually estimate using the slit lamp.

4. Lock the silt lamp and have the patient sit back outside of the slit lamp.

5. Hold the foam cushion with the collagen plugs with one hand (nondominant). Brace your hand to steady it, either using the chin rest or forehead bar of the slit lamp. Make minor hand adjustments by moving the foam cushion slightly forward or backwards to ensure clear focus.

6. Take the forceps and hold with your thumb and index finger with the other hand (dominant).

7. Look outside the slit lamp, place the tips of the forceps towards the top of the form cushion close to the punctal plugs. Brace your hand with the forceps to ensure it is steady either on the bar or chin rest of the slit lamp. Return to look through the slit lamp oculars. Slowly move the forceps to grasp the upper portion of the collagen plug and remove from the foam cushion. (**See Figures 10-1** and **10-2.**)

8. While holding the grasped plug off to the side, ask the patient to return back to the slit lamp and gently pull the lower lid to view the lower puncta with your free hand. Ensure you are clearly focused on the puncta, otherwise unlock and readjust the slit lamp. Instruct the patient to look up and away from the puncta for the duration of the insertion.

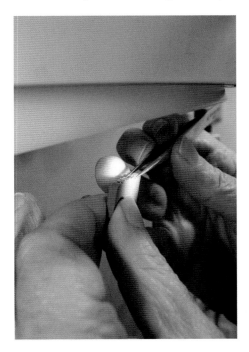

**FIGURE 10-1.** | External view of the examiner removing the temporary collagen plug from the cushion behind the slit lamp, while looking through the slit lamp oculars.

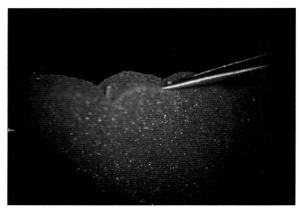

**FIGURE 10-2.** | Examiner's view of plug removal through the slit lamp oculars.

9. Look outside the slit lamp and hold the forceps with the collagen punctal plug approximately 1–1.5 cm (0.5 in) from the lower puncta bracing part of your hand either on the patient's nose, cheek or forehead (**see Figure 10-3**). Always perform this alignment externally (outside of the slit lamp oculars) to ensure safe and proper positioning with the sharp forceps.

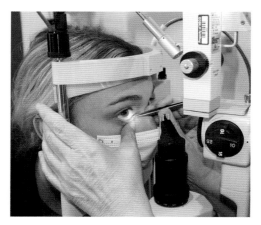

**FIGURE 10-3.** | External view of the examiner's hand and forceps positioning for plug insertion.

10. Gradually move the forceps with the collagen punctal plug to the punctum. Insert the plug vertically into the puncta part way and then release the forceps from the plug (**see Figure 10-4**). Use the tip of the closed forceps to push the plug fully into the puncta. The plug should not be visible.

11. If the collagen plug is destined to be placed horizontally in the canaliculus, gently pull the on the lower lid laterally to allow the plug to slide horizontally in the canaliculus until the plug is no longer visible.

12. Release the lower lid allowing it to resume its normal apposition. To ensure that the plug is not extruding out of the puncta, recheck several minutes after the procedure.

13. To place a collagen plug on the upper puncta, have the patient look down and direct their gaze temporally for the duration of the procedure. Gently lift and hold the upper lid (using your nondominant hand along the orbital bone). Ensure you are focused otherwise readjust the sit lamp. Repeat steps 3 through 12.

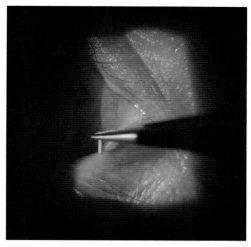

**FIGURE 10-4.** │ Examiner's view of plug insertion through the slit lamp oculars.

*External Technique Using a Magnifying Loop*

1. Ensure the patient is seated comfortably with their head against a head rest in an examination chair.

2. Don the magnifying loop and tighten as needed.

3. Use adequate overall illumination on the patient's face or light attached with the magnifying loop.

4. Instruct the patient to look up and direct their gaze temporally. Gently and slightly pull down the lower lid to locate the lower puncta.

5. Determine the size of the punctal plug to be used by either using a sterilized punctal size gauge or visually estimate using the magnifying loop.

6. Perform the following at a safe distance in space from the patient; hold the foam cushion with the collagen plugs with one hand (nondominant). Take the forceps and hold them with your thumb and index finger with the other (dominant) hand and while viewing through the magnifying loop, slowly move the forceps to grasp the upper portion of the collagen plug and remove from the foam cushion.

7. While holding the plug off to the side with your dominant hand, gently pull down the patient's lower lid with your free (nondominant) hand to view the lower puncta. Instruct the patient to look up and away from the puncta at all times during insertion.

8. Gradually move the forceps with the collagen punctal plug to the punctum. Insert the plug vertically into the puncta part way and then release the forceps from the plug. Use the tip of the closed forceps to push the plug into the puncta. Gently pull the lower lid laterally to allow the plug to slide horizontally in the canaliculus until the plug is no longer visible.

9. Release the lower lid allowing it to resume its normal apposition. To ensure that the plug is not extruding out of the puncta, recheck several minutes after the procedure with a slit lamp.

10. To use a collagen plug on the upper puncta, have the patient look down and direct their gaze temporally for the duration of the procedure. Gently lift and hold the upper lid (using your nondominant hand) along the orbital bone. Repeat steps 5 through 9.

### Recording
- Record the eye and which puncta (upper, lower).
- Record short duration intracanalicular collagen plug with the type, size, and length of plug used.
- Record how the patient tolerated the procedure.

### Examples
- Left lower puncta, intracanalicular temporary short duration collagen plug, size 0.3 mm diameter, 1.6 mm length.  In office procedure. Patient tolerated the procedure well.
- Right upper puncta, intracanalicular temporary short duration collagen plug, size 0.4 mm diameter, 2 mm length.  In office procedure. Patient tolerated the procedure well.

### Notes
- Patient cooperation is important for successful intracanalicular punctal plug insertion.
- Temporary short duration intracanalicular collagen plugs come in a variety of diameters (listed above). There are vertical intracanalicular and horizontal intracanalicular collagen plugs.
- The short duration intracanalicular collagen plugs dissolve between 5 and 14 days, the average being 7–10 days depending on what type are used.
- Intracanalicular collagen plugs reduce tear outflow by approximately 60–80%.
- Lower and or upper puncta can be occluded.
- Prophylactic topical antibiotic maybe prescribed after the procedure.
- The average time for symptoms to improve is approximately 3–5 days. If symptoms improve, consider extended duration temporary intracanalicular collagen plugs (3–6 months) or permanent plugs that partially or completely occlude the puncta and may be reversible.
- Other permanent types of punctal occlusion can be considered such as laser occlusion (punctoplasty) or electrocautery.
- Potential complications include extrusion of the punctal plug, irritation to the punctal area, epiphora, and infection in the punctal and intracanalicular area. If complication is suspected, appropriate follow up care should be performed.

## 10.3 DILATION AND IRRIGATION

### Purpose
The aim of this procedure is to determine the patency of the lacrimal excretory system, as well as to improve flow through the nasolacrimal system. Dilation/irrigation (D/I) is used to remove canalicular obstruction by dilation of the punctum followed by irrigation of the nasolacrimal system with saline injected through the lacrimal canula.

### Indications
Lacrimal D/I should be considered when a patient presents with symptoms of epiphora. Especially in cases of unilateral epiphora in the absence of acute bacterial inflammation or infection, mechanical blockage of the nasolacrimal system should be suspected, and D/I procedure would be indicated. Canalicular obstruction can occur from stenosis, mucous plugs, post-dacryocystitis/canaliculitis or small stones in the tear ducts. Dilation alone can be performed to open a stenosed punctum and allow tear drainage. Irrigation can also be performed to remove an intracanalicular (punctal) plug.

### Contraindications
Active acute infection of the lacrimal sac (dacryocystitis) or canaliculus (canaliculitis).

## Equipment

- Slit lamp (biomicroscope)
- Lacrimal dilator (double-ended stainless steel or disposable plastic)
- 19- to 27-gauge cannula (depends on the size of patient's punctum, 25-gauge is most frequently used)
- 3–5 ml syringe
- Sterile drape/field
- Sterile saline solution

## Setup

- Setup a sterile field to place equipment.
- Prepare the syringe and lacrimal cannula.
  - Open a sterile plastic disposable syringe and lacrimal cannula.
  - Attach the lacrimal cannula by twisting onto the syringe.
  - Remove the plunger and fill the syringe with sterile saline.
  - Reattach the plunger and eject any residual air by ejecting some saline with the syringe/cannula in upright position.
- Instill a drop of topical anesthetic into the inferior conjunctival sac (see Procedure 5.7) and/or soak a cotton-tipped swab with topical anesthetic and place directly over the puncta for 1–2 minutes.
- Open the sterilized or disposable dilator.
- D/I can be performed either behind the slit lamp or outside the slit lamp in "free space". A benefit of performing D/I in free space is the easier accessibility to the patient and freedom of movement. Overhead magnifiers can often be used to provide magnification in free space. A benefit of performing D/I behind the slit lamp is the increased magnification; however, it may be difficult to perform the irrigation procedure behind the slit lamp on the contralateral eye, unless the provider is ambidextrous.

## Procedure

1. Position the patient comfortably in the slit lamp (see Procedure 5.2).
2. Have the patient fixate superior-temporally, away from the puncta and evaluate the puncta.
3. Perform lacrimal sac palpation to rule out active infection, tenderness, and inflammation.
4. Start with *dilation* of the involved eye, or of the inferior punctum on the ipsilateral eye of your dominant hand if epiphora is bilateral (e.g., inferior punctum of the left eye when right-hand dominant). The puncta usually need to be temporarily enlarged in order to be able to comfortably insert a lacrimal cannula for the irrigation procedure.
   a. Using the index finger of your nondominant hand, gently pull down the lower lid to expose the punctum.
   b. Using your dominant hand, hold the dilator in a relatively vertical position with your thumb, index, and middle finger. Use your remaining fingers to brace your hand against the patient's cheek and nose.
   c. Insert the dilator into the puncta vertically and gently advance up to 2 mm into the vertical canaliculus while gently rotating the dilator clockwise and counterclockwise to expand the punctum (**see Figure 10-5**). Do not continue to insert the dilator if it meets an obstruction or resistance.
   d. Gently pull the lower lid temporally to straighten the ampulla and bring the vertical canaliculus into a more horizontal position, so that it lines up with the horizontal canaliculus (**see Figure 10-6**).

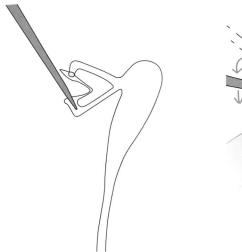

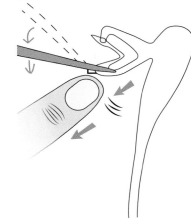

**FIGURE 10-5.** | Schematic of dilator insertion into the vertical canaliculus.

**FIGURE 10-6.** | Schematic of digital straightening of ampulla followed by rotation and advancement of dilator or cannula.

    e. Rotate the dilator and advance gently a few millimeters into the horizontal canaliculus. Again, do not force the dilator in if it meets an obstruction.

    f. Remove the dilator while continuing the rotating motion.

5. Immediately proceed with the *irrigation* portion of the procedure, as the punctum has a tendency to reclose over time.

    a. Hold the prepared syringe with your dominant hand in the same manner as the dilator but have your thumb on the plunger.

    b. Insert the lacrimal cannula vertically into the inferior punctal opening while bracing your hand in a similar fashion as with the dilator.

    c. Let the cannula slide gently downward 2 mm into the vertical canaliculus before rotating the cannula horizontally toward the nose and advancing another 3–4 mm, while holding the lower lid with your nondominant hand to bring the vertical and horizontal canaliculi into alignment. Do not continue to insert the cannula any further if met with an obstruction at any point.

    d. Advance the cannula far enough into the horizontal canaliculus so that it will stay stable during irrigation but take caution not to go too far. If you move too far horizontally toward the nose, you'll hit nasal bone and cause some discomfort for the patient.

    e. Once the cannula is stable in the horizontal canaliculus, apply a slow, gentle pressure on the plunger to inject 1–2 ml of saline and ask the patient to report when they can taste saline or feel it in their nose.

    f. Ask the patient to swallow after irrigating to avoid coughing.

    g. When the patient can feel the saline, slowly remove the cannula in a smooth gentle motion.

6. Perform D/I on the patient's other eye for both inferior and superior puncta, if indicated.

7. *If the lacrimal system is open*, the patient will feel or taste the salty saline in the back of their throat. This result indicates a successful procedure and patency of lacrimal

excretory system. In this instance, the cause of the epiphora could either be a small "easy-to-remove" blockage or it was not due to nasolacrimal duct obstruction.

8. *If the lacrimal system is blocked,* you'll feel resistance of the plunger and see regurgitation of the saline through the punctum. If saline regurgitates through either superior punctum (usually indicates that blockage is distal to the common canaliculus) or inferior punctum (usually indicates the blockage is proximal to the common canaliculus) during irrigation and the patient cannot feel the saline, it indicates a blockage in the nasolacrimal system. In this instance, have an assistant block the superior punctum with a dilator and reirrigate to attempt to release the blockage. If the blockage is not released with additional attempts to irrigate, it is possible that other intervention such as lacrimal probing is indicated. Do not apply excessive force as this can injure the tissue.

## Expected Findings
- If the procedure was uncomplicated and successful, no additional treatment is indicated. Recommended follow-up is 1–2 weeks for symptom assessment.
- In cases where the blockage was difficult to release and/or when significant irritation of the local tissue is suspected after D/I, a topical antibiotic/steroid drop can be prescribed.
- In cases when D/I was not successful, the patient needs to be referred for further assessment (lacrimal probing) and treatment.

## Recording
- Name the procedure, the eye(s), and the result, e.g., D/I was performed in-office successfully. Lacrimal system is open.

## Examples
- D/I was performed in-office on the lower and upper punctum OS. Patient tolerated procedure well. Lacrimal system is open OS.

## 10.4 INTENSE PULSED LIGHT (IPL)

### Purpose
The aim of this procedure is to treat dry eye disease from meibomian gland dysfunction (MGD), ocular inflammation, rosacea, and demodex. The technique consists of delivering a noncoherent and polychromatic light, between the wavelengths of 500–1,200 nm to the skin. Cut-off wavelength filters are utilized for the process of selective photothermolysis of the target chromophores (melanin, hemoglobin, and water) within the dermis. Total energy delivered to the skin is measured in fluence (joules/cm$^2$) and generally ranges from 10 to 16 j/cm$^2$ for the treatment of MGD. Specific energy parameters are adjusted and programmed into the instrument based on the degree of the patient's skin pigmentation. These energy parameters include the fluence, number of sub-pulses, size, and the time interval between each pulse.

Generally, for the treatment of MGD, IPL treatment is applied from tragus to tragus, including the nose and below the orbital bone. After the double pass IPL treatment, immediate meibomian gland expression has been shown to improve patient symptoms. Depending on the IPL instrument utilized, the clinician may be able to choose from preset energy parameters based on the skin pigmentation category or the instrument will require manual adjustments of the energy parameters. An initial and full IPL treatment plan consists of four sessions, held three to six weeks apart. After the conclusion of the initial full treatment, maintenance IPL sessions may be scheduled 6 to 12 months apart, or closer as needed.

## Pretreatment Patient Directions

- Prior to IPL treatment, the patient's skin pigmentation should be classified using the Fitzpatrick skin classification (I through V). This classification system can be useful in selecting the cut-off filter wavelengths and energy parameters to be programmed into the IPL device. As more melanin absorbs more energy, IPL may not be suitable for patients with a Fitzpatrick skin type V, or darker pigmented skin, as it can lead to unwanted pigmentary changes or an unsafe rise of temperature within the dermis. Though there are no set guidelines on pretreatment sun exposure, the patient is generally instructed to avoid sun exposure for approximately 72 hours prior to the treatment. The clinician should use their discretion on the timeline of sun exposure prior to IPL treatment.
- An informed consent form should be given to the patient prior to administering IPL treatment. The IPL informed consent form outlines important patient instructions, highlights any expected side effects and warns the patient about any adverse reactions that may occur as a result of IPL treatment. The patient is expected to thoroughly read and sign the informed consent form prior to treatment application.

## Equipment

- IPL flash lamp (**see Figure 10-7**)
- Cut off wavelength filters (in nm) (**see Figure 10-8**)
- Lightguide (varying sizes)
- Protective eye shields for the patient (disposable or laser-grade permanent shields may be used)
- Protective tinted eye goggles for the clinician
- Coupling ultrasound gel
- Spatula, gloves for gel application
- Hair net
- SPF 30-50 sunblock
- Anesthetic, e.g., 0.5% proparacaine (*optional*)
- Meibomian gland expressor or cotton tip applicator (*optional*)

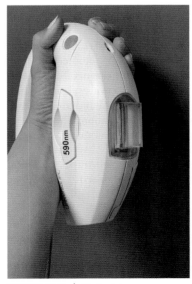

**FIGURE 10-7.** | IPL flash lamp.

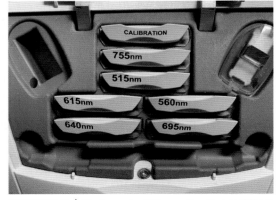

**FIGURE 10-8.** | Photograph of IPL wavelength cutoff filters.

## Setup

- Periocular area, or the treatment area, must be free from makeup, facial moisturizers or lotions. The treatment area should also be free of facial hair, or shaved, if necessary. Use a moistened face wipe or makeup remover to clean the treatment area.
- Apply the protective, opaque, eye shields over the orbital area of each eye (**see Figure 10-9**).
- Apply coupling ultrasound gel of 1-2 mm in thickness to the periocular area, or the treatment area (**see Figure 10-9**).

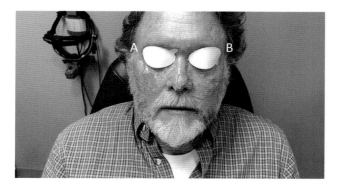

**FIGURE 10-9.** | Placement of eye shields on patient before IPL procedure. (A) Demonstrates proper placement. (B) Demonstrates improper placement of the shield. This patient also has the coupling gel on the area to be treated.

- Program the IPL device with the appropriate settings on the user interface (**see Figure 10-10**):
  - Select the appropriate light guide.

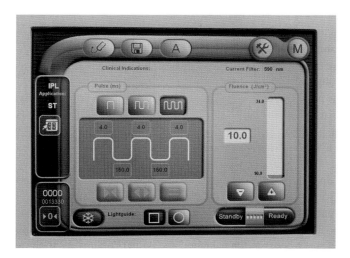

**FIGURE 10-10.** | Photograph of IPL screen. Specific energy parameters are adjusted and programmed into the instrument based on the degree of the patient's skin pigmentation. These energy parameters include the fluence, number of sub-pulses, size, and the time interval between each pulse.

- Select the appropriate cut-off filter.
- Select the appropriate energy parameters including the fluence (j/cm²) and pulse settings.
- Ensure the lightguide tip cooling feature is turned on. This can be controlled from the user interface of the IPL instrument. This feature prevents burning or blisters when applying IPL on thin skin.

## Procedure

1. Position the patient in the exam chair such that the treatment area is at the clinician's chest level. Recline the exam chair as needed.
2. Apply the appropriate cut-off filter into the instrument, as programmed.
3. Ensure the appropriate lightguide (rectangle) is in place.
4. Remove the flash lamp arm from the instrument stand.
5. Hold the lamp head with your dominant hand and position your thumb or index finger over the activation button. Use your nondominant hand for support, as needed.
6. Select "ready" mode on the instrument. This will remove the safety "standby" feature that prevents a flash application. Once in "ready" mode, the IPL will be ready for application. There may be an auditory signal to alert the clinician that the instrument is in ready mode. The clinician should maintain caution once this step is completed.
7. Begin at the tragus or preauricular area closest to you.
8. Position the distal part of the lightguide perpendicular to the skin, lightly touching the coupling gel over the skin without applying too much pressure. Position the lightguide as close to the lid margin as possible, keeping safety top of mind.
9. Press the activation button to apply the light treatment.
10. Continue to apply pulses of light over the treatment area (tragus to tragus), only overlapping the treatment area very slightly (less than 1 mm) and pausing approximately 2 seconds with each treatment pulse.
11. After a first pass of treatment, put the device in "standby" mode.
12. Place the lamp arm on the stand.
13. Reapply the coupling gel, as needed. Then, perform a second pass of treatment (repeat steps 2 through 12).
14. Remove the patient's eye shields. Dispose or clean any permanent shields as necessary.
15. Assist the patient in removal and cleanup of the coupling gel from their face.
16. Manual meibomian gland expression may be performed after the IPL treatment. Although it is not a necessary step, it has shown to improve signs and symptoms of MGD.

    a. Instill 1 drop of proparacaine 0.5% topical solution in each eye (*optional*) (see Procedure 5.7).

    b. Ask the patient to look up.

    c. Place the disinfected meibomian gland expressor or the cotton tip applicator in the pocket of space between the palpebral and bulbar conjunctiva in the area of the meibomian gland.

d. Apply gentle, but continuous pressure to the eyelid and the meibomian gland by squeezing the expressor together for approximately 20–30 seconds (or use your index finger externally and cotton tip applicator internally and squeeze together).

e. Repeat the procedure over the length of the lower eyelid.

f. Ask the patient to look down and repeat the steps c and d. Use fingers and cotton tipped applicator to press and apply pressure if it is difficult to use the meibomian gland expressor for the upper eyelid margin.

17. Apply a cold washcloth over the treated area for 5–10 minutes.

18. Apply SPF 30–50 sunblock or sunscreen over the treated area prior to leaving the office. The patient is advised to continue sunscreen application for the first month of IPL treatment.

## Notes

- The clinician may first apply a test spot to rule out any adverse reaction of the skin. The test spot is typically applied to an area of similar coloration, thickness and consistency as treatment. For example, the lateral side of the malar region, close to the temples, may be used as the test spot. It is advisable to wait 5 minutes and then check for any adverse reactions. If an adverse reaction such as a break in skin integrity, extreme redness, swelling, discoloration, sloughing or blistering of the skin is noted, then reduce the fluence by 1 j/cm² and repeat the treatment in a different test spot. Discontinue treatment if the second test spot results in an adverse reaction.
- Generally, 10–15 pulses will be needed to complete the first pass of the IPL treatment.
- If the treatment area is tanned, the IPL procedure should only be administered once the tan has faded.
- Caution should be taken to avoid treatment administration over hair.
- The patient must be instructed to avoid sun exposure for the first 48 hours after IPL treatment.
- At the beginning of each treatment, it is best practice to inquire if any adverse events related to a previous IPL treatment have occurred. If an adverse reaction has occurred, treatment should be paused until the area has healed.
- Mild discomfort during the procedure is common. The pulse delivery may produce a sensation similar to a rubber band snap on the skin.
- Side effects may include mild discomfort during application, mild redness (similar to a mild sunburn), flaking of pigmented lesions, and crusting of the skin (this may last 5–10 days).
- Although rare, adverse reactions should be described during the IPL consultation, any patient education, and listed on the informed consent form. These adverse reactions include the following:
  - permanent discoloration, scarring, and/or bruising of the treatment and adjacent tissue area;
  - prolonged redness, swelling, irritation, infection, dryness, pruritus, and blistering of treatment and adjacent tissue area;
  - herpes simplex virus outbreak; and
  - post inflammatory hypertension.

## Recording

- Record the patient's Fitzpatrick skin type, the lightguide used, the cut-off filter (in nm) used, the fluence and pulse parameters, as well as the number of pulses used.

- Note the treatment session (initial versus maintenance).
- Note any adverse reactions.

## Example
- Skin Type III, rectangle lightguide, 590 nm, 10 j/cm², 14 triple pulses. Initial IPL session 1 of 4. No adverse reactions.

## 10.5 EYELASH EPILATION

### Purpose
The aim of this procedure is to manually/mechanically remove eyelash(es) or cilium/cilia that are misdirected and/or contact the ocular surface resulting in ocular irritation.

### Indications
Epilation may be performed in conditions such as trichiasis, distichiasis, and entropion.

### Equipment
- Slit lamp (biomicroscope)
- Sterilized or disposable surgical forceps, e.g., Jeweler's forceps or cilia forceps
- Magnifying loop
- Anesthetic e.g., 0.5% proparacaine

### Setup
Slit lamp setup is the same as Procedure 5.2 with the following specifications:
- Adjust the slit beam to a medium width parallelepiped, low to moderate intensity and set the illumination arm of the biomicroscope approximately 30–45°. Use low magnification of 6× to 10×.
- Disinfect the forceps according to manufacturer and CDC guidelines (or other local legal requirements if outside the United States).
- Instill a drop of a topical anesthetic into the eye to be examined (*optional*) (see Procedure 5.7).

### Procedure
*Slit Lamp Technique*
1. Ensure the patient is comfortably seated, and properly position the patient in the slit lamp with their forehead and chin positioned firmly against the rests.
2. Isolate the misdirected lash/cilium. If located on the lower lid, direct the patient to look up and direct their gaze away from the misdirected lash(es). Pull the lower lid down slightly and gently.
3. Lock the silt lamp and look outside the slit lamp. Take the forceps and hold it between your thumb and index finger.
4. Position and hold the forceps approximately 1–1.5 cm (0.5 in) away from the lower lid and ensure the lower portion of your hand is steady and supported on the patient's face (cheek or nose) or on the bar of the slit lamp. Always perform this alignment externally (outside of the slit lamp oculars) to ensure safe and proper positioning with the sharp forceps.
5. Return to look through the slit lamp oculars holding the forceps positioning steady. Move the forceps toward the base of the lash (against the skin of the lid). **See Figure 10-11**.
6. Firmly grasp the base of the lash and gently pull the lash from the follicle (epilation). **See Figure 10-12**.

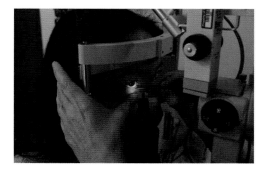

**FIGURE 10-11.** | External view of examiner's hand and forceps positioning for eyelash epilation.

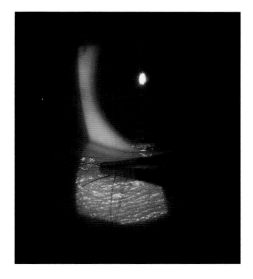

**FIGURE 10-12.** | Examiner's view of grasped eyelash for epilation through slit lamp oculars.

7. Repeat steps 4–6, if there is more than one lash to epilate.
8. Rescan the lid margin at the end of epilation.
9. If the lash is located on the upper lid, have the patient look down and direct their gaze away from the area of mis-directed lash(es). Gently lift and hold (using your nondominant hand) the upper lid along the orbital bone. Ensure you are focused otherwise readjust the sit lamp. Repeat steps 2–8.

*External Technique Using a Magnifying Loop*
1. Ensure the patient is seated comfortably with their head against the head rest on an examination chair.
2. Use adequate overall illumination on the patient's face or with the light attached to the magnifying loop.
3. Isolate the misdirected lash/cilium. If located on the lower lid, instruct the patient to look up and direct their gaze away from the direction of the misdirected lashes.
4. Take the forceps and hold them between your thumb and index finger.

5. Ensure part of your hand is steady and supported on the patient's face (cheek or nose) and hold the forceps approximately 1–1.5 cm (0.5 in) away from the lower lid initially and gradually move the forceps towards the base of the lashes (against the skin of lid).

6. Firmly grasp the base of the lash and pull the lash from the follicle (epilation).

7. If the lash is located on the upper lid, have the patient look down. Gently hold with one hand (nondominant hand) and lift the upper lid along the orbital bone. Repeat steps 2–6.

8. Reassess the lid when epilation is completed.

### Recording
- Record the eye on which the epilation was performed.
- Record epilation and location and number of lash(es) removed.

### Examples
- Left lower lid close to medial canthus, 5 in-turning lashes epilated without complication.
- Right upper lid close to the lateral canthus, 1 in-turning lash epilated without complication.

### Notes
- Patient cooperation is important for successful epilation.
- Topical anesthetic (e.g., 0.5% proparacaine) can be used prior to the procedure depending on the patient's level of comfort.
- Prophylactic topical ophthalmic antibiotic may be considered post epilation.
- Manual/mechanical epilation is best when removing a few isolated lashes. For repeated epilation of lashes, consider referral for more permanent techniques that can destruct the hair follicle such as electrolysis, cryotherapy, or laser ablation.

## 10.6 FOREIGN BODY (FB) REMOVAL

### Purpose
The aim of this procedure is to remove nonpenetrating ocular FBs. FB removal techniques vary depending on the type and location of the entrapped foreign object. Superficial FB may be loosely embedded in either the cornea, palpebral, or bulbar conjunctiva and typically can be removed with irrigation and/or moistened cotton-tip applicator. Deeper embedded FB in the cornea will require special instruments. The goal of FB removal is to disrupt as little ocular tissue as possible while removing the foreign object.

### Indications
Presence of FB in the eye (conjunctiva or cornea) requires immediate ophthalmologic evaluation. Corneal FB may be visible outside of the slit lamp or may require anterior segment examination with the slit lamp to be visualized. FB may also be entrapped behind the lid, and thus, would require lid eversion to be located. In the majority of cases, presence of ocular FB is associated with symptoms of pain, FB sensation, tearing, photophobia, and blurred vision. Risks of corneal infection or scarring increase when embedded FB is left for a longer duration and therefore, timely removal of a corneal FB is highly advised.

### Contraindications
Intraocular and/or penetrating FB or suspected penetrating ocular injury require immediate ophthalmologic referral. Signs of penetrating injury may include positive Seidel sign (indication of corneal or scleral perforation), a shallow anterior chamber, hyphema, iris/pupillary irregularity, a break in Descemet's membrane, or a traumatic cataract. Magnetic resonance imaging is contraindicated in cases that involve metallic FB. Other

contraindications include uncooperative patients or patients with unsteady fixation. In addition, deeply embedded corneal metallic or organic FB that are at risk of penetrating or significant scarring may warrant an immediate referral to a cornea specialist.

## Equipment
- Slit lamp with a cobalt blue filter or a Burton lamp with a similar filter
- Topical sodium fluorescein or fluorescein strips
- Topical anesthetic drops, e.g., 0.5% proparacaine
- Sterile drape/field
- Sterile saline
- pH strips
- Sterile cotton-tipped applicators
- Nylon loop
- Sterilized or disposable Jeweler's forceps
- Magnetic spud
- FB spuds: dull spuds (golf club) and sharp spuds (lance/chisel)
- Needles: 19-gauge to 27-gauge
- Syringe (1–10 ml): can be used as a needle holder
- Rotating ophthalmic burr tool (e.g., Alger brush)

## Setup
- Review patient history and mechanism of ocular injury.
- Review indications/contraindications to perform the procedure.
- Obtain the Informed Consent outlining risks, benefit, and alternatives.
- Confirm with patient any allergies, systemic and ocular medications.
- Perform an external examination and a thorough slit lamp examination with and without sodium fluorescein (see Procedures 5.2 and 5.8).
- Locate FB and estimate its depth.
- Perform lid eversion to rule out hidden debris behind the upper lid of the involved eye(s).
- Assess for Seidel sign. Positive Seidel indicates intraocular penetration and is considered to be a contraindication for the procedure; the patient should be immediately referred for ophthalmologic assessment.
- Setup sterile field with sterile equipment.
- Setup slit lamp with low to medium magnification (10× to 16×).

## Procedure
*Ocular Irrigation*
1. Indicated when the patient received a chemical (basic or acidic) splash to the eye(s) and when there is no penetrating or suspected penetrating FB.
2. Immediately start gently but copiously irrigating they eye(s) with sterile saline.
3. Test pH of the eye by placing a pH strip to the lower palpebral conjunctiva. If the pH is neutral (7.0–7.4) and remains neutral 5 minutes after irrigation, you may stop the irrigation. If the pH is acidic or basic, continue to irrigate and repeat.
4. If necessary, use 1 or 2 drops of topical anesthetic and lid retractors.
5. Evert upper and lower eyelids to ensure you irrigate everywhere.
6. Take history while continuing to irrigate. Do not stop to take visual acuity until the pH is neutral.
7. The end goal of the procedure is to achieve neutral pH in the eye(s).
8. After completion of the procedure, evaluate corneal and conjunctival surface for any chemical damage and treat accordingly.

*Superficial FB*

1. Instill 2 drops of topical anesthetic in both eyes.
2. Gently irrigate the eye to possibly dislodge the FB.
3. If irrigation is not sufficient, stabilize the patient's head at the slit lamp. It may be helpful to identify a target for the patient to look at to ensure stable fixation.
4. Use a saline-moistened sterile cotton-tipped applicator to elevate the FB from the surface by using a rolling motion. The examiner may choose to use a finer instrument for less tissue disruption (see below).
5. Once the superficial FB is removed, evaluate corneal and conjunctival surface for any damage and treat accordingly.

*Corneal or Conjunctival Embedded FB*

1. Instill 2 drops of topical anesthetic in both eyes.
2. Choose the instrument for FB removal according to your preference: a spud or a 25- or 27-gauge needle. The needle may be attached to a small syringe for ease of handling.
   a. The type of instrument you use depends in part on the depth of the FB, patient co-operation, and doctor's personal choice. You must use common sense and clinical judgment when making these decisions. **See Figure 10-13** for various FB removal instruments.

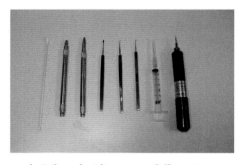

**FIGURE 10-13.** │ Variety of tools used for FB removal.

   b. When deciding upon different instruments, here are some general suggestions:
   - If the corneal FB appears large, regular, and deep, you may attempt to "scoop" it out with a spud or spatula type FB remover.
   - If the FB appears fine or irregular and shallow, you can attempt to remove it with a fine gauge needle. One of the benefits of this instrument is that you can be very precise. However, you must take great care due to the sharpness of the instrument and its ability to penetrate the cornea into the anterior chamber. Orient the needle tangential to the surface and brace your hand so that you do not accidentally puncture the cornea. The bevel of the needle should be facing away from the patient (or toward the examiner).
   - For a child or a patient with unsteady fixation, you may opt for a loop, which is semi-rigid and flexible with no sharp edges. One potential drawback of the loop is that it is less precise and tends to cause a larger area of corneal disruption. It also works best on shallow foreign bodies. However, if safety is an issue, you should become familiar with using this tool.

3. Hold the instrument as you would hold a pencil. Position the patient comfortably in the slit lamp and give them a target to look at to keep their fixation steady. Focus the slit lamp on the FB to be removed.
4. Brace your hand and arm on the slit lamp (or patent's face) for stability.

5. To initially position the instrument, introduce it from the side, while looking from outside the slit lamp. Always perform this alignment externally (outside of the slit lamp oculars) to ensure safe and proper positioning with sharp instruments.

6. Once the instrument is braced in place in front of the eye, keep the instrument tangential to the eye and move behind the oculars of the slit lamp.

7. Under magnification, orient the instrument so that the tip of the spud/spatula or the bevel of the needle is toward you.

8. While keeping the instrument tangential to the globe, gently place the tip of the instrument under the FB and attempt to lift or flick it off the surface of the cornea or conjunctiva.

9. You may need to repeat this procedure several times to fully remove the FB while attempting to damage as little ocular tissue as possible.

10. This technique can also remove some superficial rust rings.

11. If the FB has been dislodged but remains on the surface of the eye, try irrigation to rinse it away or use one of the same removal tools used to remove the FB.

12. Post-procedurally, treat the same way as a corneal abrasion choosing a topical antibiotic with coverage that considers the material of the FB. *Note:* Some practitioners also choose to instill a loading dose of the topical antibiotic at the start of the procedure.

*Rust Ring Removal*

1. Instill 2 drops of topical anesthetic to aid in patient comfort and adjust them so that their chin and forehead are firmly in the rests of the slit lamp.

2. Set the slit lamp to low or medium magnification (10× to 16×).

3. Set the beam width to a wide parallelepiped and use direct illumination.

4. Ask the patient to look at a specific target to keep their fixation steady.

5. Turn on the Alger brush, hold it in your dominant hand, and stabilize the arm of your dominant hand on the slit lamp base, using a prop if necessary.

   a. If the affected eye is situated in front of your dominant hand (left eye/right hand, right eye/left hand), stabilize your hand by placing your wrist on the chinrest of the slit lamp and/or resting your lower fingers on the temporal aspect of the patient's face.

   b. If the affected eye is situated in front of your nondominant hand (right eye/right hand, left eye/left hand), stabilize your hand by bracing your hand on the forehead rest of the slit lamp or gently across the bridge of the patient's nose.

6. Begin by introducing the Alger brush so that it is oriented tangential to the cornea and sighting from outside the slit lamp. Always perform this alignment externally (outside of the slit lamp oculars) to ensure safe and proper positioning.

7. Once the burr of the Alger brush is in front of the eye, view from behind the slit lamp oculars.

8. Keeping the burr of the Alger brush tangential to the cornea at all times, gently touch the burr to the rust ring. Do not apply too much pressure.

   a. Older styles of Alger brushes have a weak motor that will stop if it contacts Bowman's membrane. This type is preferable as there is little chance of penetrating the cornea. If the burr stops, you must restart it and reduce the amount of pressure you are applying to the cornea.

   b. Newer styles of Alger brushes have stronger motors. You must be extra careful when using these that you apply as little pressure as necessary and have good hand control.

   c. At any time, you may stop the rotation of the Alger brush burr by holding down the rotating arm with your finger at the base where the arm meets the handle.

9. The end goal of the procedure is to remove the rust from the cornea, leaving a clean corneal abrasion.

10. Post-procedurally, treat the same way as a corneal abrasion including the use of a prophylactic topical ophthalmic antibiotic.

## Recording
Write down the following:
- Procedure performed and tools used.
- Location: OD/OS and location on the ocular tissue from which the FB was removed.
- Ocular tissue integrity post-procedure, e.g., size of remnant abrasion.
- Proper post-procedural in-office and home care instruction (medications instilled or to be used, etc.) and when patient should return to clinic (RTC).

## Examples
Following slit lamp documentation:
- Superficial metallic FB removed with informed consent from inferior temporal cornea OD using 25-gauge needle, without complication. Rust ring removed with Alger brush. Small, 1 mm abrasion of inferior temporal cornea with no rust remaining. Instilled 1 drop of moxifloxacin in office OD and patient to continue drops QID OD until follow up. RTC next day for reevaluation, sooner if symptoms worsen.

## 10.7 CHALAZION REMOVAL

### Purpose
A chalazion is a chronic lipogranulomatous inflammation of a meibomian gland in the eyelid. The aim of the chalazion removal procedure is to remove the lesion with consideration for protecting the globe and maintaining eyelid integrity. Usually, suturing is not indicated as the wound closes via secondary intention. However, the surgeon may choose to close the incision site with sutures for large chalazion lesions.

### Indications
Chronic chalazions may alter eyelid anatomy, can be unsightly, and in some cases can cause additional infection or alter refractive error. Surgical interventions are acceptable after reasonable attempts to eradicate the lesion via nonsurgical methods such as consistent use of warm compresses, topical or oral antibiotics, hypochlorous sprays, or lid wipes have proven ineffective. Two such surgical interventions are incision and curettage and steroid injection into the lesion (such as triamcinolone). Surgical concerns as to which procedure to employ include age of the patient, pigmentation of the skin, location of the lesion, and not to be overlooked, patient apprehension and preference. Patients should be monitored for postoperative healing, recurrence, and/or complications.

### Contraindications
Contraindications include acutely inflamed chalazia (hordeolum), location of chalazion near the lacrimal puncta and allergy or sensitivity to anesthesia.

### Equipment
- Sterile scalpel (#15 blade shown in **Figure 10-14**)
- Meyerhoefer Chalazion Curette
- Hunt Chalazion Clamp (12 mm diameter shown in **Figure 10-14**)

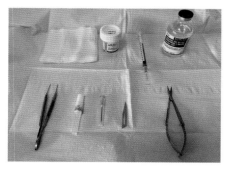

**FIGURE 10-14.** | Sterile field setup prior to chalazion removal.

- 1 cc syringe contains:
  - 27–32-gauge needle (32-gauge needle shown in **Figure 10-14**)
  - Anesthetic (2% Lidocaine/Epinephrine 1:100,000 is shown in **Figure 10-14**)
- Povidone-iodine solution 5% or alcohol prep pads
- Antibiotic ointment
- Sterile saline
- Gauze 4 × 4
- Surgical marker (to mark chalazion)
- Blood pressure cuff and stethoscope
- Sterile drape(s)
- Corneal shield (*optional*)
- Surgical fine cautery (*optional*)
- Additional needles and sutures (*optional*)
- Cotton tipped applicator (*optional*)

### Setup
- Review patient history and indications to perform the procedure.
- Obtain the Informed Consent including discussion of risks, benefits, and alternatives.
- Record preoperative diagnosis and the proper operating eyelid.
- Confirm with patient allergies, systemic, and ocular medications.
- Explain the purpose of the procedure to the patient.
- Measure blood pressure and pulse prior to the start of the procedure (see Procedure 7.2).
- Recline the patient to a comfortable position and confirm that their head is firmly supported by the headrest.
- Perform hand hygiene, don proper personal protective equipment (PPE) including gloves and follow necessary infection control guidelines (see Procedure 2.2).
- Setup sterile field with sterile equipment, surgical tools, and sutures.
- Confirm type of materials and correct sizing.
- Open and prepare supplies with sterile technique.
- Prepare ophthalmic povidone-iodine and ophthalmic anesthesia (such as 2% Lidocaine/Epinephrine 1:100,000) *Note:* Injection training, certification, and/or licensure is a prerequisite for all advanced procedures that require injections.

### Procedure
1. Clean the skin area with povidone-iodine or alcohol prep pads.
2. Mark chalazion by outlining its shape with a marker.
3. Anesthetize wound area by injecting 0.3–0.5 ml of 2% Lidocaine/Epinephrine 1:100,000 using preloaded syringe (intradermal injection in the area adjacent to the chalazion, and on both sides of chalazion).
4. Apply digital massage to spread anesthesia.

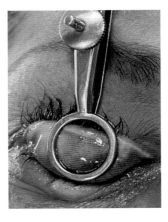

**FIGURE 10-15.** | Clamp placed on the upper eyelid demonstrating positioning against the upper tarsal plate.

5. Apply chalazion clamp and appropriately evert eyelid, if indicated. **See Figures 10-15 and 10-16** for appropriate positioning of the chalazion clamp for upper and lower lids, respectfully.
6. Using scalpel, make a vertical incision through the center of chalazion following the direction of the meibomian glands (see **Figure 10-16**).
7. Remove the capsular content with curette.
8. Identify and remove fibrotic capsule.
9. Apply pressure in order to achieve hemostasis. Can be done with a sterile cotton tipped applicator (**Figure 10-16**).
10. Palpate to be certain that the mass is fully excised.
11. Rinse lesion with sterile saline.
12. Remove clamp from the eyelid and return all instruments to tray. Dispose of soiled materials following infection control protocols using biohazard containers and puncture resistant biohazard containers for sharps.
13. Apply topical ophthalmic antibiotic ointment and pressure patch which may be worn for several hours post procedurally or overnight.
14. Monitor the patient post-procedurally and provide home care instructions.

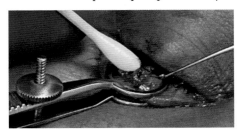

**FIGURE 10-16.** | Clamp placed on lower lid while lesion is incised via scalpel. The surgeon is maintaining control of curette and controlling bleeding with a q-tip.

## Recording
For charting purposes, the following needs to be documented following the procedure:
- Needle safety was maintained.
- Aseptic technique was maintained.
- Which eyelid the procedure was performed.
- How the patient tolerated the procedure.
- Patient disposition post-treatment.
- Proper postoperative home care instructions (medications, pressure patch removal, etc.)
- When the patient should RTC.

### Example

- Example of recording for the patient in Figures 10-15 and 10-16:
  "Excision: chalazion, multiple, different lids, right lower lid, right upper lid.
  Diagnosis: Chalazia upper and lower lids, right eye.
  Anesthesia: Intradermal.
  Prep: Povidone-iodine scrub.
  Procedure: Prior to treatment, the risks/benefits/alternatives were discussed. The patient wished to proceed with the procedure. Local anesthesia was applied, and the lid was prepped. The lid was clamped exposing the posterior surface of the eyelid. The chalazia were incised and removed with a curette. Bleeding was controlled and the clamp was removed. The eye was pressure patched with antibiotic ointment. Patient tolerated the procedure well. There were no complications. Post procedure instructions given and to RTC within 1 week for follow up."

### Acknowledgment

Special acknowledgment to Alex Martin, OD, Cornea Specialist Vinny Keshav, MD, and Oculoplastic Specialist John J. Lee, MD, MPH of Boston Vision for additional consultation, procedure development, and photography during surgery.

## 10.8 SUTURING, EXCISION, AND BIOPSY

### Purpose

Eyelid excision is performed for removal of benign or malignant lesions with minimal damage to the eyelid and adnexa. To obtain a biopsy of the desired lesion, a tissue sample of the lesion is collected via eyelid excision and sent to a laboratory for histological analysis. The purpose of suturing is to provide adequate wound closure without tension, allowing careful approximation of both sides of the laceration, so tissue can heal by primary intention. The goal is to approximate the wound edges without strangulating the tissue. The wound edges should be closed with slight eversion to promote ideal wound healing.

### Indications

Suturing and microsurgical procedures represent an opportunity for eye care practitioners to positively impact patient cosmesis and detect potential malignancies. Lesions around the eyelid are common (approximately 5–10% of all skin malignancies) and represent abnormal tissue growth which arises from various cancers, viruses, or anatomical changes. Lesions should be removed and biopsied if there is any concern for malignancy or recurrence. Additionally, lesion removal would be indicated regardless of malignancy status if it obstructs vision or the patient is symptomatic. The patient may also choose to remove the lesion for cosmetic reasons on an out-of-pocket basis. Due to increased ultraviolet exposure, lesions should be biopsied to detect malignancies. Any lesion removed by excision should be biopsied.

It is important to decide on a strategy for excision which involves minimal tissue alteration. One should consider planning of the wound and subsequent closure in order to optimize cosmesis using surrounding existing facial lines and skin tension lines. If moderate or large amounts of tissue need to be altered or removed, and the resulting wound or sutures are likely to cause anatomical changes such as changes to the eyelid's ability to open and close, referral to an oculoplastic specialist is necessary. The practitioner should always err on the side of caution and confirm a lesion is benign via a pathology report.

Suturing is indicated in some cases to achieve primary closure of skin lacerations for deep wounds (extending through the dermis), large wounds (>3–4 mm) and when scarring is likely if wound edges are not properly opposed. Two of the most common suture types used in ocular surgery are plain gut or polyglactin 910 (absorbable) and nylon (nonabsorbable). Practitioners will select absorbable sutures in situations where follow up for suture removal would not be indicated or tissue healing will follow a natural process such as in most eyelid procedures. Nonabsorbable sutures are ideal in other situations in eye care surgical management such as corneal procedures where sutures can be permanent or must be removed at various time points. Additionally, size of the suture is important based on the tissue or the surgical technique involved; size 6-0 sutures are common in skin closure while a size 10-0 is preferable in corneal surgery. In many procedures that involve small wounds or lesions of the conjunctiva, closure by secondary intention may be preferred.

As with any kind of surgical procedure, postoperative complications can happen. The eye care practitioner who provides surgical intervention to the patient also has the burden of providing or co-managing postoperative care. It is critical to ensure that the lesion, wound, or sutures are healing, anatomical function is unchanged, and there are no signs of postoperative infection. Any serious complications may require additional referral.

## Equipment
**See Figure 10-17** for equipment setup.
- Ophthalmic scissors (e.g., Westcott)
- Ophthalmic needle holder (e.g., Castroviejo) with lock
- Ophthalmic needle holder without lock
- Toothed forceps 0.3 mm with tying platform
- Suture (commonly absorbable 6-0 plain gut or nonabsorbable 6-0 prolene)
- 1 mL syringe
- 32-gauge needle
- #11 or #15 Scalpel
- Povidone-iodine solution
- Gauze 4 × 4
- Surgical marker (to mark operative eye/site)
- Scleral shells
- Blood pressure cuff and stethoscope
- Topical antibiotic ophthalmic ointment
- 1 cc syringe filled with an anesthetic (such as 2% Lidocaine/Epinephrine 1:100,000)
- Specimen bag (not pictured)
- Biopsy specimen cup
- Pathology requisition sheet (not pictured)
- Sterile drape

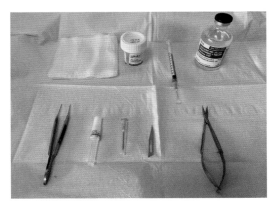

**FIGURE 10-17.** | Sterile field setup prior to suturing, excision, and biopsy.

## Setup

- Review patient history and indications to perform the procedure.
- Obtain the Informed Consent including discussion of risks, benefits, and alternatives.
- Record preoperative diagnosis and the proper operating eyelid.
- Confirm with patient allergies, systemic, and ocular medications.
- Explain the purpose of the procedure to the patient.
- Measure blood pressure and pulse prior to the start of the procedure (see Procedure 7.2).
- Recline the patient to a comfortable position and confirm that their head is firmly supported by the headrest.
- Perform hand hygiene, don proper PPE including gloves and follow necessary infection control guidelines (see Procedure 2.2).
- Setup sterile field with sterile equipment, surgical tools, and sutures.
- Confirm the type of materials and correct sizing.
- Open and prepare supplies with sterile technique.
- Prepare ophthalmic povidone-iodine and ophthalmic anesthesia (such as 2% Lidocaine/Epinephrine 1:100,000). *Note:* Injection training, certification, and/or licensure is a prerequisite for all advanced procedures that require injections.

## Procedure

1. Sterilize the area around the lesion with povidone-iodine (or can use alcohol as an alternative).
2. Inspect the area around the lesion to ensure no FB, dirt, etc.
3. Anesthetize immediate area by performing an intradermal injection of 2% Lidocaine/Epinephrine 1:100,000, on each side of lesion avoiding injecting directly into the lesion (**Figure 10-18**). Apply digital massage to enhance penetration.

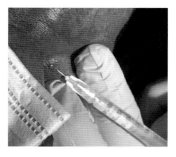

FIGURE 10-18. | Injection of anesthetic around the lesion before excision.

4. Adhere a sterile drape prior to starting the procedure (*optional*).
5. If lesion is stalk-like or pedunculated (**Figure 10-19**):
   a. Grasp lesion with toothed forceps and use Westcott scissors to excise the lesion at its base. Careful not to cut too deep and cut into deep layers (muscle, etc.).

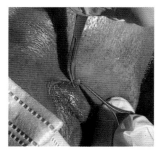

FIGURE 10-19. | Excisional biopsy of epidermal inclusion cyst with toothed forceps, exposing the base for excision via Westcott scissors.

6. If the lesion is flat within the skin and/or minimally raised:

   a. A shave (excision of the lesion with a scalpel or a razor) should be performed forming a pattern slightly larger than the lesion. There are other techniques and surgical tools that can be used as well, such as punch biopsy that is done with a hollow circular scalpel (a punch). A snip biopsy/excision may be used for pedunculated lesions; whereas shave biopsy is usually done for mildly elevated lid lesions. Another important consideration when choosing the best biopsy/excision technique is the cosmetic outcome of the procedure. Epidermal lesions are generally excised at the dermo-epidermal junction to minimize residual scarring. Therefore, shave biopsy usually produces a better cosmetic outcome than a deeper wedge elliptical excision which may leave a scar in the eyelid. Large residual wounds (after excision) should be sutured with respect to existing facial lines and skin tension lines to improve cosmesis.

7. If the lesion is on the lid margin:

   a. The incision should be made flush with the surrounding tissue. A chalazion clamp can be placed with the lid margin and lesion centered within the clamp window (see Procedure 10.7). A #15 blade is then run along the lid margin to remove the lesion.

8. Place specimen in the specimen container and label both container and paperwork to send to the lab.

9. Once the lesion is removed and bleeding has been controlled, return all instruments into the tray. Dispose of soiled materials following infection control protocols using biohazard containers and puncture resistant biohazard containers for sharps.

10. For wounds that require suturing, perform the following:

    a. Open sutures and properly load needle into the needle driver/holder.

    b. Hold suture needle at 2/3 of the length from the needle point.

    c. Simple Interrupted Suture:

       i. Position the first suture ~2–3 mm from the laceration margin.

       ii. Needle should be introduced at a 90-degree angle from the skin surface.

       iii. Advance through the tissue following the curvature of the needle exiting on the other side of laceration ~2–3 mm away from the laceration margin.

       iv. Pull the suture/thread through until about 5–10 cm (2–4 in) is left on the other side.

       v. Perform surgeon's knot: the first throw (2–3 squares), then the second throw (1 square), then the final throw (1 square).

       vi. Cut the thread leaving ~8 mm tails in place.

       vii. Perform as many interrupted sutures as needed approximately ~5 mm distance from each other to ensure the two sides of laceration come in close proximity to each other. *Note:* make sure not to tighten sutures too much as it may result in tissue ischemia and necrosis.

    d. As an alternative, simple running suture can be performed (example demonstrated in **Figure 10-20A–C.**)

    e. Once the wound is properly closed, dispose needle into the sharps container and return all instruments into the tray.

11. Apply antibiotic ointment in office.

12. Monitor the patient post-procedurally and provide home care instructions.

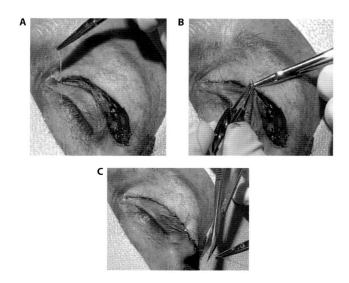

**FIGURE 10-20.** | Continuous suture during blepharoplasty procedure to fix dermatochalasis of the upper lid left eye. (A) First suture demonstrating surgeon's knot to start closing open wound. (B) Midway of running suture demonstrating control of the suture to be at equal depth on both sides of the skin that is to close. (C) Final surgeon's knot being cut to close the wound and running suture.

## Recording

Write down the following:
- Sharps safety was maintained.
- Aseptic technique was maintained.
- Which eyelid the procedure was performed.
- How patient tolerated the procedure.
- Patient disposition post-treatment.
- Proper postoperative home care instruction (medications, etc.)
- When patient should RTC.

## Example

- Example of recording for Excisional Biopsy procedure (**Figures 10-18 and 10-19**):
  "Procedure Note: Excision of Eyelid lesion, left upper lid.
  Diagnosis: Other benign neoplasm of the skin of the eyelid.
  Anesthesia: Intradermal.
  Prep: Povidone-iodine scrub.
  Prior to treatment, the risks/benefits/alternatives were discussed. The patient wished to proceed with the procedure. Local anesthetic was given. The eyelid was prepped and draped for the procedure. The lesion was excised and removed. Patient tolerated the procedure well. There were no complications. Post procedure instructions given and to RTC within 1 week for follow up."

## Acknowledgment

Special acknowledgment to Alex Martin, OD and Oculoplastic Specialist John J. Lee, MD, MPH of Boston Vision for additional consultation, procedure development, and photography during surgery.

## 10.9 ANTERIOR SEGMENT LASERS

### Purpose

The aim of this procedure is to use laser energy to treat a wide range of eye diseases. Most laser procedures are relatively painless and are performed on an outpatient basis. The combination of safety, accuracy, and relative low cost make lasers useful ophthalmic tools for treatment of anterior and posterior segment diseases.

LASER is an acronym for "Light Amplification by Stimulated Emission of Radiation" and is used commonly as a noun, "laser". Lasers emit light that is monochromatic (single wavelength), coherent (the waves are in phase in space and time), and collimated (narrow beam in a specific direction with minimal divergence). The purpose of a laser is to transfer emitted laser energy into a different form of energy within the target tissue. It is the combination of specific laser parameters and target tissue properties that will determine the final effect on the target tissue.

*Laser Parameters*

Ophthalmic lasers range from ultraviolet (UV) to infra-red (IR) wavelengths. Laser wavelength plays a significant role in how laser light interacts with the target tissue and its pigment. The wavelength also determines how far the laser wave will be traveling within the eye (Example: Excimer laser [193 nm] can travel a short distance and thus used for the cornea versus Neodymium-doped Yttrium Aluminum Garnet [Nd:YAG] laser [1,064 nm] has the ability to reach the posterior pole of the eye). Some lasers are pigment-dependent (pigment is required to transfer energy from the laser to the tissue), and some are pigment-independent (laser does not need pigment to affect the target tissue). There are other laser variables such as spot size, pulse duration, and energy level that all factor into the overall energy delivered to the target tissue. As a general rule, use the lowest energy settings, the least number of shots, and the lowest duration to accomplish the desired effect.

*Types of Laser-Tissue Interactions*

- Photochemical (photoablation): Excimer laser interacts with tissue by the process of photoablation. In this process, laser energy is used to change the shape of proteins inside the target tissue, thus changing (or activating) tissue's biological processes.
- Photothermal (photocoagulation): Argon laser or frequency-doubling Nd:YAG laser interact with tissue by the process of photocoagulation. This is a pigment-dependent laser-tissue interaction in which laser energy is absorbed by pigment and is transferred into heat.
- Ionizing (photodisruption): Nd:YAG laser interacts with tissue by the process of photodisruption. This is a pigment-independent laser-tissue interaction in which laser energy is delivered in strong short pulses, causing acoustic shockwaves and optical breakdown of molecules, reducing tissue to plasma.

For the purposes of this text, the focus will be on three types of ophthalmic anterior segment laser procedures: Selective Laser Trabeculoplasty (SLT), Laser Peripheral Iridotomy (LPI) and Neodymium-doped Yttrium Aluminum Garnet (Nd:YAG) Capsulotomy.

### Indications

*Selective Laser Trabeculoplasty (SLT)*

The SLT procedure is used for the purposes of lowering intraocular pressure (IOP) by increasing aqueous outflow through the trabecular meshwork (TM). SLT is indicated for treatment of primary open-angle glaucoma, ocular hypertension, normal tension glaucoma, pigment dispersion syndrome or pigmentary glaucoma, pseudoexfoliation syndrome, and pseudoexfoliation glaucoma.

SLT is contraindicated in narrow angles or angle closure where TM is not visible. Also, SLT is not recommended in inflammatory glaucoma, neovascular glaucoma, angle recession glaucoma, juvenile glaucoma, significant corneal endothelial disease, and prior failure of SLT procedure.

*Laser Peripheral Iridotomy (LPI)*

The LPI procedure is used for the purposes of equalizing the pressure between anterior and posterior chambers by creating a bypass mechanism (hole in the iris) that allows aqueous fluid to free flow from behind the iris to the anterior chamber. LPI is indicated for treatment of pupil block in primary angle closure (PAC) suspect, PAC, PAC glaucoma, PAC crisis, and plateau iris. LPI is also used preoperatively or intraoperatively when surgical situations where pupillary block is likely: phakic intraocular lens (IOL), iris fixated IOL, or endothelial keratoplasty.

LPI is contraindicated in secondary angle closures that do not involve pupil block, significant corneal opacity that reduces the view of the iris, and in cases when the anterior chamber is very shallow.

*Neodymium-Doped Yttrium Aluminum Garnet (Nd:YAG) Capsulotomy*

The Nd:YAG Capsulotomy (or YAG Capsulotomy) procedure is used for the treatment of subjective visual complaints, increased glare, and reduced BCVA caused by posterior capsular opacification (PCO). PCO occurs when remaining residual natural lens epithelial cells migrate and spread along the inner surface of the capsule after cataract extraction. YAG Capsulotomy is indicated when PCO is dense enough to cause reduction in BCVA of 20/40 or worse or when subjective complaints of reduced vision and/or glare impact activities of daily living. YAG Capsulotomy is also indicated in capsular contraction syndromes and can be used for refractive shifts in plate haptic or pseudo-accommodating IOLs, as well as prior to refractive enhancements in pseudo-phakic patients.

YAG Capsulotomy is contraindicated when significant corneal opacities reduce the view of the PCO, during active intraocular inflammation or in patients with high risk for intraocular inflammation or retinal detachment. Absolute contraindications include glass IOL implants and significant calcification of IOL surface that can be seen in older silicon and hydrogel IOL materials. Prior to performing YAG Capsulotomy it is also advised to ensure that reduction in best-corrected visual acuity (BCVA) is due to formation of PCO, rather than other (non-PCO related) treatable ocular pathology. It is also important to know that IOL exchange is more challenging and has more risk after a capsulotomy has been done. IOL issues should be ruled out prior to YAG (patients who are not happy with multifocal IOL, scratches or defects on the IOL).

## Equipment

- Nd:YAG laser device
- Ophthalmic lenses for SLT (required for SLT procedure)
- Ophthalmic lenses for Iridotomy and Capsulotomy (*optional* for these procedures)

   *Note:* The use of lenses during the procedure has several advantages: (1) the lens helps to stabilize the eye and minimize eye movements; (2) the lens helps to focus and concentrate laser energy; (3) the lens can be used to apply pressure to the eye to control hyphema, in case this rare complication occurs.

- Lubricating gel or ointment (if ophthalmic lenses are used)
- Laser-grade safety glasses
- Preoperative medications: alpha-agonist, proparacaine, dilating medication (if indicated) and pilocarpine (if indicated). *Note:* Any use of drugs, including eyedrops, requires the examiner to have an awareness of the contraindications and side effects of the selected drug (see Procedure 5.7).

## Setup

- Review patient history and indications to perform the procedure.
- Obtain the Informed Consent including discussion of risks, benefits, and alternatives.

- Record preoperative diagnosis and the proper operating eye.
- Confirm with patient allergies, systemic, and ocular medications.
- Explain the purpose of the procedure to the patient.

## Procedure

*Selective Laser Trabeculoplasty (SLT)*

1. Preoperative care:

   a. Perform gonioscopy to locate the TM, assess the amount of pigmentation and check for indications and contraindications (see Procedure 5.18).

   b. Instill preoperative drops ~15–30 minutes prior to the procedure: one or two drops of alpha-agonist (such as brimonidine 0.1–0.2% or apraclonidine 1%) into the operating eye. In some cases, pilocarpine 1% may be instilled in the operating eye to open up TM (optional.)

   c. Instill preoperative drops immediately prior to the procedure: proparacaine in both eyes.

2. Setup appropriate laser mode and settings (**see Table 10-1**).

| TABLE 10-1. SLT Laser Setup and Specs | | |
|---|---|---|
| **Selective Laser Trabeculoplasty (SLT)** | | |
| **Laser** | FD Nd:YAG (532 nm) | • *Pre-Op Meds:* 1–2 gtts alpha agonist, anesthetic OU, and 1% pilocarpine (pilocarpine is optional) |
| **Tissue reaction** | Photocoagulation: Sublethal photostimulation pigment dependent | • Aim for TM, burns next to each other<br>• Usually ~50–60 shots per 180 degrees |
| **Initial Energy/ Power** | 0.8–1.0 mJ<br><0.8 for heavy pigmented TM;<br>>1.0 for light pigmented TM | • More pigmented TM = less power<br>• Aim for energy <50 mJ<br>• *Post-Op Meds:* 1-2 gtts alpha agonist in office |
| **Spot Size** | Fixed (400 µm) | • Rx 1% prednisolone acetate ophthalmic suspension QID × 3 days or ophthalmic |
| **Duration** | Fixed (3 ns) | NSAID QID × 3 days |
| **Off-set** | 0 | • *Follow-up:* 1 hr IOP check; 1 week; 1 month |

*Note:* The listed pre-op and post-op medications, quantities, and length of time are listed as examples. Clinicians should use their own judgement based on the patient's history and severity of condition to determine best treatment.

3. Laser shot counter should be reset to its initial ("zero") position.

4. Keep laser on "inactive" mode.

5. Slit-lamp settings:

   a. Magnification 16× (can range 12.5× to 20×).

   b. Illumination tower: variable. Some surgeons recommend having illumination on the opposite side of the mirror for the clearest and brightest views of the angle.

6. Apply small amount of cushioning agent (artificial tear gel or ointment) to the SLT laser lens.

7. Place the lens on patient's anesthetized eye. Make a mental note of where you are starting to treat based on the position of the lens and the mirror.

8. Engage laser to its "active" mode.

9. Position aiming beam over the entire width of TM (**see Figure 10-21**).

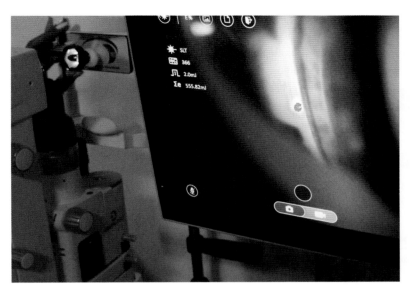

**FIGURE 10-21.** | Laser placement on TM for SLT procedure.

10. Laser pulses are applied to the mirror followed by rotating the lens to the next rotation.
11. Apply laser pulses next to each other moving in the clockwise direction.
12. Desired tissue reaction: appearance of bubbles at least 50–75% of the time.
13. Rotate the lens clockwise to the next direction.
14. Perform the procedure over 360°. Studies showed less efficacy when SLT was performed over 90° or 180° versus 360°. For highly pigmented TM, 180° versus 360°, may be considered.
15. Approximately 100 nonoverlapping laser pulses for 360° or 50 for 180°.
16. Disengage the laser to the proper post treatment setting, the "inactive" mode.
17. Postoperative care:
    a. Instill postoperative drops immediately after the procedure: one or two drops of alpha-agonist (such as brimonidine 0.1–0.2% or apraclonidine 1%) into the operating eye.
    b. IOP should be checked ~30–60 minutes after the procedure and treated if significant rise in IOP is noted. If IOP increase is >10 mmHg, oral acetazolamide should be used in office, topical IOP lowering medications should be used in office and prescribed.
    c. Prescribe topical steroid (1% prednisolone acetate ophthalmic suspension) or topical NSAID for 3–4 days to the operating eye(s).
18. Complete recording in the chart (see section "Recording").
19. One-week follow-up: check IOP and anterior chamber assessment for inflammation.
20. Four to six-week follow-up: in addition to checking IOP and anterior chamber, assess effectiveness of the procedure; it will take between 4 and 12 weeks to see IOP reduction.

*Laser Peripheral Iridotomy (LPI)*
1. Preoperative care:
    a. Perform gonioscopy to assess indications and contraindications (see Procedure 5.18).
    b. Instill preoperative drops ~15–30 minutes prior to the procedure: one or two drops of alpha-agonist (such as brimonidine 0.1–0.2% or apraclonidine 1%) into the operating eye. Instill pilocarpine 1% in the operating eye to increase iris tonicity.

c. Instill preoperative drops immediately prior to the procedure: proparacaine in both eyes.

2. Setup appropriate laser mode and settings (**see Table 10-2**).

3. Laser shot counter should be reset to its initial ("zero") position.

| TABLE 10-2. YAG Laser Peripheral Iridotomy Setup and Specs | | |
|---|---|---|
| **Laser Peripheral Iridotomy (LPI)** | | |
| **Laser** | Nd:YAG (1,064 nm) | • *Pre-Op Meds:* 1-2 gtts alpha agonist, anesthetic OU, and 1% pilocarpine |
| **Tissue reaction** | Photodisruption, pigment independent | • Aim for crypt at 11:00/1:00 or 3:00/9:00 • ~2/3 or more from the pupil frill |
| **Initial Energy/ Power** | 2.0–6.0 mJ, single or double shot  Max energy: <150 mJ | • Allow time between shots, watch for plume • ~0.5 mm opening • *Post-Op Meds:* 1-2 gtts alpha agonist in office |
| **Spot Size** | Fixed (~10 µm) | • Rx 1% prednisolone acetate ophthalmic suspension 1% QID × 3–4 days |
| **Duration** | Fixed (3–4 ns) | • *Follow-up:* 1 hr IOP check; 1 week; 1 month |
| **Off-set** | 0 | |

*Note:* The listed pre-op and post-op medications, quantities, and length of time are listed as examples. Clinicians should use their own judgement based on the patient's history and severity of condition to determine best treatment.

4. Keep laser on "inactive" mode.

5. Slit-lamp settings:

   a. Magnification 12.5× to 16× (medium).

   b. Illumination tower: variable.

6. It is optional to use the iridotomy lens. If using the lens, apply small amount of cushioning agent to the laser lens and place the lens on patient's anesthetized eye.

7. Engage laser to its "active" mode.

8. Beam position on the iris: traditionally the beam is positioned 2/3 from the pupil, closer to the limbus at the 11:00 or 1:00 o'clock position. Studies show less dysphotopsia when LPI is done at 3:00 or 9:00 o'clock position (**see Figure 10-22**). The goal is to position the beam in the crypt or thinner area of the iris avoiding iris blood vessels. Also avoid placing LPI at 12:00 o'clock position.

9. With target area centered at the button of the Iridotomy lens, the initial shots should be placed in exactly the same position.

10. Desired tissue reaction: appearance of plume of pigment when penetration is achieved.

11. If hyphema is noted, pause the procedure and apply moderate pressure to the eye with the lens for 30–60 seconds or until iris bleeding stops.

12. It is important to watch the total energy used during the procedure. Higher postoperative complications have been associated with high total energy that exceeded 150 mJ.

13. The end goal of the procedure is a patent PI approximately 0.25–0.50 mm in diameter

14. Disengage the laser to the proper post treatment setting, the "inactive" mode.

15. Postoperative care:

   a. Perform thorough assessment of the anterior chamber and PI without the lens.

   b. Instill postoperative drops immediately after the procedure: one or two drops of alpha-agonist (such as brimonidine 0.1–0.2% or apraclonidine 1%) into the operating eye.

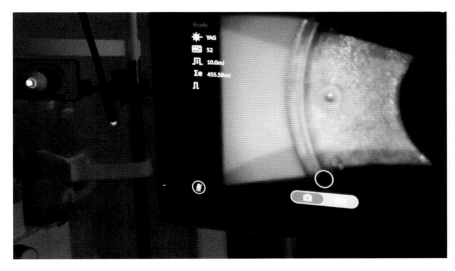

**FIGURE 10-22.** | Laser performed at 9 o'clock position for LPI placement. Continuation of shots to ensure iridotomy patency.

    c. IOP should be checked ~30–60 minutes after the procedure and treated if significant rise in IOP is noted. If IOP increase is >10 mmHg, oral acetazolamide should be used in office, topical IOP lowering medications should be used in office and prescribed.

    d. Prescribe topical steroid (1% prednisolone acetate ophthalmic suspension) or topical NSAID for 3–4 days to the operating eye(s).

16. Complete recording in the chart (see section "Recording").

17. One-week follow-up: check IOP and anterior chamber assessment for inflammation.

18. Four to six-week follow-up: in addition to checking IOP and anterior chamber, assess effectiveness of the procedure, patency of LPI and perform gonioscopy; it may take between 2 and 6 weeks to see the effect. Patency of LPI can be confirmed by positive retroillumination or by performing Anterior Segment OCT (see Procedure 9.4).

*YAG Capsulotomy*

1. Preoperative care:

    a. Measure pre-dilation pupil size to establish the minimum diameter of capsulotomy opening (see Procedure 2.15).

    b. Instill dilating drops into the operating eye and perform dilated exam (see Procedures 5.7, 5.20, and 5.22).

    c. Instill preoperative drops ~15–30 minutes prior to the procedure: one or two drops of alpha-agonist (such as brimonidine 0.1–0.2% or apraclonidine 1%) into the operating eye.

    d. Instill preoperative drops immediately prior to the procedure: proparacaine in both eyes.

2. Setup appropriate laser mode and settings (**see Table 10-3**).

3. Laser shot counter should be reset to its initial ("zero") position.

4. Off-set should be setup (see **Table 10-3**). To avoid damage to the surrounding structures, the center of the shockwave is typically offset from the plane of focus.

5. Keep laser on "inactive" mode.

| TABLE 10-3. YAG Capsulotomy Laser Setup and Specs | | |
|---|---|---|
| **YAG Capsulotomy** | | |
| Laser | Nd:YAG (1,064 nm) | • *Pre-Op Meds:* 1-2 gtts alpha agonist, dilation, anesthetic OU |
| Tissue reaction | Photodisruption, pigment independent | • Cruciate, octagon or "can opener" pattern<br>• First shot should be away from visual axis |
| Initial Energy/ Power | 1.3–1.8 mJ, single shot | • Usually ~15–50 shots in total, average ~40 |
| | Max energy: 60–80 mJ | • Aim for total energy <50 mJ |
| Spot Size | Fixed | • *Post-Op Meds:* 1-2 gtts alpha agonist in office |
| Duration | Fixed | • Rx 1% prednisolone acetate ophthalmic suspension 1% or topical NSAID QID × 1–2 weeks |
| Off-set | Posterior Capsulotomy: ~100–250 posterior off-set; | • *Follow-up:* 1 hr IOP check; 1–2 weeks |
| | Anterior Capsulotomy: ~0–100 anterior off-set | |

*Note:* The listed pre-op and post-op medications, quantities, and length of time are listed as examples. Clinicians should use their own judgement based on the patient's history and severity of condition to determine best treatment.

6. Slit-lamp settings:

    a. Magnification 12.5× to 16× (medium).

    b. Illumination tower: variable.

7. It is optional to use the Capsulotomy lens. If using the lens, apply small amount of cushioning agent to the laser lens and place the lens on patient's anesthetized eye.

8. Instruct the patient to fixate on a specific target in front of them and to hold steady.

9. Engage laser to its "active" mode.

10. Focus aiming beams on the PCO.

11. It is recommended that the initial shot should be some distance away from the visual axis.

12. Fire shots in a pattern (**see Figure 10-23**). It can be a cruciate pattern (starting at 12:00, proceeding to 6:00, then horizontally on each side, forming octagon shape) or a "can opener" pattern (starting at 7:00 and moving clockwise till round opening is formed).

13. Any remaining posterior capsular striae or folds should be treated.

14. Typical number of laser shots is ~15–50 depending on the density of PCO with typical total energy being ~30–40 mJ. Higher postoperative complications have been associated with high total energy that exceeded 60–80 mJ.

15. The end goal of the procedure is an opening diameter that is larger than the undilated pupil size and not bigger than 1.0–1.5 mm distance from the edge of the IOL optic.

16. Disengage the laser to the proper post treatment setting, the "inactive" mode.

17. Postoperative care:

    a. Instill postoperative drops immediately after the procedure: one or two drops of alpha-agonist (such as brimonidine 0.1–0.2% or apraclonidine 1%) into the operating eye.

    b. IOP should be checked ~30–60 minutes after the procedure and treated if significant rise in IOP is noted. If IOP increase is >10 mmHg, oral acetazolamide should be used in office, topical IOP lowering medications should be used in office and prescribed.

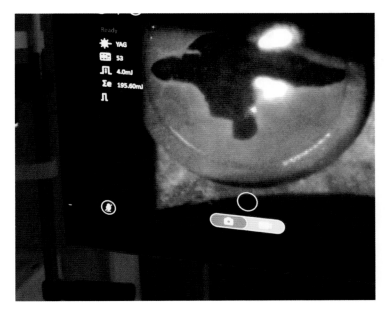

**FIGURE 10-23.** | Laser continuation of cruciate pattern for YAG capsulotomy.

    c. May consider prescribing topical steroid (1% prednisolone acetate ophthalmic suspension) or topical NSAID for 1–2 weeks to the operating eye(s).

18. Complete recording in the chart (see section "Recording").
19. One to two-week follow-up: check IOP, anterior chamber assessment for inflammation and capsular opening assessment.

## Recording
Write down the following:
- Procedure performed.
- Location: eye (and degrees for SLT).
- Number of laser shots, energy per shot, and total energy used.
- How patient tolerated the procedure.
- Patient disposition post-treatment.
- Proper postoperative home care instructions (medications, etc.)
- When patient should RTC.

## Examples
- Preoperatively one drop of topical brimonidine 0.2% was instilled into the right eye. Topical proparacaine was used immediately prior to the procedure in both eyes. Laser Nd:YAG Iridotomy was performed at 11 o'clock position in the right eye. Total amount energy: 90 mJ, total number of laser shots performed: 15 with 3.0 mJ double shots used. Procedure was completed without incidents, patient tolerated procedure well. Postoperatively one drop of topical brimonidine 0.2% was instilled into the right eye. IOP before and after the procedure was normal OU. Rx prednisolone acetate ophthalmic suspension 1% QID × 3–4 days. RTC 1 week.

## Acknowledgment
Special acknowledgment to Cornea, Cataract, and Refractive Surgeon Jason Brenner, MD of Boston Vision for additional consultation and procedure development.

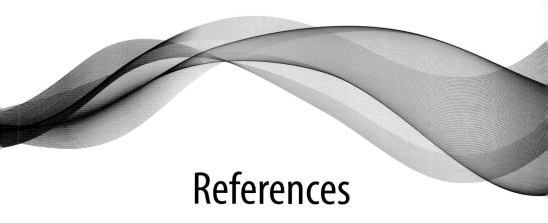

# References

## Chapter 1: Patient Communication

### General References

1. Dean S, Mathers JM, Calvert M, et al. "The patient is speaking": discovering the patient voice in ophthalmology. *Br J Ophthalmol.* 2017;101(6):700–708.
2. Hausman A. Taking your medicine: relational steps to improving patient compliance. *Health Mark Q.* 2001;19(2):49–71.
3. Llyod M, Bor R, Noble LM. *Clinical Communication Skills for Medicine.* 4th ed. Edinburgh, Scotland: Elsevier; 2018.
4. Wanzer MB, Booth-Butterfield M, Gruber K. Perceptions of health care providers' communication: relationships between patient-centered communication and satisfaction. *Health Commun.* 2004;16(3):363–383.

### Technique-Specific References

#### 1.2 Patient Privacy

5. Chen JQ, Benusa A. HIPAA security compliance challenges: the case for small healthcare providers. *International Journal of Healthcare Management.* 2017;10(2):135–146.
6. Eap SH. *Optometry Law.* Denver, CO: Outskirts Press; 2012.
7. Sterling R. Defend your practice against HIPAA violations. *Med Econ.* 2015;92(5):52–57.
8. U.S. Department of Health and Human Services, Center for Disease Control and Prevention, https://www.cdc.gov/phlp/publications/topic/hipaa.html. Accessed July 21, 2021.
9. U.S. Department of Health and Human Services, Health Information Privacy, https://www.hhs.gov/hipaa/for-professionals/compliance-enforcement/index.html Accessed July 21, 2021.

#### 1.3 Case History

10. Ettinger ER. *Professional Communications in Eye Care.* Boston, MA: Butterworth-Heinemann; 1993.
11. Makoul G, Zick A, Green M. An evidence-based perspective on greetings in medical education. *Arch Intern Med.* 2007;167(11):1172–1176.
12. Maguire P, Pitceathly C. Key communication skills and how to acquire them. *BMJ.* 2002;325(7366):697–700.
13. Pace C. Communication skills in optometry – case history and case disposition. In: Rosenfield M, Logan N, eds. *Optometry: Science, Techniques, and Clinical Management.* 2nd ed. Butterworth-Heinemann; 2009:419–430.

#### 1.4 Presenting Examination Results to a Patient

14. Cooke S, Wakefield A, Chew-Graham C, Boggis C. Collaborative training in breaking bad news to patients. *J Interprof Care.* 2003;17(3):307–309.
15. Dawn AG, Santiago-Turla C, Lee PP. Patient expectations regarding eye care: focus group results. *Arch Ophthalmol.* 2003;121(6):762–768.

#### 1.5 Verbal Presentation of Your Patient to a Colleague, Preceptor, or Attending Supervisor

16. Chan MY. The oral case presentation: toward a performance-based rhetorical model for teaching and learning. *Med Educ Online.* 2015;20:28565.
17. Rodin R, Rohailla S, Detsky AS. The oral case presentation: time for a "refresh". *J Gen Intern Med.* 2021;36(12):3659–3664.
18. Wiese J, Saint S, Tierney LM. Using clinical reasoning to improve skills in oral case presentation. *Semin Med Pract.* 2002;5(3):29–36.

#### 1.6 Writing an Assessment and Plan

19. Pearce PF, Ferguson LA, George GS, Langford CA. The essential SOAP note in an EHR age. *The Nurse Practitioner.* 2016;41(2):29–36.
20. Sundling V, Stene HA, Eide H, Ofstad EH. Identifying decisions in optometry: a validation study of the decision identification and classification taxonomy for use in medicine (DICTUM) in optometric consultations.

*Patient Education and Counseling.* 2019;102(7):1288–1295.

21. Weed LL. Medical records, patient care, and medical education. *Ir J Med Sci.* 1964;462:271–282.

**1.7 Writing a Consultancy, Communication, or Referral Letter**

22. Davey CJ, Scally AJ, Green C, Mitchell ES, Elliott DB. Factors influencing accuracy of referral and the likelihood of false positive referral by optometrists in Bradford, United Kingdom. *J Optom.* 2016;9(3):158–165.

23. Elliott DB. Communication Skills. In: Elliott DB. *Clinical Procedures in Primary Eye Care.* 5th ed. Elsevier; 2020:11–25.

24. Evans BJW, Edgar DF, Jessa Z, et al. Referrals from community optometrists to the hospital eye service in England. *Ophthalmic Physiol Opt.* 2020;41(2):365–377.

25. Scully ND, Chu L, Siriwardena D, Wormald R, Kotecha A. The quality of optometrists' referral letters for glaucoma. *Ophthalmic Physiol Opt.* 2009;29(1):26–31.

**1.8 Reporting Abuse**

26. Elner VM. Ocular manifestations of child abuse. *Arch Ophthalmol.* 2008;126(8):1141–1142.

27. Moore B. *Eye Care for Infants and Young Children.* Boston, MA: Butterworth-Heinemann; 1997.

28. Smith SK. Child abuse and neglect: a diagnostic guide for the optometrist. *J Am Optom Assoc.* 1988;59(10):760–765.

29. U.S. Department of Health and Human Services, Child Welfare Gateway, https://www.childwelfare.gov/. Accessed May 4, 2022.

30. U.S. Department of Health and Human Services, Administration for Community Living, https://acl.gov/programs/elder-justice/elder-justice-coordinating-council-ejcc. Accessed April 14, 2022.

31. U.S. Department of Health and Human Services, National Center on Elder Abuse, https://ncea.acl.gov/. Accessed April 14, 2022.

**1.9 Writing a Prescription for Medication**

32. Gabay M. Federal controlled substances act: dispensing requirements, electronic prescriptions, and fraudulent prescriptions. *Hosp Pharm.* 2014;49(3):244–246.

33. Sheikh D, Mateti UV, Kabekkodu S. Sanal T. Assessment of medication errors and adherence to WHO prescription writing guidelines in a tertiary care hospital. *Future Journal of Pharmaceutical Sciences.* 2017;3(1):60–64.

**Chapter 2: Entrance Tests**

*General References*

34. Benjamin WJ. *Borish's Clinical Refraction.* 2nd ed. Boston, MA: Butterworth-Heinemann; 2006.

35. Elliott DB. *Clinical Procedures in Primary Eye Care.* 5th ed. Elsevier; 2020.

36. Eskridge JB, Amos JF, Bartlett JD. *Clinical Procedures in Optometry.* Philadelphia, PA: Lippincott; 1991.

37. Grosvenor T. *Primary Care Optometry: A Clinical Manual.* 5th ed. Boston, MA: Butterworth-Heinemann; 2007.

38. Rosenfield M, Logan N. *Optometry: Science, Techniques and Clinical Management.* 2nd ed. Boston, MA: Butterworth-Heinemann/Elsevier; 2009.

39. Scheiman M, Wick B. *Clinical Management of Binocular Vision: Heterophoric, Accommodative and Eye Movement Disorders.* 4th ed. Philadelphia, PA: Lippincott, Williams & Williams; 2014.

40. von Noorden GK. *Binocular Vision and Ocular Motility: Theory and Management of Strabismus.* 6th ed. London: CV Mosby; 2002.

41. Weissberg EM. *Essentials of Clinical Binocular Vision.* Boston, MA: Butterworth-Heinemann; 2004.

*Technique-Specific References*

**2.2 Infection Control**

42. Fernandes P, Oyong K, Terashita D. Understanding infection prevention practices in optometry clinics. *Optom Vision Sci.* 2020;97:24–27.

43. Hart KM, Stapleton F, Carnt N, Arundel L, Lian K-Y. Optometry Australia's infection control guidelines 2020. *Clin Exp Optometry.* 2021;104(3):267–284.

44. Tyhurst KN, Hettler DL. Infection control guidelines-an update for the optometric practice. *Optometry.* 2009;80(11):613–620.

**2.3 External Observation**

45. Bell FC. The external eye examination. In: Walker HK, Hall WD, Hurst JW. 3rd ed. *Clinical Methods: The History, Physical, and Laboratory Examinations.* Boston, MA: Butterworths; 1990.

**2.4 Visual Acuity: Minimum Legible (Snellen)**

46. Elliott DB, Yang KCH, Whitaker D. Visual acuity changes throughout adulthood in normal, healthy eyes: seeing beyond 6/6. *Optom Vis Sci.* 1995;72:186–191.

47. Grosvenor T. The preliminary examination—Part 2: visual acuity. *Optom Weekly.* 1977:36–39.

48. Holliday JT. Visual acuity measurements. *J Cataract Refract Surg.* 2004:30:287–290.

49. Kaiser PK. Prospective evaluation of visual acuity assessment: a comparison of Snellen versus ETDRS charts in clinical practice. *Trans Am Ophthalmol Soc.* 2009;107:311.

50. Pitts DG. Visual acuity as a function of age. *J Am Optom Assoc.* 1982;53:117–124.

51. Velasco e Cruz AA. Historical roots of 20/20 as a (wrong) standard value of normal visual acuity. *Optom Vis Sci.* 1990;67:661.

**2.5 Visual Acuity: Minimum Legible Using a LogMAR Chart**

52. Bailey IL, Lovie JE. New design principles for visual acuity letter charts. *Am J Optom Physiol Opt.* 1976;53:740–745.
53. Bailey IL, Lovie-Kitchin JE. Visual acuity testing. From the laboratory to the clinic. *Vision Res.* 2013;90:2–9.
54. Brown B, Lovie-Kitchin J. Repeated visual acuity measurement: establishing the patient's own criterion for change. *Optom Vis Sci.* 1993;70:45–53.
55. Carkeet A. Modeling logMAR visual acuity scores: effects of termination rules and alternative forced-choice options. *Optom Vis Sci.* 2001;78:529–538.
56. Ferris FL III, Freidlin V, Kassoff A, Green SB, Milton RC. Relative letter and position difficulty on visual acuity charts from the early treatment diabetic retinopathy study. *Am J Ophthalmol.* 1993;116:735–740.
57. Ferris FL, Bailey I. Standardizing the measurement of visual acuity for clinical research studies. *Ophthalmology.* 1996;103:181–182.
58. Kaiser PK. Prospective evaluation of visual acuity assessment: a comparison of Snellen versus ETDRS charts in clinical practice. *Trans Am Ophthalmol Soc.* 2009;107:311.
59. Lovie-Kitchin JE, Brown B. Repeatability and intercorrelations of standard vision tests as a function of age. *Optom Vis Sci.* 2000;77:412–420.
60. Ricci F, Cedrone C, Cerulli L. Standardized measurement of visual acuity. *Ophthalmol Epidemiol.* 1997;5:41–53.
61. Siderov J, Tiu AL. Variability of measurements of visual acuity in a large eye clinic. *Acta Ophthalmol Scand.* 1999;77:673–676.
62. Wood JM, Bullimore MA. Interocular differences in visual function in normal subjects. *Ophthalmol Physiol Opt.* 1996;16:507–512.

**2.6 Visual Acuity: Minimum Legible Using the Massachusetts Visual Acuity Test**

63. Anstice NS, Thompson B. The measurement of visual acuity in children: an evidence-based update. *Clin Exp Optom.* 2014;97:3–11.
64. Becker R, Hubsch S, Graf MH, Kaufmann H. Examination of young children with Lea symbols. *Br J Ophthalmol.* 2002;86:513–516.
65. Hyvarinen L, Nasanen R, Laurinen P. New visual acuity test for pre-school children. *Acta Ophthalmol.* 1980;58:507–511.

**2.7 Pinhole Visual Acuity**

66. Kleinstein R. Use of the pinhole test. *Optom Monthly.* 1982:171–173.
67. Kumar RS, Rackenchath MV, Sathidevi AV, et al. Accuracy of pinhole visual acuity at an urban Indian hospital. *Eye.* 2019;33:335–337.
68. Takahashi E. The use and interpretation of the pinhole test. *Optom Weekly.* 1965:83–86.

**2.8 Color Vision**

69. Bailey JE, Neitz M, Tait DM, Neitz J. Evaluation of an updated HRR color vision test. *Vis Neurosci.* 2004;21(03):431–436.
70. Cole BL, Llan KY, Lakkis C. The new Richmond HRR pseudoisochromatic for colour vision is better than the Ishihara test. *Clin Exp Optom.* 2006;89(2):73–80.
71. Chioran G, Sheedy J. Pseudoisochromatic plate design—Macbeth or tungsten illumination? *Am J Optom Physiol Opt.* 1983;60:204–215.
72. Diez MA, Luque MJ, Capilla P, et al. Detection and assessment of color vision anomalies and deficiencies in children. *J Pediatr Ophthalmol Strab.* 2001;38:195–205.
73. Duckman RH. *Visual Development, Diagnosis, and Treatment of the Pediatric Patient.* [Electronic Resource]. Lippincott Williams & Wilkins; 2006.
74. Fanlo Zarazaga A, Gutiérrez Vásquez J, Pueyo Royo V. Review of the main colour vision clinical assessment tests. *Arch Soc Esp Oftalmol.* 2019;94(1):25–32.
75. Huna-Baron R, Glovinsky Y, Habot-Wilner Z. Comparison between Hardy-Rand-Rittler 4th edition and Ishihara color plate tests for detection of dyschromatopsia in optic neuropathy. *Graefes Arch Clin Exp Ophthalmol.* 2013;251(2):585–589.
76. Rodgin S. Acquired color vision defects. *N Engl J Optom.* 1986;38:11–24.
77. Somerfield M, Long G, Tuck JP, Gillard ET. Effects of viewing conditions on standard measures of acquired and congenital color defects. *Optom Vis Sci.* 1989;66:29–33.
78. Thiadens AA, Hoyng CB, Polling JR, Bernaerts-Biskop R, van den Born LI, Klaver CC. Accuracy of four commonly used color vision tests in the identification of cone disorders. *Ophthalmic Epidemiol.* 2013;20(2):114–121.

**2.9 Cover Test**

79. Daum KM. Heterophoria and heterotropia. In: Eskridge JB, Amos JF, Bartlett JD. *Clinical Procedures in Optometry.* Philadelphia, PA: Lippincott; 1991:72–89.
80. Eskridge J. The complete cover test. *J Am Optom Assoc.* 1973;44:602–609.

81. Evans BJW. *Pickwell's Binocular Vision Anomalies*. 6th ed. Elsevier; 2021.

82. Rabbetts RB. *Bennett and Rabbett's Clinical Visual Optics*. Oxford, England: Butterworth-Heinemann Ltd; 2007.

83. Rainey BB, Schroeder TL, Goss DA, Grosvenor TP. Reliability of and comparisons among three variations of the alternating cover test. *Ophthalmol Physiol Optom*. 1998;18:430–437.

84. Scheiman M, Wick B. *Clinical Management of Binocular Vision; Heterophoric, Accommodative, and Eye Movement Disorders*. 5th ed. Wolters Kluwer/Lippincott Williams & Wilkins; 2019.

85. Sheedy JE, Saladin JJ. Exophoria at near in presbyopia. *Am J Optom Physiol Opt*. 1975;52:474–481.

86. Von Noorden GK. *Binocular Vision and Ocular Motility: Theory and Management of Strabismus*. London: CV Mosby; 2002.

87. Sloan P. The cover test in clinical practice. *Am J Optom Arch Am Acad Optom*. 1954;31:311.

**2.10 Stereopsis**

88. Antona B, Barrio A, Sanchez I, Gonzalez E, Gonzalez G. Intraexaminer repeatability and agreement in stereoacuity measurements made in young adults. *Int J Ophthalmol*. 2015;8(2):374–381.

89. Ciner EB, Ying GS, Kulp MT, et al. VIP Study Group. Stereoacuity of preschool children with and without vision disorders. *Optom Vis Sci*. 2014;91:351–358.

90. Glaholt T, Spivak T, Sacripanti B. Evaluation of clinical stereopsis tests for use in aircrew vision assessment DRDC – Toronto Research Centre Prepared For: Col. Morrissette RCAF Surgeon Defence Research and Development Canada Scientific Report DRDC-RDDC-2017-R032 June 2017.

91. Heron G, Dholakia S, Collins DE, McLaughlan H. Stereoscopic threshold in children and adults. *Am J Optom Physiol Opt*. 1985;62:505–515.

92. Piano M, Tidbury L, O'Connor A. Normative values for near and distance clinical tests of stereoacuity. *Strabismus*. 2016;24(4),169–172.

93. Random Dot 3 Stereo Test Manual. Vision Assessment Corporation. https://www.visionassessment.com/random-dot-3-s. Accessed June 29, 2021.

94. Saladin, J. Phorometry and Stereopsis. In: Benjamin WJ. *Borish's Clinical Refraction*. 2nd ed. Butterworth-Heinemann -Elsevier. 2006:899–960.

95. Simons K. Stereoacuity norms in young children. *Arch Ophthalmol*. 1981;99(3):439–445.

**2.11 Near Point of Convergence (NPC)**

96. Adler P, Cregg M, Viollier A, Woodhouse J. Influence of target type and RAF rule on the measurement of near point of convergence. *Ophthalmic Physiol Opt*. 2007;27(1):22–30.

97. Haynes G, Cohen B, Rouse M, De Land PN. Normative values for the nearpoint of convergence of elementary schoolchildren. *Optom Vis Sci*. 1998;75(7):506–512.

98. Jimenez R, Perez M, Garcia J, Gonzalez M. Statistical normal values of visual parameters that characterize binocular function in children. *Spain Ophthal. Physiol. Opt*. 2004;24:528–542.

99. Maples W, Hoenes R. Near point of convergence norms measured in elementary school children. *Optom Vis Sci*. 2007;84(3):224–228.

100. Mohindra I, Molinari J. Convergence insufficiency: its diagnosis and management - part I. *J. Optom Mon* 1980;71(3):38–43.

101. Mohindra I, Molinari J. The subjective measurement of the near point of convergence and its significance in the diagnosis of convergence insufficiency. *Am Orthopt J*. 1952;2:40–42.

102. Pang Y, Gabriel H, Frantz KA, Saeed F. A prospective study of different test targets for the near point of convergence. *Ophthalmic Physiol Opt*. 2010;30:298–303.

103. Rous, MW, Hyman L, CIRS Study Group. How do you make the diagnosis of convergence insufficiency? Survey results. *J Optom Vis Devel*. 1997;28:91–97.

104. Siderov J, Chiu SC, Waugh SJ. Differences in the near point of convergence with target type. *Ophthalmic Physiol Opt*. 2001;21:356–360.

105. Scheiman M, Gallaway M, Frantz KA, Peters RJ, Hatch S, Cuff M, Mitchell GL. Nearpoint of convergence: test procedure, target selection, and normative data. *Optom Vis Sci*. 2003;80(3):214–225.

106. Scheiman M, Wick B. *Clinical Management of Binocular Vision: Heterophoric, Accommodative, and Eye Movement Disorders*. 4th ed. Philadelphia: Wolters Kluwer/Lippincott Williams & Wilkins; 2013.

107. Von Noorden GK, Brown DJ and Parks M. Associated convergence and accommodative insufficiency. *Doc Ophthal*. 1973;34:393–403.

108. Wick B, Amos JF. Horizontal deviations. In: Amos JF. *Diagnosis and Management in Vision Care*. Butterworth-Heinemann;1987:473.

**2.12 Hirschberg Test and Krimsky Test**

109. Eskridge JB, Wick B, Perrigin D. The Hirschberg test: a double-masked clinical evaluation. *Am J Optom Physiol Opt*. 1988;65:745–750.

110. Gräf M. The Brückner test revisited. In: Lorenz B, Brodsky MC (eds). *Pediatric Ophthalmology, Neuro-Ophthalmology, Genetics. Essentials in Ophthalmology*. Springer; 2010.

111. Choi Y, Kushner B. The accuracy of experienced strabismologists using the Hirschberg and Krimsky tests. *Ophthalmology.* 1998;105(7):1301–1316.

112. Scheiman M. Hirschberg, Krimsky, Brückner tests. In: Eskridge JB, Amos JF, Bartlett JD, eds. *Clinical Procedures in Optometry.* Lippincott; 1991.

113. Scheiman M, Wick B. *Clinical Management of Binocular Vision; Heterophoric, Accommodative, and Eye Movement Disorders.* 5th ed. Wolters Kluwer/Lippincott Williams & Wilkins; 2019.

**2.13 Brückner Test**

114. Gräf M. The Brückner test revisited. In: Lorenz B, Brodsky MC (eds). *Pediatric Ophthalmology, Neuro-Ophthalmology, Genetics. Essentials in Ophthalmology.* Springer; 2010.

115. Gräf M, Alhammouri Q, Vieregge C, Lorenz B. The Brückner transillumination test: limited detection of small-angle esotropia. *Ophthalmology.* 2011;118(12):2504–2509.

116. Gräf M, Jung A. The Brückner test: extended distance improves sensitivity for ametropia. *Graefes Arch Clin Exp Ophthalmol.* 2008;246:135–141.

117. Griffin JR, Cotter SA. The Brückner test: evaluation of clinical usefulness. *Am J Optom Physiol Opt.* 1986;63:957.

118. Kothari MT. Can the Brückner test be used as a rapid screening test to detect significant refractive errors in children? *Indian J Ophthalmol.* 2007;55(3);213.

**2.14 Extraocular Motilities (EOMs)**

119. Eskridge J. Evaluation and diagnosis of incomitant ocular deviations. *J Am Optom Assoc.* 1989;60:375–388.

120. Eskridge J, Wick B, Perrigin D. The Hirschberg test: a double-masked clinical evaluation. *Am J Optom Physiol Opt.* 1988;65:745–750.

121. Genco L. Testing extraocular muscles and visual skills. *Optom Monthly.* 1979;70:261–266.

122. Gray L. Doctor I see double. *Rev Optom.* March 1985:41–49.

123. Dell-Osso LF, Daroff RB. Eye movement characteristics and recording techniques. In: Jaeger E, Tasman W. *Duane's Ophthalmology.* Vol. 2, 2nd ed. Lippincott Williams & Wilkins; 2013.

124. Koene AR, Erklens CJ. Properties of 3D rotations and their relation to eye movement control. *Biol Cybern.* 2004;90:410–417.

125. Leigh RJ, Zee DS. *The Neurology of Eye Movements.* 4th ed. New York, NY: Oxford University Press; 2006.

126. Rush JA, Younge BR. Paralysis of cranial III, IV, and VI. Cause and prognosis in 1000 cases. *Arch Ophthalmol.* 1981;99:76–79.

127. Sharpe JA. Neurophysiology and neuroanatomy of smooth pursuit: lesion studies. *Brain Cogn.* 2008;68:241–254.

128. Sheni D, Remole A. Variation of convergence limits with change in direction of gaze. *Am J Optom Physiol Opt.* 1988;65:76–83.

**2.15 Pupils**

129. Bremner FD. Pupil assessment in optic nerve disorders. *Eye (Lond).* 2004;18(11):1175–1181.

130. Carter J. Diagnosis of pupillary anomalies. *J Am Optom Assoc.* 1979;50:671–680.

131. Chang DS, Xu L, Boland MV, Friedman DS. Accuracy of pupil assessment for the detection of glaucoma: a systematic review and meta-analysis. *Ophthalmology.* 2013;120(11):2217–2225.

132. Gray L. The five-step pupil evaluation. *Rev Optom.* February 1981:38–44.

133. Hsu JL, Weikert MP, Foroozan R. Modified upgaze technique for pupil examination. *J Neuroophthalmol.* 2010;30(4):344–346.

134. Hwang JM, Kim C, Kim JY. Relative afferent pupillary defect in patients with asymmetric cataracts. *J Cataract Refract Surg.* 2004;30(1):132–136.

135. Kawasaki A, Miller NR, Kardon R. Pupillographic investigation of the relative afferent pupillary defect associated with a midbrain lesion. *Ophthalmology.* 2010;117(1):175–179.

136. Nyman J, Nyman N. Pupillary examination. *J Am Optom Assoc.* 1977;48:1375–1380.

137. Slamovits TL, Glaser JS, Mbekeani JN. The pupils and accommodation. In: Jaeger E, Tasman W. *Duane's Ophthalmology.* Vol. 2, 2nd ed. Lippincott Williams & Wilkins; 2013.

138. Thompson HS. Pupillary signs in the diagnosis of optic nerve disease. *Trans Ophthalmol Soc UK.* 1976;96:377–381.

139. Thompson HS, Pilley SF. Unequal pupils. A flowchart for sorting out the anisocorias. *Surv Ophthalmol.* 1976;21:45–48.

140. Walsh TJ. Pupillary abnormalities. In: Walsh TJ, ed. *Neuro-ophthalmology: Clinical Signs and Symptoms.* Philadelphia, PA: Lea & Febiger; 1992.

141. Wilhelm H, Peters T, Lüdtke H, Wilhelm B. The prevalence of relative afferent pupillary defects in normal subjects. *J Neuroophthalmol.* 2007;27(4):263–267.

142. Wilhelm H. The pupil. *Curr Opin Neurol.* 2008;21(1):36–42.

**2.16 Finger Counting Visual Fields**

143. Anderson AJ, Shuey NH, Wall LM. Rapid confrontation screening for peripheral visual field defects and extinction. *Clin Exp Optom.* 2009;92(1)45–48.

144. Bass SJ, Cooper J, Feldman J, Horn D. Comparison of an automated confrontation testing device

versus finger counting in the detection of field loss. *Optometry.* 2007;78(8):390–395.

145. Genco L. Visual losses and perimetry. *Optom Monthly.* 1979;70:621–626.

146. Grosvenor T. The preliminary examination, part 10. Visual field screening. *Optom Weekly.* 1978;64:111–116.

147. Kerr NM, Chew SS, Eady EK, Gamble GD, Danesh-Meyer HV. Diagnostic accuracy of confrontation visual field tests. *Neurology.* 2010;74(15):1184–1190.

148. Pandit RJ, Gales K, Griffiths PG. Effectiveness of testing visual fields by confrontation. *Lancet.* 2001;358(9290):1339–1340.

149. Prasad S, Cohen AB. Diagnostic accuracy of confrontation visual field tests. *Neurology.* 2011;76(13):1192–1193.

150. Reader A, Harper D. Confrontation visual-field testing. *JAMA.* 1976;236:250.

151. Trobe JD, Acosta PC, Krischer JP, et al. Confrontation visual field techniques in the detection of anterior visual pathway lesions. *Ann Neurol.* 1981;10:28–34.

152. Wirtschafter J, Hard-Boberg A, Coffman S. Evaluating the usefulness in neuro-ophthalmology of visual field examinations peripheral to 30 degrees. *Trans Am Ophthalmol Soc.* 1984;82:329–357.

## Chapter 3: Refraction

### General References

153. Benjamin WJ. *Borish's Clinical Refraction.* 2nd ed. Boston, MA: Butterworth-Heinemann; 2006.

154. Edwards K, Llewellyn R. *Optometry.* Boston, MA: Butterworth; 1988.

155. Grosvenor T. *Primary Care Optometry: A Clinical Manual.* 2nd ed. Chicago, IL: Professional Press; 1989.

156. Kurtz, D. The perfect eye: a novel model for teaching the theory of refraction. *J Optom Ed.* 1999;24:91–95.

157. Michaels D. *Visual Optics and Refraction: A Clinical Approach.* 3rd ed. St Louis, MO: Mosby; 1985.

158. Michaels David D. *Basic Refraction Techniques.* New York,: Raven Press; 1988.

159. Zadnik K, ed. *The Ocular Examination: Measurements and Findings.* Philadelphia, PA: Saunders; 1997.

### Technique-Specific References

#### 3.2 Interpupillary Distance (PD)

160. Brooks CW, Borish I. Measuring the interpupillary distance. In: *System for Ophthalmic Dispensing. 3rd ed.* Philadelphia, PA: Butterworth-Heinemann; 2007:26–38.

161. Brown WL. Interpupillary distance, In: Eskridge JB, Amos JF, Bartlett JD. *Clinical Procedures in Optometry.* Philadelphia, PA: Lippincott; 1991:39–52.

162. Gupta VP, Sodhi PK, Pandey RM. Normal values for inner intercanthal, interpupillary, and outer intercanthal distances in the Indian population. *Int J Clin Pract.* 2003;57(1):25–29.

163. Holland BJ, Siderov J. Repeatability of measurements of interpupillary distance. *Ophthalm Physiol Opt.* 1999;19:74–78.

164. Murphy WK, Laskin DM. Intercanthal and interpupillary distance in the black population. *Oral Surg Oral Med Oral Pathol.* 1990;69(6):676–680.

165. Pointer JS. The interpupillary distance in adult Caucasian subjects, with reference to 'readymade' reading spectacle centration. *Ophthalmic and Physiological Optics.* 2012;32:324–331.

#### 3.3 Lensometry

166. Bhootra AK. Lensometry. In: *Clinical Refraction Guide. 2nd ed.* Kathmandu, Nepal: Jaypee Brothers Medical Publishers Ltd.; 2019:74–79.

167. Brooks CW, Borish I. Ordering and verification. In: *System for Ophthalmic Dispensing. 3rd ed.* Philadelphia, PA: Butterworth-Heinemann; 2007:89–119.

168. Fannin TE, Grosvenor T. *Clinical Optics.* Boston, MA: Butterworth; 1987.

#### 3.4 Introduction to the Manual Phoropter

169. Reichert Technologies, Ametek Ultra Precision Technologies. *Reichert Phoroptor user guide.* Ametek. 2015.

170. OptiUSA. *Phoropter instruction manual.* OptiUSA. https://www.optiusa.com/files/pdfs/Manual_INS-11010.pdf. Accessed March 25, 2022.

#### 3.5 Static Retinoscopy

171. Corboy JM. *The Retinoscopy Book: An Introductory Manual for Eye Care Professionals.* Thorofare, NJ: Slack; 2003.

172. Jones R. Physiological pseudomyopia. *Optom Vis Sci.* 1990;67:610.

173. Mutti DO. Sources of normal and anomalous motion in retinoscopy. *Optom Vis Sci.* 2004;81(9):663–672.

174. Mutti DO, Zadnik K. Refractive error. In: Zadnik K, ed. *The Ocular Examination: Measurements and Findings.* Philadelphia, PA: Saunders, 1997:64–74.

175. Roorda A, Bobier WR. Geometrical technique to determine the influence of monochromatic aberrations of retinoscopy. *J Opt Soc Am.* 1996;13:3–11.

176. Roorda A, Bobier WR. Retinoscopic reflexes: theoretical basis and effects of monochromatic aberrations. *J Opt Soc Am.* 1996;6:610–618.

### 3.6 Routine Distance Subjective Refraction with the Manual Phoropter

177. Atchison DA, Charman WN, Woods RL. Subjective depth-of-focus of the eye. *Optom Vis Sci.* 1997:74:511–520.

178. Bannon RE. *Clinical Manual on Refraction with the AO Ultramatic Rx Master Phoropter.* Buffalo, NY: American Optical Corporation; 1975.

179. Borish IL, Benjamin WJ. Monocular and binocular subjective refraction. In: Benjamin WJ, ed. *Borish's Clinical Refraction.* Philadelphia, PA: WB Saunders; 2006:790–898.

180. Cooper J, Citek K, Feldman JM. Comparison of refractive error measurements in adults with Z-View aberrometer, Humphrey autorefractor, and subjective refraction. *Optometry.* 2011;82:231–240.

181. Hung L-F, Ramamirtham R, Wensveen JM, Harwerth RS, Smith EL III. Objective and subjective refractive error measurements in monkeys. *Optom Vis Sci.* 2012;89:168–177.

182. Johnson BL, Edwards JS, Goss DA, et al. A comparison of three subjective tests for astigmatism and their interexaminer reliabilities. *J Am Optom Assoc.* 1996;67:590–598.

183. Layton A. A supplementary technique for balancing refraction. *Am J Optom Physiol Opt.* 1975;52:125–127.

184. Luo HD, Gazzard G, Liang Y, Shankar A, Tan DTH, Saw SM. Defining myopia using refractive error and uncorrected logMAR visual acuity >0.3 from 1334 Singapore school children ages 7-9 years. *Br J Ophthalmol.* 2006;90(3):362–366.

185. Marcos S, Moreno E, Navarro R. The depth-of-field of the human eye from objective and subjective measurements. *Vision Res.* 1999;39:2039–2049.

186. Milder B, Rubin ML. *The Fine Art of Prescribing Glasses Without Making a Spectacle of Yourself.* 2nd ed. Gainesville, FL: Triad Scientific; 1991.

187. Miller AD, Kris MJ, Griffiths AC. Effect of small focal errors on vision. *Optom Vis Sci.* 1997;74:521–526.

188. Mutti DO, Zadnik K. Refractive error. In Zadnik, K. ed. *The Ocular Examination: Measurements and Findings.* Philadelphia, PA: Saunders; 1997:74–81, Chap 4.

189. Polasky M. Monocular subjective refraction. In: Eskridge J B Amos J B, Bartlett J D (eds) *Clinical Procedures in Optometry.* Philadelphia, PA: Lippincott; 1991:174–188.

190. Rabbetts RB. *Bennett & Rabbetts' Clinical Visual Optics.* Edinburgh; New York: Elsevier/Butterworth Heinemann, 2007.

191. Reinecke RD, Herm RJ. *Refraction: A Programmed Text.* 2nd ed. New York, NY: Appleton-Century-Crofts; 1976.

192. Rosenfield M. Subjective refraction. In: Rosenfield M, Logan N. eds. *Optometry: Science, Techniques and Clinical Management.* Edinburgh: Elsevier; 2009:209–228.

193. Rosenfield M, Chiu NN. Repeatability of subjective and objective refraction. *Optom Vis Sci.* 1995;72:577–579.

194. Smith K, Weissberg E, Travison TG. Alternative methods of refraction: a comparison of three techniques. *Optom Vis Sci.* 2010;87(3):176–182.

195. Ward PA, Charman WN. An objective assessment of the effect of fogging on accommodation. *Am J Optom Physiol Opt.* 1987;64:762–767.

### 3.7 Use of the Trial Frame to Modify a Prescription

196. Howell-Duffy C, Umar G, Ruparelia N, Elliott DB. What adjustments, if any, do UK optometrists make to the subjective refraction result prior to prescribing? *Ophthalmic Physiol Opt.* 2010;30(3):225–239.

197. Segura F, Sanchez-Cano A, Lopez de la Fuente C, Fuentes-Broto L, Pinilla I. Evaluation of patient visual comfort and repeatability of refractive values in non-presbyopic healthy eyes. *Int J Ophthalmol.* 2015;8(5):1031–1036.

### 3.8 Clock Chart (Sunburst Dial)

198. Perches S, Collados MV, Ares J. Retinal image simulation of subjective refraction techniques. *PLoS ONE.* 2016;11(3):e0150204.

### 3.9 Jackson Cross Cylinder Check Test for Uncorrected Astigmatism

199. Brookman KE. The Jackson crossed cylinder: historical perspective. *Optom Vis Sci.* 1993;64:329–331.

200. Murphy PJ, Beck AJ, Coll EP. An assessment of the orthogonal astigmatism test for the subjective measurement of astigmatism. *Ophthalmic Physiological Opt.* 2002;22:194–200.

201. O'Leary D, Yang PH, Yeo CH. Effect of cross cylinder power on cylinder axis sensitivity. *Am J Optom Physiol Opt.* 1987;64:367–369.

202. Rabbetts RB. *Bennett & Rabbetts' Clinical Visual Optics.* Edinburgh; New York: Elsevier/Butterworth Heinemann, 2007.

### 3.10 Ocular-Dominance Testing

203. Walls GL. A theory of ocular dominance. *AMA Arch Ophthalmol.* 1951;45:387–412.

204. Zeri F, DeLuca M, Spinelli D, Zoccolotti P. Ocular dominance stability and reading skill: a controversial relationship. *Optom Vis Sci.* 2011;88(11):1353–1362.

### 3.11 Trial Frame Refraction

205. Bailey IL. Low vision refraction. In: Amos JF, Bartlett JD, Eskridge JB. *Diagnostic Procedures in Optometry.* Philadelphia,PA:Lippincott; 1991:762–768.

206. Bailey IL. Refracting low-vision patients. *Optom Monthly*. May 1978:131–135.

207. DeCarlo DK, McGwin G Jr, Searcey K, et al. Trial frame refraction versus autorefraction among new patients in a low-vision clinic. *Invest Ophthalmol Vis Sci*. 2013;54(1):19–24.

208. Momeni-Moghaddam H, Goss DA. Comparison of binocular balancing techniques. *Clin Exp Optom*. 2014;97:422–425.

**3.12 Cycloplegic Refraction**

209. Amos D. Cycloplegic refraction. In: Bartlett J, Jaanus S, eds. *Ocular Pharmacology*. Boston, MA: Butterworth; 1984:469–482.

210. Chung I. Topical ophthalmic drugs and the pediatric patient. *Optometry*. 2000;71:511–518.

211. Farhood, QK. Cycloplegic refraction in children with cyclopentolate versus atropine. *J Clin Exp Ophthalmol*. 2012;3(7):1–6.

212. Fotedar R, Rochtchina E, Morgan I, Wang JJ, Mitchell P, Rose KA. Necessity of cycloplegia for assessing refractive error in 12-year-old children: a population-based study. *Am J Ophthalmology*. 2007;144:307–309.

213. Kleinstein RN, Mutti DO, Manny RE, et al. Cycloplegia in African-American children. *Optom Vis Sci*. 1999;76:102–107.

214. Lahdes KK, Huupponen RK, Kaila RJ. Ocular effects and systemic absorption of cyclopentolate eyedrops after canthal and conventional application. *Acta Ophthalmol*. 1994;72:698–702.

215. Manny RE, Fern KD, Zervas HJ, et al. 1% cyclopentolate hydrochloride: another look at the time course of cycloplegia using an objective measure of the accommodative response. *Optom Vis Sci*. 1993;70:651–665.

216. Manny RE, Scheiman M, Kurtz D, et al. and The COMET Study Group. Tropicamide 1%: an effective cycloplegic agent for myopic children. *Invest Ophthalmol Vis Sci*. 2001;42:1728–1735.

217. Mutti DO, Zadnik K. Refractive error. In: Zadnik K, ed. *The Ocular Examination: Measurements and Findings*. Philadelphia, PA: Saunders; 1997:Chap 4, 82–84.

218. Smith D. Point: the usefulness of cycloplegic retinoscopy. *Opt Vis Dev*. 2013;1:8–9.

219. Guo X, Shakarchi AF, Block SS, Friedman DS, Repka MX, Collins ME. Non-cycloplegic compared with cycloplegic refraction in a Chicago school-aged population. *Ophthalmology*. 2022;S0161-6420(22)00166-X.

**3.13 Delayed Subjective Refraction**

220. Grosvenor T. How to keep your patient from accommodating. *Optom Weekly*. 1976:44–46.

221. Satgunam PN. Relieving accommodative spasm: two case reports. *Optometry Visual Performance*. 2018;6(5):207–212.

**3.14 Determining the Add for a Presbyope**

222. Antona B, Barra F, Barrio A, Gutierrez A, Piedrahita E, Martin Y. Comparing methods of determining addition in presbyopes. *Clin Exp Optom*. 2008;91(3):313–318.

223. Blystone PA. Relationship between age and presbyopic addition using a sample of 3,645 examinations from a single private practice. *J Am Optom Assoc*. 1999;70:505–508.

224. Iyamu E, Iyamu JE, Oghovwerha L. Anthropometry, amplitude of accommodation, and spherical equivalent refractive error in a Nigerian population. *ISRN Ophthalmol*. September 5, 2012:295613 (published online).

225. Kurtz D. Presbyopia. In Brookman KE, ed. *Refractive Management of Ametropia*. Boston, MA: Butterworth-Heinemann; 1996:145–179.

226. Leffler CT, Davenport B, Rentz J, Miller A, Benson W. Clinical predictors of the optimal spectacle correction for comfort performing desktop tasks. *Clin Exp Optom*. 2008;91:530–537.

227. Pointer JS. The presbyopic add. I. Magnitude and distribution in a historical context. *Ophthalmol Physiol Optom*. 1995;15:235–240.

228. Pointer JS. The presbyopic add. III. Influence of the distance refractive type. *Ophthalmol Physiol Optom*. 1995;15:249–253.

**3.15 Writing a Spectacle Prescription**

229. Brooks CW, Borish I. Ordering and verification. In: *System for Ophthalmic Dispensing. 3rd ed.* Philadelphia, PA: Butterworth-Heinemann; 2007:89–119.

**3.16 Keratometry**

230. Fam HB, Lim KL. Validity of the keratometric index: large population-based study. *J Cataract Refract Surg*. 2007;33:686–691.

231. Olsen T, Arnarsson A, Sasaki H, Sasaki K, Jonasson F. On the ocular refractive components: the Reykjavik Eye Study. *Acta Ophthalmol Scand*. 2007;85:361–366.

## Chapter 4: Functional Tests

*General References*

232. Benjamin WJ. *Borish's Clinical Refraction*. 2nd ed. Boston, MA: Butterworth-Heinemann; 2006.

233. Griffith JR, Grisham JD. *Binocular Anomalies: Diagnosis and Vision Therapy*. 4th ed. Chicago, IL: Professional Press; 2002.

234. Grosvenor T. *Primary Care Optometry: A Clinical Manual*. 5th ed. Boston, MA: Butterworth-Heinemann; 2007.

235. Rosenfield M, Logan N. *Optometry: Science, Techniques and Clinical Management*. 2nd ed. Boston, MA: Butterworth-Heinemann; 2009.

236. Scheiman M, Wick B. *Clinical Management of Binocular Vision; Heterophoric, Accommodative,*

*and Eye Movement Disorders.* 5th ed. Wolters Kluwer/Lippincott Williams & Wilkins; 2019.

237. Schor CM, Ciuffreda KJ. *Vergence Eye Movements: Basic and Clinical Aspects.* Boston, MA: Butterworth; 1983.

## Technique-Specific References

### 4.2 Distance Lateral and Vertical Deviations by von Graefe (VG) Technique

238. Calvin H, Rupnow P, Grosvenor T. How good is the estimated cover test at predicting the von Graefe phoria measurement? *Optom Vis Sci.* 1996;73:701–706.

239. Casillas EC, Rosenfield M. Comparison of subjective heterophoria testing with a phoropter and trial frame. *Optom Vis Sci.* 2006;83(4):237–241.

240. Goss DA, Moyer BJ, Teske MC. Comparison of dissociated phoria test findings with von Graefe phorometry & modified Thorington testing. *JBO.* 2008;19(6):145–149.

241. Kromeier M, Schmitt C, Bach M, Kommereli G. Heterophoria measured with white, dark-grey and dark-red Maddox rods. *Graefes Arch Clin Exp Ophthalmol.* 2001;239:937–940.

242. Oh KK, Cho HG, Moon B-Y, Kim S-Y, Yu D-S. The effect of dissociating prism on lateral phoria in von Graefe and Howell phoria card test. *J Korean Ophthalmic Opt Soc.* 2018;23(2):143–149.

243. Robertson KM. Symptoms, signs, and diagnostic testing of vertical misalignment. *Prob Optom.* 1992;4:541–555.

244. Saladin JJ, Sheedy JE. Population study of fixation disparity, heterophoria, and vergence. *Am J Optom Physiol Opt.* 1992;55:744–750.

245. Schroeder TL, Rainey BB, Goss DA, Grosvenor TP. Reliability of and comparisons among methods of measuring dissociated phoria. *Optom Vis Sci.* 1996;73:389–397.

246. Walline JJ, Mutti DO, Zadnik K, Jones L. Development of phoria in children. *Optom Vis Sci.* 1998;75:605–610.

### 4.3 Near Lateral and Vertical Deviations by von Graefe (VG) Technique

247. Escalante JB, Rosenfield M. Effect of heterophoria measurement technique on the clinical accommodative convergence to accommodation ratio. *Optometry.* 2006;77(5):229–234.

248. Kim J, Shim J. Comparison of amount of at distance and near phoria in dominant eye and non-dominant eye by von Graefe method. *J Korean Ophthalmic Opt Soc.* 2018;23(2):111–116.

249. Maples W, Savoy R, Harville J. Comparison of distance and near heterophoria by two clinical methods. *Optometry and Vision Development.* 2009;40(2):100–106.

250. Sanker N, Prabhu A, Ray A. A comparison of near-dissociated heterophoria tests in free space. *Clin Exp Optom.* 2012;95(6):638–642.

251. Yu DS, Ha EM. Comparisons of phoria test among prism settings of Von Graefe technique. *Korean Ophthalmic Opt Soc.* 2015;20(2):211–218.

### 4.4 Distance Horizontal Step and Smooth Vergences

252. Antona B, Barrio A, Barra F, Gonzalez E, Sanchez, I. Repeatability and agreement in the measurement of horizontal fusional vergences. *Ophthalmic Physiol Opt.* 2008;28(5):475–491.

253. Feldman J, Cooper J, Carniglia P, et al. Comparison of fusional ranges measured by Risley prisms, vectograms, and computer orthopter. *Optom Vis Sci.* 1989;66:375–382.

254. Gall R, Wick B, Bedell H. Vergence facility: establishing clinical utility. *Optom Vis Sci.* 1998;75:731–742.

255. Goss DA. Effect of test sequence on fusional vergence ranges. *N Engl J Optom.* 1995;47:39–42.

256. Jackson TW, Goss DA. Variation and correlation of standard clinical phoropter tests of phorias, vergence ranges, and relative accommodation. *J Am Optom Assoc.* 1991;62:540–547.

257. Lança CC, Rowe FJ. Measurement of fusional vergence: a systematic review. *Strabismus.* 2019;27(2):88–113.

258. Penisten DK, Hofstetter HW, Goss DA. Reliability of rotary prism fusional vergence ranges. *Optometry.* 2001;72:117–122.

259. Saladin JJ, Sheedy JE. Population study of fixation disparity, heterophoria, and vergence. *Am J Optom Physiol Opt.* 1978;55:744–750.

260. Scheiman M, Herzberg H, Frantz K, et al. A normative study of step vergences in elementary schoolchildren. *J Am Optom Assoc.* 1989;60:276–280.

261. Sheedy JE, Saladin JJ. Association of symptoms with measures of oculomotor deficiencies. *Am J Physiol Opt.* 1978;55:670–676.

262. Tuff LC, Firth AY, Griffiths HJ. Prism vergence measurements following adaptation to a base out prism. *Brit Orthop J.* 2000;57:42–44.

### 4.5 Distance Vertical Step and Smooth Vergences

263. Lança CC, Rowe FJ. Measurement of fusional vergence: a systematic review. *Strabismus.* 2019;27(2):88–113.

### 4.6 Near Horizontal Step and Smooth Vergences

264. Antona B, Barrio A, Barra F, Gonzalez E, Sanchez I. Repeatability and agreement in the measurement of horizontal fusional vergences. *Ophthalmic Physiol Opt.* 2008;28(5):475–491.

265. Fry G. An analysis of the relationships between phoria, blur, break and recovery findings at the

near point. *Am J Optom Arch Am Acad Optom.* 1941;18:393–402.

266. Goss D, Becker E. Comparison of near fusional vergence ranges with rotary prisms and with prism bars. *Optometry.* 2011;82(2):104–107.

267. Rowe FJ. Fusional vergence measures and their significance in clinical assessment. *Strabismus.* 2010;18(2):48–57.

**4.7 Near Vertical Step and Smooth Vergences**

268. Fry G. An analysis of the relationships between phoria, blur, break and recovery findings at the near point. *Am J Optom Arch Am Acad Optom.* 1941;18:393–402.

**4.8 Amplitude of Accommodation (Amps)**

269. Atchison DA, Capper EJ, McCabe KL. Critical subjective measurement of amplitude of accommodation. *Optom Vis Sci.* 1994;71:699–706.

270. Chen A, O'Leary DJ. Validity and repeatability of the modified push-up method for measuring the amplitude of accommodation. *Clin Exp Optom.* 1998;81:63–71.

271. Koslowe K, Glassman T, Tzanani-Levi C, Shneor E. Accommodative amplitude determination: pull-away versus push-up method. *OVD.* 2010;41(1):28–32.

272. Taub MB, Shallo-Hoffmann J. A comparison of three clinical tests of accommodation amplitude to Hofstetter's norms to guide diagnosis and treatment. *OVD.* 2012;43(4):180.

**4.9 Fused Cross Cylinder (FCC)**

273. Antona B, Barra F, Barrio A, Gutierrez A, Piedrahita E, Martin Y. Comparing methods of determining addition in presbyopes. *Clin Exp Optom.* 2008;91(3):313–318.

274. Benzoni JA, Collier JD, McHugh K, Rosenfield M, Portello JK. Does the dynamic cross cylinder test measure the accommodative response accurately? *Optometry.* 2009;80(11):630–634.

275. Bittencourt L, Alves M, Dantas D, Rodrigues P, Santos-Neto E. An evaluation of estimation methods for determining addition in presbyopes. *Arq Bras Oftalmol.* 2013;76(4):218–220.

276. Rosenfield M, Logan N. *Optometry: Science, Techniques and Clinical Management.* 2nd ed. Boston, MA: Butterworth-Heinemann; 2009.

277. Wee SH, Yu DS, Moon BY, Cho HG. Comparison of presbyopic additions determined by the fused cross-cylinder method using alternative target background colours. *Ophthalmic Physiol Opt.* 2010;30(6):758–765.

**4.10 Negative Relative Accommodation/Positive Relative Accommodation (NRA/PRA)**

278. Antona B, Barra F, Barrio A, Gutierrez A, Piedrahita E, Martin Y. Comparing methods of determining addition in presbyopes. *Clin Exp Optom.* 2008;91(3):313–318.

279. Bittencourt L, Alves M, Dantas D, Rodrigues P, Santos-Neto E. An evaluation of estimation methods for determining addition in presbyopes. *Arq Bras Oftalmol.* 2013;76(4):218–220.

280. García A, Cacho P, Lara F. Evaluating relative accommodations in general binocular dysfunctions. *Optom Vis Sci.* 2002;79(12):779–787.

281. Yekta A, Hashemi H, Khabazkhoob M, et al. The distribution of negative and positive relative accommodation and their relationship with binocular and refractive indices in a young population. *J Curr Ophthalmol.* 2017;29(3), 204–209.

**4.11 Binocular Accommodative Facility (BAF) & Monocular Accommodative Facility (MAF)**

282. Eskridge J. Clinical objective assessment of the accommodative response. *J Am Optom Assoc.* 1989;60:272–274.

283. McKenzie K, Kerr S, Rouse M. Study of accommodative facility testing reliability. *Am J Optom Physiol Opt.* 1987;64:186–194.

284. Rouse M, Hutter R. A normative study of the accommodative lag in elementary school children. *Am J Optom Physiol Opt.* 1984;61:693–697.

285. Scheiman M, Herzberg H, Frantz K, et al. Normative study of accommodative facility in elementary schoolchildren. *Am J Optom Physiol Opt.* 1988;65:127–134.

286. Siderov J, Johnston AW. The importance of the test parameters in the clinical assessment of accommodative facility. *Optom Vis Sci.* 1990;67:551–557.

287. Wick B, Yothers T, Morse S. Clinical testing of accommodative facility: part I. A critical appraisal of the literature. *Optometry.* 2002;73(1):11–23.

288. Yothers T, Wick B, Morse SE. Clinical testing of accommodative facility: part II. Development of an amplitude-scaled test. *Optometry.* 2002;73(2):91–102.

289. Zellers JA, Alpert TL, Rouse MW. A review of the literature and a normative study of accommodative facility. *J Am Optom Assoc.* 1984;55:31–37.

**4.12 Dynamic Retinoscopy: Monocular Estimation Method (MEM)**

290. Antona B, Barra F, Barrio A, Gutierrez A, Piedrahita E, Martin Y. Comparing methods of determining addition in presbyopes. *Clin Exp Optom.* 2008;91(3):313–318.

291. Eskridge J. Clinical objective assessment of the accommodative response. *J Am Optom Assoc.* 1989;60:272–274.

292. Goss DA, Rana S, Ramolia J. Accommodative response/stimulus by dynamic retinoscopy: near add guidelines. *Optom Vis Sci.* 2012;89(10):1497–1506.

293. Goss D, Sobhani M. Accommodative response under monocular and binocular conditions as a function of phoria in symptomatic and asymptomatic subjects. *Clin Experimental Optometry.* 2014;97(1):36–42.

294. Koslowe KC. The dynamic retinoscopies. *JBO.* 2010;21(3):63–67.

295. Locke LC, Somers W. A comparison study of dynamic retinoscopy techniques. *Optom Vis Sci.* 1989;66:540–544.

296. Rouse M, Hutter R. A normative study of the accommodative lag in elementary school children. *Am J Optom Physiol Opt.* 1984;61:693–697.

297. Tarczy-Hornoch K. Modified bell retinoscopy: measuring accommodative lag in children. *Optom Vis Sci.* 2009;86(12):1337.

**4.13 Modified Thorington (MT)**

298. Cebrian JL, Antona B, Barrio A, Gonzalez E, Gutierrez A, Sanchez I. Repeatability of the Modified Thorington card used to measure far heterophoria. *Optom Vis Sci.* 2014;91(7):786–792.

299. Facchin A, Maffioletti S. Comparison, within-session repeatability and normative data of three phoria tests. *J Optom.* 2021;14(3):263–274.

300. Lyon DW, Goss DA, Horner D, Downey JP, Rainey, B. Normative data for modified Thorington phorias and prism bar vergences from the Benton-IU study. *Optometry.* 2005;76(10):593–599.

301. Newman-Toker DE, Rizzo III JF. Subjectively quantified Maddox rod testing improves diagnostic yield over alternate cover testing alone in patients with diplopia. *J Clin Neurosci.* 2010;17(6):727–730.

**4.14 Maddox Rod (MR)**

302. Casillas Casillas E, Rosenfield M. Comparison of subjective heterophoria testing with a phoropter and trial frame. *Optom Vis Sci.* 2006;83(4):237–241.

303. Newman-Toker DE, Rizzo III JF. Subjectively quantified Maddox rod testing improves diagnostic yield over alternate cover testing alone in patients with diplopia. *J Clin Neurosci.* 2010;17(6):727–730.

**4.15 Gradient Accommodative Convergence to Accommodation (AC/A) Ratio**

304. Escalante J, Rosenfield M. Effect of heterophoria measurement technique on the clinical accommodative convergence to accommodation ratio. *Optometry.* 2006;77(5):229–234.

305. Johnston MS, Firth AY. Non-linearity of the response accommodative convergence to accommodation ratio. *Strabismus.* 2013;21(3):175–182.

306. Murray M, Newsham D. The normal accommodative convergence/accommodation (AC/A) ratio. *J Binocul Vis Ocul Motil.* 2018;68(4):140–147.

307. Scheiman M, Wick B. *Clinical Management of Binocular Vision; Heterophoric, Accommodative, and Eye Movement Disorders.* 5th ed. Wolters Kluwer/Lippincott Williams & Wilkins; 2019.

**4.16 Associated Phoria**

308. Carter D. Fixation disparity and heterophoria following prolonged wearing of prisms. *Am J Optom Arch Am Acad Optom.* 1965;42: 141–152.

309. Eskridge JB. Adaptation to vertical prism. *Am J Optom Physiol Opt.* 1988;65:371–376.

310. London R, Crelier R. Fixation disparity analysis: sensory and motor approaches. *Optometry.* 2006;77(12):590–608.

311. Otto J, Bach M, Kommerell G. The prism that aligns fixation disparity does not predict the self-selected prism. *Ophthalmic Physiol Opt.* 2008;28(6):550–557.

312. Otto JM, Kromeier M, Bach M, Kommerell G. Do dissociated or associated phoria predict the comfortable prism? *Graefes Arch Clin Exp Ophthalmol.* 2008;246(5):631–639.

313. Rutstein R, Eskridge J. Studies in vertical fixation disparity. *Am J Optom Physiol Opt.* 1986;63:639–644.

314. Sheedy JE. Actual measurement of fixation disparity and its use in diagnosis and treatment. *J Am Optom Assoc.* 1980;51:1079–1084.

**4.17 Worth 4 Dot (W4D)**

315. Bak E, Yang K, Hwang J. Validity of the Worth 4 dot test in patients with red-green color vision defect. *Optometry Vis Scie.* 2017;94:5.

316. Etezad R, Najaran M, Moravvej R, Ansari A, Azimi A. Correlation between Worth four dot test results and fusional control in intermittent exotropia. *J Ophthalmic Vis Res.* 2012;7(2):134–138.

317. Lueder G, Arnoldi K. Does "Touching Four" on the Worth 4-dot test indicate fusion in young children? A computer simulation. *Ophthalmology.* 1996;103:8,1237–1240.

318. Roper-Hall G. The "worth" of the Worth four dot test. *Am Orth J.* 2004;54(1):112–1119.

319. Von Noorden GK. *Binocular Vision and Ocular Motility: Theory and Management of Strabismus.* London: CV Mosby; 2002.

**4.18 Four Prism Diopter Base Out Test (4Δ BO Test)**

320. Frantz KA, Cotter SA, Wick B. Re-evaluation of the four prism diopter base-out test. *Optom Vis Sci.* 1992;69:777–786.

321. Savino G, Di Nicola D, Bolzani R, Dickmann A. Four diopters prism test recording in small angle esotropia: a quantitative study using a magnetic search coil. *Strabismus.* 1998;6(2):59.

322. Tomaç S. The Irvine prism test: does the positive response indicate suppression scotoma? *Int Ophthalmol.* 2005;26(1–2):67–72.

**4.19 Pursuits and Saccades**

323. Bilbao C, Pinero DP. Objective and subjective evaluation of saccadic eye movement in healthy children and children with neurodevelopmental disorders. *Vision.* 2021;5(2):28.

324. Maples WC. NSUCO oculomotor test. Santa Ana, CA: Optometric Extension Program. 1995.

325. Maples WC, Ficklin TW. Interrater and test-retest reliability of pursuits and saccades. *J Am Optom Assoc.* 1988;59(7):549–552.

**Chapter 5: Ocular Health Assessment**

*General References*

326. Bartlett JD, Jaanus SD, eds. *Clinical Ocular Pharmacology.* 5th ed. Butterworth-Heinemann; 2008.

327. Budenz DL, McSoley J. Evaluating patients for glaucoma: a history- and examination-driven method. *Prac Optom.* 2002;13:6–12.

328. Casser L, Fingeret M, Woodcome HT. *Atlas of Primary Eyecare Procedures.* 2nd ed. Norwalk, CT: Appleton & Lange; 1997.

329. Catania L. *Primary Care of the Anterior Segment.* 2nd ed. Norwalk, CT: Appleton & Lange; 1994.

330. Duane T. *Clinical Ophthalmology.* Philadelphia, PA: Lippincott; 1988.

331. Eskridge JB, Amos JF, Bartlett JD. *Clinical Procedures in Optometry.* Philadelphia, PA: Lippincott; 1991.

332. Thomann KH, Marks ES, Adamczyk DT. *Primary Eyecare in Systemic Disease.* 2nd ed. New York: McGraw-Hill; 2001.

*Technique-Specific References*

**5.2 Biomicroscopy (Slit Lamp)**

333. Chaong R, Simpson T, Fonn D. The repeatability of discrete and continuous anterior segment grading scales. *Optom Vis Sci.* 2000;77:244–251.

334. Clover J. Slit-Lamp Biomicroscopy. *Cornea.* 2018;37 Suppl 1:S5–S6.

335. Garston M. Turn up the light Part II. How to see more with your slit lamp. *Rev Optom.* September 15, 2002:75–78.

336. Martonyi CL, Bahn CF, Meyer RF. *Slit Lamp: Examination and Photography.* 3rd ed. Time One Ink; 2007;1–149.

**5.3 Examination of the Anterior Chamber**

337. Jabs DA, Nussenblatt RB, Rosenbaum JT. Standardization of uveitis nomenclature for reporting clinical data. Results of the first international workshop. *Am J Ophthalmol.* 2005;140:509–516.

338. Martin R. Cornea and anterior eye assessment with slit lamp biomicroscopy, specular microscopy, confocal microscopy, and ultrasound biomicroscopy. *Indian J Ophthalmol.* 2018;66(2):195–201.

**5.4 Specular Reflection Technique**

339. Ong Tone S, Jurkunas U. Imaging the corneal endothelium in Fuchs corneal endothelial dystrophy. *Seminars in Ophthalmol.* 2019;34(4):340–346.

**5.5 Sclerotic Scatter Technique**

340. Denion E, Béraud G, Marshall M-L, Denion G, Lux A-L. Sclerotic scatter. *J Français d'Ophtalmologie.* 2018;41(1):62–77.

341. Hayashi H, Maeda N, Ikeda Y, Nishida K, Watanabe H, Tano Y. Sclerotic scattering illumination during phototherapeutic keratectomy for better visualization of corneal opacities. *Am J Ophthlamol.* 2003;135(4):559–561.

**5.6 Eversion of the Upper Eyelid**

342. Stevens S. Ophthalmic practice. *Community Eye Health/International Centre for Eye Health.* 2005;18(55):109–110.

**5.7 Instillation of Drops**

343. Gupta R, Patil B, Shah BM, Bali SJ, Mishra SK, Dada T. Evaluating eye drop instillation technique in glaucoma patients. *J Glaucoma.* 2012;21(3):189–192.

344. Lahdes KK, Huupponen RK, Kaila RJ. Ocular effects and systemic absorption of cyclopentolate eyedrops after canthal and conventional application. *Acta Ophthalmologica.* 1994;72:698–702.

345. Smith SE. Eyedrop instillation for reluctant children. *Br J Ophthalmol.* 1991;75:480–481.

**5.8 Corneal or Conjunctival Staining**

346. Bron AJ, Evans VE, Smith JA. Grading of corneal and conjunctival staining in the context of other dry eye tests. *Cornea.* 2003;22(7):640–650.

347. Dundas M, Walker A, Woods RL. Clinical grading of corneal staining of non-contact lens wearers. *Ophthalmol Physiol Opt.* 2001;21:30–35.

348. Manning FJ, Wehrly SR, Foulks GN. Patient tolerance and ocular surface staining characteristics of lissamine green versus rose Bengal. *Ophthalmology.* 1995;102:1953–1957.

349. Wolffsohn JS, Arita R, Chalmers R, et al. TFOS DEWS II diagnostic methodology report. *Ocul Surf.* 2017;15(3):539–574.

**5.9 Tear Breakup Time (TBUT)**

350. Abelson MB, Ousler GW, Nally LA, Wlch D, Krenzer K. Alternative reference values for tear film break up time in normal and dry eye populations. *Adv Exp Med Biol.* 2002;506:1121–1125.

351. Bron AJ. Diagnosis of dry eye. *Surv Ophthalmol.* 2001;45(2):S221–S226.

352. Johnson ME, Murphy PJ. Measurement of ocular surface irritation on a linear interval scale with the ocular comfort index. *Invest. Ophthalmol. Vis. Sci.* 2007;48(10):4451–4458.

353. Korb DR. Survey of preferred tests for the diagnosis of the tear film and dry eye. *Cornea.* 2000;19:483–486.

354. Korb DR, Greiner JV, Herman J. Comparison of fluorescein break-up time measurement reproducibility using standard fluorescein strips versus the Dry Eye Test (DET) method. *Cornea.* 2001;20:811–815.

355. Lee JS, Salapatek A, Patel P, Soong F. Comparison of non-invasive tear break up times (NIBUT) assessed with video-corneal topography to the standard invasive TBUT as studied in patients after exposure to low humidity environment (LHE). *Invest. Ophthalmol. Vis. Sci.* 2009;50(13):525.

356. Mooi JK, Wang MTM, Lim J, Müller A, Craig JP. Minimising instilled volume reduces the impact of fluorescein on clinical measurements of tear film stability. *Cont Lens Anterior Eye.* 2017;40(3):170–174.

357. Pflugfelder SC, Scheffer CG, Tseng SC, et al. Evaluation of subjective assessments and objective diagnostic tests for diagnosing tear-film disorders known to cause ocular irritation. *Cornea.* 1998;17:38–56.

358. Sweeney DF, Millar TJ, Raju SR. Tear film stability: a review. *Exp Eye Res.* 2013;117:28–38.

359. Wang MT, Murphy PJ, Blades KJ, Craig JP. Comparison of non-invasive tear film stability measurement techniques. *Clin Exp Optom* 2018;101:13–17.

360. Wang MTM, Craig JP. Comparative evaluation of clinical methods of tear film stability assessment: a randomized crossover trial. *JAMA Ophthalmol.* 2018;136(3):291–294.

361. Wolffsohn JS, Arita R, Chalmers R, et al. TFOS DEWS II diagnostic methodology report. *Ocul Surf.* 2017;15(3):539–574.

**5.10 Schirmer Tests: Schirmer #1 Test and Basic Lacrimation Test**

362. de Monchy I, Gendron G, Miceli C, Pogorzalek N, Mariette X, Labetoulle M. Combination of the Schirmer I and phenol red thread tests as a rescue strategy for diagnosis of ocular dryness associated with Sjögren's syndrome. *Invest Ophthalmol Vis Sci.* 2011;52(8):5167–5173.

363. Li N, Deng XG, He MF. Comparison of the Schirmer I test with and without topical anesthesia for diagnosing dry eye. *Int J Ophthalmol* 2012;5:478–481.

364. Serin D, Karsloğlu S, Kyan A, Alagöz G. A simple approach to the repeatability of the Schirmer test without anesthesia: eyes open or closed? *Cornea.* 2007;26(8):903–906.

365. Tsubota K, Kaido M, Yagi Y, et al. Diseases associated with ocular surface abnormalities: the importance of reflex tearing. *Br J Ophthalmol.* 1999;83:89–91.

**5.11 Phenol Red Thread Test (Cotton Thread Test)**

366. Doughty MJ, Whyte J, Li W. The phenol red thread test for lacrimal volume: does it matter if the eyes are open or closed? *Ophthalmic Physiol Opt* 2007;27:482–489.

367. Masmali A, Alqahtani TA, Alharbi A, El-Hiti TA. Comparative study of repeatability of phenol red thread test versus Schirmer test in normal adults in Saudi Arabia. *Eye Contact Lens.* 2014;40:127–131.

368. Patel S, Farrell J, Blades KJ, Grierson DJ. The value of a phenol red impregnated thread for differentiating between the aqueous and non-aqueous deficient dry eye. *Ophthalmic Physiol Opt.* 1998;18:471–476.

369. Pult H, Purslow C, Murphy PJ. The relationship between clinical signs and dry eye symptoms. *Eye (Lond)* 2011;25:502–510.

370. Tomlinson A, Blades KJ, Pearce EI. What does the phenol red thread test actually measure? *Optom Vis Sci* 2001;78:142–146.

371. Yokoi N, Kinoshita S, Bron AJ, et al. Tear meniscus changes during cotton thread and Schirmer testing. *Invest Ophthalmol Vis Sci.* 2000;41:3748–3753.

**5.12 Fluorescein Clearance Test (or "Fluorescein Dye Disappearance Test")**

372. Cuthbertson FM, Webber S. Assessment of functional nasolacrimal duct obstruction--a survey of ophthalmologists in the southwest. *Eye (Lond).* 2004;18(1):20–23.

373. Kashkouli MB, Mirzajani H, Jamshidian-Tehrani M, Pakdel F, Nojomi M, Aghaei GH. Reliability of fluorescein dye disappearance test in assessment of adults with nasolacrimal duct obstruction. *Ophthalmic Plast Reconstr Surg.* 2013;29(3):167–169.

374. Kashkouli MB, Mirzajani H, Jamshidian-Tehrani M, Shahrzad S, Sanjari MS. Fluorescein dye disappearance test: a reliable test in assessment of success after dacryocystorhinostomy procedure. *Ophthalmic Plast Reconstr Surg.* 2015;31(4):296–299.

375. Roh JH, Chi MJ. Efficacy of dye disappearance test and tear meniscus height in diagnosis

and postoperative assessment of nasolacrimal duct obstruction. *Acta Ophthalmologica.* 2010;88(3):73–77.

376. Zappia RJ, Milder B. Lacrimal drainage function: the fluorescein dye disappearance test. *Am J Ophthalmol.* 1972;74(1):160–162.

**5.13 Jones #1 (Primary Dye) Test**

377. Guzek JP, Yoon PS, Stephenson CB, et al. Lacrimal testing: the dye disappearance test & the Jones test. *An Ophthalmol.* 1996;28:357–363.

378. Flachs A. The fluorescein appearance test for lacrimal obstruction. *Ann Ophthalmol.* 1979;237–242.

379. Jones L, Linn M. The diagnosis of the causes of epiphora. *Am J Ophthalmol.* 1969;67:751–754.

380. Paramanathan N, Nemet A, Lee SE, Benger RS. A modified Jones test: lacrimal scintigram correlation. *Ophthalmic Plast Reconstr Surg.* 2011;27(2):81–86.

**5.14 Goldmann Applanation Tonometry (GAT)**

381. Agudelo LM, Molina CA, Alvarez DL. Changes in intraocular pressure after laser in situ kera-tomileusis for myopia, hyperopia, and astigmatism. *J Refract Surg.* 2002;18:472–474.

382. Blumenthal EZ. Aligning the Goldmann tonometer tip by means of the "precontact whitish rings". *Surv Ophthalmol.* 1999;44:171–172.

383. Burvenich H, Sallet G, DeClercq J. The correlation between IOP measurement, central corneal thickness and corneal curvature. *Bull Soc Belge Ophthalmol.* 2000;276:23–26.

384. Doughty MJ, Zamen ML. Human corneal thickness and its impact on intraocular pressure measures: a review and meta-analysis approach. *Surv Ophthalmol.* 2000;44:367–408.

385. Faucher A, Gregoire J, Blondeau P. Accuracy of Goldmann tonometry after refractive surgery. *J Cataract Refract Surg.* 1997;23:832–838.

386. Gimeno JA, Munoz LA, Valenzuela LA, et al. Influence of refraction on tonometric readings after photorefractive keratectomy and laser assisted in situ keratomileusis. *Cornea.* 2000;19:512–516.

387. Holladay J, Allison M, Prager T. Goldmann applanation tonometry in patients with regular corneal astigmatism. *Am J Ophthalmol.* 1983;96:90–93.

388. Moses R. The Goldmann applanation tonometer. *Am J Ophthalmol.* 1958;46:865–869.

389. Motolko MA, Feldman F, Hyde M, Hudy D. Sources of variability in the results of applanation tonometry. *Can J Ophthalmol.* 1982;17:93–95.

390. Park SJK, Ang GS, Nicholas S, Wells AP. The effect of thin, thick and normal corneas on Goldmann intraocular pressure measurements

and correction formulae in individual eyes. *Ophthalmology.* 2012;119:443–449.

**5.15 Noncontact Tonometry (NCT)**

391. Bhartiya S, Bali SJ, Sharma R, et al. Comparative evaluation of TonoPen AVIA, Goldmann applanation tonometry and non-contact tonometry. *Int Ophthalmol.* 2011;31:297.

392. Cook JA, Botella AP, Elders A, et al. Systematic review of the agreement of tonometers with Goldmann applanation tonometry. *Ophthalmology;* 2012;119:1552–1557.

393. Hsu SY, Sheu MM, Hsu AH, et al. Comparisons of intraocular pressure measurements: Goldmann applanation tonometry, noncontact tonometry, Tono-Pen tonometry, and dynamic contour tonometry. *Eye.* 2009;23:1582–1588.

**5.16 Rebound Tonometry**

394. Davies LN, Bartlett H, Mallen EAH, Wolffsohn JS. Clinical evaluation of rebound tonometer. *Acta Ophthalmologica Scandinavica.* 2006;84:206–209.

395. Iliev ME, Goldblum D, Katsoulis K, et al. Comparison of rebound tonometry with Goldmann applanation tonometry and correlation with central corneal thickness. *Br J Ophthalmol.* 2006;90:833–835.

396. Lambert SR, Melia M, Buffen AN, Chiang MF, Simpson JL, Yang MB. Rebound tonometry in children: a report by the American Academy of Ophthalmology. *Ophthalmology.* 2013;120(4):e21–e27.

397. Martinez-de-la-Casa JM, Garcia-Feijoo J, Castillo A, Garcia-Sanchez J. Reproducibility and clinical evaluation of rebound tonometry. *Invest. Ophthalmol Vis Sci.* 2005;46(12):4578–4580.

**5.17 Pachymetry**

398. Hoffmann EM, Lamparter J, Mirshahi A, et al. Distribution of central corneal thickness and its association with ocular parameters in a large central European cohort: The Gutenberg Health Study. *PLoS One.* 2013;8(8):1–9.

399. Maresca N, Fabrizio Z, Palumbo P, Calossi A. Agreement and reliability in measuring central corneal thickness with a rotating Scheimpflug–Placido system and ultrasound pachymetry. *Cont Lens Anterior Eye.* 2014;37(6):442–446.

400. Sanchis-Gimeno J, Sanchez-Zuriaga D, Martinez-Soriano F. White-to-white corneal diameter, pupil diameter, central corneal thickness and thinnest corneal thickness values of emmetropic subjects. *Surg Radiol Anat.* 2012;34(2):167–170.

**5.18 Gonioscopy**

401. Cockburn D. A new method for gonioscopic grading of the anterior chamber angle. *Am J Optom Physiol Opt.* 1980;57:258–261.

402. Fisch BM. *Gonioscopy and the Glaucomas.* Boston, MA: Butterworth-Heinemann; 1993.
403. Fisch BM, Scott C. Gonioscopy in optometric practice: how to perform the examination, what to look for. *Contemp Optom.* 1987;6:27–34.
404. Gray L. Fundamentals of gonioscopy. *Rev Optom.* 1977:51–60.
405. Gray L. Fundamentals of gonioscopy, part 2. *Rev Optom.* 1978:47–55.
406. Johnson TV, Ramulu PY, Quigley HA, Singman EL. Low sensitivity of the Van Herick method for detecting gonioscopic angle closure independent of observer expertise. *Am J Ophthalmol.* 2018;195:63–71.
407. Penisten, D. Get a better angle on the gonio exam. *Rev Optom.* 1998:135:63–9.
408. Prokopich CL, Flanagan JG. Gonioscopy: evaluation of the anterior chamber angle. Part I. *Ophthalmic Physiol Opt.* 1996;16:S39–S42.
409. Prokopich CL, Flanagan JG. Gonioscopy: evaluation of the anterior chamber angle. Part II. *Ophthalmic Physiol Opt.* 1997;17:S9–S13.
410. Williams KC, Barnebey HS. Meeting the challenge of secondary glaucomas. *Rev Optom.* 1998:74–91.

**5.19 Direct Ophthalmoscopy**

411. Casser L, Fingeret M, Woodcome HT. In: *Atlas of Primary Eyecare Procedures.* 2nd ed. Stamford: Appleton & Lange; 1997:220–223.
412. Fingeret M, Medeiros FA, Remo, S, Weinreb RN. Five rules to evaluate the optic disc and retinal nerve fiber layer for glaucoma. *Optometry.* 2005;76:661–668.
413. Grosvenor TP. The Ocular health examination. In: *Primary Care Optometry.* 5th ed. St. Louis, MO: Butterworth-Heinemann/Elsevier; 2007:147–149.
414. Mackay DD, Garza PS, Bruce BB, Newman NJ, Biousse V. The demise of direct ophthalmoscopy: A modern clinical challenge. *Neurol Clin Pract.* 2015;5(2):150–157.

**5.20 Binocular Indirect Ophthalmoscopy (BIO)**

415. Chung I. Topical ophthalmic drugs and the pediatric patient. *Optometry.* 2000;71:511–518.
416. Denial A, Hanley M. Safe exposure times for slit lamp fundus biomicroscopy with high plus lenses. *Optometry.* 2000;72:45–51.
417. Garston M. Turn up the light on your diagnosis: part 1. *Rev Optom.* August 14, 2002:71–74.
418. Kornberg DL, Klufas MA, Yannuzzi NA, Orlin A, D'Amico DJ, Kiss S. Clinical utility of ultra-widefield imaging with the Optos Optomap compared with indirect ophthalmoscopy in the setting of non-traumatic rhegmatogenous retinal detachment. *Semin Ophthalmol.* 2016;31(5)505–512.
419. Mizuguchi T, Horiguchi M, Tanikawa A, Sakurai R. Asymmetric extent of distortion measured using the Watzke-Allen Test in patients with macular hole. *Heliyon.* 2021;7(9):e08059.
420. Potter J, Semes L, Cavallerano A, et al. *Binocular Indirect Ophthalmoscopy.* Boston, MA: Butterworth; 1988.
421. Siegel D. Beyond binocular indirect. *Rev Optom.* 1990:64–71.

**5.21 Scleral Depression**

422. Casser L, Fingeret M, Woodcome HT. Scleral indentation. In: *Atlas of Primary Eyecare Procedures.* Stamford, CT: Appleton & Lange, 1997:234–237.
423. Tran KD, Schwartz SG, Smiddy WD, Flynn Jr HW. The role of scleral depression in modern clinical practice. *Am J Ophthalmol.* 2018;195:PXVIII–XIX.

**5.22 Fundus Biomicroscopy**

424. Ansari-Shahrezaei S, Maar N, Biowski R, Stur M. Biomicroscopic measurement of the optic disc with a high-power positive lens. *Invest Ophthalmol Vis Sci.* 2001;42:153–157.
425. Besada E. Examination of retinal lesions using binocular indirect ophthalmoscopy and non-contact lens biomicroscopy. *Prac Optom.* 2002;13:162–174.
426. Garway-Heath DF, Rudnicka AR, Lowe T, et al. Measurement of optic disc size: equivalence of methods to correct for ocular magnification. *Br J Ophthalmol.* 1998;82:643–649.
427. Houston G. Fundus photography using the Volk 90 diopter lens. *So J Optom.* 1988;6:23–26.
428. Hrynchak P, Hutchings N, Jones D, Simpson T. A comparison of cup-to-disc ratio evaluation in normal subjects using stereo biomicroscopy and digital imaging of the optic nerve head. *Ophthalmic Physiol Opt.* 2004;24(6):543–550.
429. Jackson J, Fisher M. Evaluation of the posterior pole with a 90D lens and the slit-lamp biomicroscope. *So J Optom.* 1987;5:80–83.
430. Tanner V, Williamson TH. Watzke-Allen slit beam test in macular holes confirmed by optical coherence tomography. *Arch Ophthalmol.* 2000;118:1059–1063.
431. Volk Optical/Tech Optics, Inc. *Volk Double Aspheric 90D BIO Lens Instruction Manual.* Mentor, OH: Volk Tech Optics; 1985.
432. Walling PE, Pole J, Karpecki P, Colatrella N, Varanelli J. Condensing lenses: sharpen your skills in choosing and using. *Rev Optom.* March 2017.
433. Watzke RC, Allen L. Subjective slitbeam sign for macular disease. *Am J Ophthalmol.* 1969;68:449–453.

434. Wing J, Barker F. Wide field fundus biomicroscopy lenses—a comparative study. *J Am Optom Assoc.* 1990;61:544–547.

**5.23 Amsler Grid**

435. Marmor MF. A brief history of macular grids: from Thomas Reid to Edvard Munch and Marc Amsler. *Surv Ophthalmol.* 2000;44:343–353.

436. Saito Y, Hirata Y, Hayashi A, et al. The visual performance and metamorphopsia of patients with macular holes. *Arch Ophthalmol.* 2000;118:41–46.

**5.24 Tangent Screen**

437. Bruce BB, Newman NJ. Functional visual loss. *Neurol Clin.* 2010;28(3):789–802.

438. Egan RA, LaFrance WC. Functional vision disorder. *Semin Neurol.* 2015;35(5):557–563.

439. Lai HC, Lin KK, Yang ML, Chen HS. Functional visual disturbance due to hysteria. *Chang Gung Med J.* 2007;30(1):87–91.

440. Walsh TJ. Functional visual loss. In: *Visual Fields: Examination and Interpretation.* New York, NY: Oxford University Press; 2010:293–297.

**5.25 D-15 Color Test**

441. Evans BEW, Rodriguez-Carmona M, Barbur JL. Color vision assessment-1: Visual signals that affect the results of the Farnsworth D-15 test. *Color Res Appl.* 2021;46(1):7–20.

442. Oliphant D, Hovis JK. Comparison of the D-15 and City University (second) color vision tests. *Vision Res.* 1998;38:3461–3465.

**5.26 Photostress Recovery Time Test**

443. Glaser J, Savino P, Sumers K, McDonald S, Knighton R. The photostress recovery test in the clinical assessment of visual function. *Am J Ophthalmol.* 1977;2:255–260.

444. Karampatakis V, Almaliotis D, Papadopoulou EP, Almpanidou S. Design of a novel smartphone based photostress recovery time test for detecting abnormalities in the macula. A cross-sectional study. *Ann Med Surg.* 2022;77.

**5.27 Red Desaturation Test**

445. Liu GT, Volpe NJ, Galetta SL. *Neuro-ophthalmology: Diagnosis and Management.* Philadelphia, PA: Saunders; 2001:7–40.

446. Modica PA. *Neuro-ophthalmic System: Clinical Procedures.* Boston, MA: Butterworth-Heinemann; 1999:139–140.

447. Skarf B, Glaser JS, Trick GL, et al. Neuro-ophthalmic examination: the visual system. In: Glaser JS, ed. *Neuro-ophthalmology.* 3rd ed. Philadelphia, PA: Lippincott, Williams & Wilkins; 1999:7–4.

448. Skarf B, Glaser JS, Trick GL, et al. Neuro-ophthalmologic examination: the visual sensory system. In: Tasman W, Jaeger EA, eds. *Duanes' Clinical Ophthalmology;* Vol 2. Philadelphia, PA: Lippincott, Williams & Wilkins. 2000:1–46.

449. Townsend JC. Brightness and color comparison. In: Eskridge JB et al., eds. *Clinical Procedures in Optometry.* Philadelphia, PA: Lippincott; 1991:493–497.

**5.28 Exophthalmometry**

450. Chang AA, Bank A, Francis IC, Kappagoda MB. Clinical exophthalmometry: a comparative study of the Luedde and Hertel exophthalmometers. *Aust NZ J Ophthalomol.* 1995;23:315–318.

451. Drews LC. Exophthalmometry. *Am J Ophthalmol.* 1957;43:37–58.

452. Kozaki A, Rishu I, Komoto N, et al. Proptosis in dysthroid ophthalmopathy: a case series of 10,931 Japanese cases. *Optom Vis Sci.* 2010;87(3):200–204.

453. Luedde WH. An improved transparent exophthalmometer. *Am J Ophthalmol.* 1938;21:426.

454. Migliori ME, Gladstone GJ. Determination of the normal range of exophthalmometric values for black and white adults. *Am J Ophthalmol.* 1984;98:438.

455. Mourits MP, Lombardo SHC, van der Sluijs FA, Fenton S. Reliability of exophthalmos measurement and the exophthalmometry value distribution in a health Dutch population and in Graves' patients. An exploratory study. *Orbit.* 2004;23(3):161–168.

## Chapter 6: Contact Lenses

*General References*

456. Bennett ES, Henry VA. *Clinical Manual of Contact Lenses* [Internet]. 5th ed. Philadelphia, PA: Wolters Kluwer Health/Lippincott Williams & Wilkins; 2020.

457. Bennett ES, Weissman BA, eds. *Clinical Contact Lens Practice.* Philadelphia, PA: Lippincott; 2004.

458. Efron N. *Contact Lens Practice.* 2nd ed. Butterworth-Heinemann; 2010.

459. Hom MM, Bruce AS. *Manual of Contact Lens Prescribing and Fitting.* Boston, MA: Butterworth-Heinemann; 2006.

460. Mandell RB. *Contact Lens Practice.* 4th ed. Springfield, IL: Thomas; 1988.

461. Mannis MJ, Zadnik K. *Contact Lenses in Ophthalmic Practice.* New York, NY: Springer; 2004.

462. Phillips AJ, *Speedwell L. Contact Lenses.* 5th ed. Boston, MA: Butterworth-Heinemann; 2006.

*Technique-Specific References*

**6.2 Contact Lens Case History**

463. Bennett ES, Perrigin JM, Watanabe RK, Begley CG. Preliminary evaluation. In: Bennett ES, Henry VA. eds. *Clinical Manual of Contact Lenses*. 4th ed. Philadelphia, PA: Lippincott Williams & Wilkins; 2014:2–4.

464. Edrington TB, Schornack JA. Initial evaluation. In: Bennett ES, Weissman BA, eds. *Clinical Contact Lens Practice*. Philadelphia, PA: Lippincott; 2004:197–203.

465. Jurkus JM. Patient selection for contact lens wear. In: Hom MM, Bruce AS. eds. *Manual of Contact Lens Prescribing and Fitting*. Boston, MA: Butterworth-Heinemann; 2006:89–97.

**6.3 External Examination of a Contact Lens Patient**

466. Bennett ES, Perrigin JM, Watanabe RK, Begley CG. Preliminary evaluation. In: Bennett ES, Henry VA. eds. *Clinical Manual of Contact Lenses*. 4th ed. Philadelphia, PA: Lippincott Williams & Wilkins; 2014:4–18.

467. Edrington TB, Schornack JA. Initial evaluation. In: Bennett ES, Weissman BA, eds. *Clinical Contact Lens Practice*. Philadelphia, PA: Lippincott; 2004:203–210.

468. Veys J, Meyler J, Davies I. Patient selection and pre-screening for contact lens wear. In: Veys J, Meyler J, Davies I, eds. *Essential Contact Lens Practice*. Oxford, England: Butterworth-Heinemann; 2002:1–7.

**6.4 Inspection and Verification of Soft Contact Lenses**

469. Biddle SP, Janoff LE. Verification of hydrogel lenses. In: Bennett ES, Henry VA, eds. *Clinical Manual of Contact Lenses*. Philadelphia, PA: Lippincott Williams & Wilkins, 2000:303–312.

470. Gasson A, Morris J. Soft lens specification and verification. In: Gasson A, Morris J. eds. *The Contact Lens Manual: A Practical Guide to Fitting*. 4th ed. Boston, MA: Butterworth Heinemann; 2010:235–240.

471. Patel S. Soft lens measurement. In: Efron N, ed. *Contact Lens Practice*. 2nd ed. Boston, MA: Butterworth Heinemann; 2010:100–108.

**6.5 Application (Insertion) and Removal of Soft Contact Lenses**

472. Gasson A, Morris J. Insertion and removal by the practitioner. In: Gasson A, Morris J, eds. *The Contact Lens Manual: A Practical Guide to Fitting*. 4th ed. Boston, MA: Butterworth Heinemann; 2010:55–56.

473. Henry VA, Do OK. Soft lens care and patient education. In: Bennett ES, Henry VA, eds. *Clinical Manual of Contact Lenses*. 4th ed. Philadelphia, PA: Lippincott Williams & Wilkins; 2014:301–303.

474. Weissbarth RE, Henderson B. Hydrogel lens care regimens and patient education. In: Bennett ES, Weissman BA, eds. *Clinical Contact Lens Practice*. Philadelphia, PA: Lippincott; 2004:408–409.

**6.6 Fit Assessment of Soft Contact Lenses**

475. Bruce AS, Little SA. Soft lens design, fitting, and physiologic response. In: Hom MM, Bruce AS. eds. *Manual of Contact Lens Prescribing and Fitting*. Boston, MA: Butterworth-Heinemann; 2006:284–285.

476. Henry VA. Soft lens fitting and evaluation. In: Bennett ES, Henry VA. eds. *Clinical Manual of Contact Lenses*. 4th ed. Philadelphia, PA: Lippincott Williams & Wilkins; 2014:279–281.

477. Veys J, Meyler J, Davies I. Soft contact lens fitting. In: Veys J, Meyler J, Davies I, eds. *Essential Contact Lens Practice*. Oxford, England: Butterworth-Heinemann, 2002:29–36.

478. Yeung KK, Weissman BA. Soft contact lens application. In: Bennett ES, Weissman BA, eds. *Clinical Contact Lens Practice*. Philadelphia, PA: Lippincott; 2004:372–375.

**6.7 Phoropter-Based Over-Refraction of Spherical or Toric Contact Lenses**

479. Bennett ES. Basic fitting. In: Bennett ES, Weissman BA, eds. *Clinical Contact Lens Practice*. Philadelphia, PA: Lippincott; 2004:267–272.

480. Bennett ES, Sorbara L, Kojima R. Gas permeable lens design, fitting and evaluation. In: Bennett ES, Henry VA, eds. *Clinical Manual of Contact Lenses*. 4th ed. Philadelphia, PA: Lippincott Williams & Wilkins; 2014:142–146.

481. Roberts CM, Hom MM. Gas-permeable lens design and fitting. In: Hom MM, Bruce AS, eds. *Manual of Contact Lens Prescribing and Fitting*. Boston, MA: Butterworth-Heinemann; 2006:145–148.

**6.8 Loose Lens Over-Refraction of Spherical or Toric Contact Lenses**

482. Bennett ES. Basic fitting. In: Bennett ES, Weissman BA, eds. *Clinical Contact Lens Practice*. Philadelphia, PA: Lippincott; 2004:267–272.

483. Bennett ES, Sorbara L, Kojima R. Gas permeable lens design, fitting and evaluation. In: Bennett ES, Henry VA, eds. *Clinical Manual of Contact Lenses*. 4th ed. Philadelphia, PA: Lippincott Williams & Wilkins, 2014:142–146.

484. Roberts CM, Hom MM. Gas-permeable lens design and fitting. In: Hom MM, Bruce AS, eds. *Manual of Contact Lens Prescribing and*

Fitting. Boston, MA: Butterworth-Heinemann, 2006:145–148.

**6.9 Evaluation of the Multifocal Contact Lens Patient**

485. Bennett ES, Henry VA. Bifocal contact lenses. In: Bennett ES, Henry VA, eds. *Clinical Manual of Contact Lenses.* 4th ed. Philadelphia, PA: Lippincott Williams & Wilkins; 2014:395–422.

486. Bennett ES, Jurkus JM. Presbyopic correction. In: Bennett ES, Weissman BA, eds. *Clinical Contact Lens Practice.* Philadelphia, PA: Lippincott; 2004:536–547.

487. Gromacki SJ. Monovision and bifocal contact lenses. In: Hom MM, Bruce AS, eds. *Manual of Contact Lens Prescribing and Fitting.* Butterworth-Heinemann; 2006:473–494.

488. Kame RT, Hom MM. Translating bifocals. In: Hom MM, Bruce AS, eds. *Manual of Contact Lens Prescribing and Fitting.* Butterworth-Heinemann; 2006:499–502.

**6.10 Loose-Lens Over-Refraction of Multifocal Contact Lenses**

489. Mannis MJ, Zadnik K. *Contact Lenses in Ophthalmic Practice.* New York, NY: Springer; 2004.

**6.11 Evaluation of the Monovision Patient**

490. Bennett ES, Henry VA. Bifocal contact lenses. In: Bennett ES, Henry VA, eds. *Clinical Manual of Contact Lenses.* 4th ed. Philadelphia, PA: Lippincott Williams & Wilkins; 2014:422–423.

491. Bennett ES, Jurkus JM. Presbyopic correction. In: Bennett ES, Weissman BA, eds. *Clinical Contact Lens Practice.* Philadelphia, PA: Lippincott; 2004:533–536.

492. Gromacki SJ. Monovision and bifocal contact lenses. In: Hom MM, Bruce AS, eds. *Manual of Contact Lens Prescribing and Fitting.* Butterworth-Heinemann; 2006:471–473.

493. Mandell RB. Presbyopia. In: Mandell RB, ed. *Contact Lens Practice.* 4th ed. Springfield, IL: Thomas; 1988:787–790.

**6.12 Inspection and Verification of Corneal and Scleral Gas Permeable Contact Lenses**

494. Henry VA. Verification of gas-permeable lenses. In: Bennett ES, Henry VA. eds. *Clinical Manual of Contact Lenses.* 4th ed. Philadelphia, PA: Lippincott Williams & Wilkins; 2014:187–199.

495. Henry VA, Bennett ES. Inspection and verification of gas-permeable contact lenses. In: Bennett ES, Weissman BA, eds. *Clinical Contact Lens Practice.* Philadelphia, PA: Lippincott; 2004:295–305.

**6.13 Base Curve (BC) Radius Measurement**

496. Paugh JR, Hom MM. Modification and verification. In: Hom MM, Bruce AS, eds.

*Manual of Contact Lens Prescribing and Fitting.* Boston, MA: Butterworth-Heinemann; 2006:224–225.

**6.14 Back Vertex Power and Optical Quality**

497. Bennett ES, Henry VA. *Clinical Manual of Contact Lenses* [Internet]. Fifth edition. Wolters Kluwer Health/Lippincott Williams & Wilkins; 2020. Accessed May 24, 2022.

498. Paugh JR, Hom MM. Modification and verification. In: Hom MM, Bruce AS, eds. *Manual of Contact Lens Prescribing and Fitting.* Boston, MA: Butterworth-Heinemann; 2006:224–225.

**6.15 Application (Insertion), Removal, and Recentering of Gas Permeable Contact Lenses**

499. Bennett ES, Wagner H. Rigid lens care and patient education. In: Bennett ES, Weissman BA, eds. *Clinical Contact Lens Practice.* Philadelphia, PA: Lippincott; 2004:285–287.

500. Bennett ES, Wagner H. Gas-permeable lens care and patient education. In: Bennett ES, Henry VA. eds. *Clinical Manual of Contact Lenses.* 4th ed. Philadelphia, PA: Lippincott Williams & Wilkins; 2014:163–168.

501. Gasson A, Morris J. Insertion and removal by the practitioner. In: Gasson A, Morris J, eds. *The Contact Lens Manual: A Practical Guide to Fitting.* 4th ed. Boston, MA: Butterworth Heinemann; 2010:54–55.

**6.16 Fit Assessment of Corneal Gas Permeable Contact Lenses**

502. Bennett ES, Sorbara L, Kojima R. Gas-permeable lens design, fitting and evaluation. In: Bennett ES, Henry VA. eds. *Clinical Manual of Contact Lenses.* 4th ed. Philadelphia, PA: Lippincott Williams & Wilkins; 2014:112–123.

503. Bennett ES. Basic fitting. In: Bennett ES, Weissman BA, eds. *Clinical Contact Lens Practice.* Philadelphia, PA: Lippincott; 2004:255–261.

504. Hom MM, Bruce AS, Watanabe R. Gas-permeable fluorescein patterns. In: Hom MM, Bruce AS. eds. *Manual of Contact Lens Prescribing and Fitting.* Butterworth-Heinemann; 2006:167–190.

505. Veys J, Meyler J, Davies I. Rigid contact lens fitting. In: Veys J, Meyler J, Davies I, eds. *Essential Contact Lens Practice.* Oxford, England: Butterworth-Heinemann; 2002:37–45.

**6.17 Fit and Assessment of Orthokeratology Lenses**

506. Bennett ES, Henry VA. *Clinical Manual of Contact Lenses* [Internet]. Fifth edition. Wolters Kluwer Health/Lippincott Williams & Wilkins; 2020. Accessed April 24, 2022.

507. Vincent SJ, Cho P, Chan KY, et al. CLEAR - Orthokeratology. *Cont Lens Anterior Eye.* 2021;44(2):240–269.

**6.18 Application (Insertion) and Removal of Scleral Contact Lenses**

508. DeNaeyer GW, Jedlicka J, Schornack MM. Scleral lenses. In: Bennett ES, Henry VA. eds. *Clinical Manual of Contact Lenses.* 4th ed. Philadelphia, PA: Lippincott Williams & Wilkins; 2014:624–625.

509. Pullum KW. Scleral lenses. In: Bennett ES, Weissman BA, eds. *Clinical Contact Lens Practice.* Philadelphia, PA: Lippincott; 2004:633.

**6.19 Fit Assessment of Scleral Contact Lenses**

510. DeNaeyer GW, Jedlicka J, Schornack MM. Scleral lenses. In: Bennett ES, Henry VA. eds. *Clinical Manual of Contact Lenses.* 4th ed. Philadelphia, PA: Lippincott Williams & Wilkins; 2014:609–624.

511. Pullum KW. Scleral lenses. In: Bennett ES, Weissman BA, eds. *Clinical Contact Lens Practice.* Philadelphia, PA: Lippincott; 2004:630–638.

512. Van der Worp E. Fitting scleral lenses – a five step fitting approach. In: Van der Worp E, ed. *A Guide to Scleral Lens Fitting* [monograph online]. Scleral Lens Education Society, 2010:23–37.

**6.20 Writing a Contact Lens Prescription**

513. Bennett ES, Henry VA. *Clinical Manual of Contact Lenses* [Internet]. Fifth edition. Wolters Kluwer Health/Lippincott Williams & Wilkins; 2020. Accessed May 24, 2022.

## Chapter 7: Systemic Health Screening

*General References*

514. Casser L, Fingeret M, Woodcome HT. *Atlas of Primary Eyecare Procedures.* 2nd ed. Stamford, CT: Appleton & Lange; 1997.

515. Shein DM, Druckenbrod RC, eds. *Clinical Medicine for Optometrists.* Wolters Kluwer Health/Lippincott Williams & Wilkins; 2021.

*Technique-Specific References*

**7.2 Blood Pressure Evaluation (Sphygmomanometry)**

516. Chobanian AV, Backris GL, Black HR, et al. The Seventh report of the Joint National Committee on prevention, detection, evaluation, and treatment of high blood pressure. *JAMA.* 2003;289:2560–2571.

517. Grubb N, Sprati J, Bradbury A. The cardiovascular system. In: Douglas G, Nicol F, Robertson C, eds. *Macleod's Clinical Examination.* 13th ed. Edinburgh, Scotland: Churchill Livingtsone; 2013:106–153.

518. Handler J. The importance of accurate blood pressure measurement. *Perm J.* 2009;13(3):51–54.

519. James PA, Oparil S, Carter BL, et al. Evidence-based guideline for the management of high blood pressure in adults: report from the panel members appointed to the Eighth Joint National Committee (JNC 8). *JAMA.* 2014;311:507–520.

520. Moyer VA. Screening for primary hypertension in children and adolescents: U.S. Preventive Services Task Force recommendation statement. *Pediatrics.* 2013;132:907–914.

521. Muntner P, Carey RM, Gidding S, et al. Potential US population impact of the 2017 ACC/AHA high blood pressure guideline. *Circulation.* 2018;137(2):109–118.

522. Muntner P, Shimbo D, Carey RM, et al. Measurement of blood pressure in humans: a scientific statement from the American Heart Association. *Hypertension.* 2019;73(5): e35–e66.

523. Navar-Boggen AM, Pencina MJ, Sniderman AD, Peterson ED. Proportion of US adults potentially affected by the 2014 hypertension guidelines. *JAMA.* 2014;311:1424–1429.

524. Shein DM, Druckenbrod RC, Freddo TF. Hypertension. In: Shein DM, Druckenbrod RC, eds. *Clinical Medicine for Optometrists.* Wolters Kluwer Health/Lippincott Williams & Wilkins; 2021:17–46.

525. Whelton PK, Carey RM, Aronow WS, et al. 2017 ACC/AHA/AAPA/ABC/ACPM/AGS/ APhA/ASH/ASPC/NMA/PCNA Guideline for the prevention, detection, evaluation, and management of high blood pressure in adults: A report of the American College of Cardiology/ American Heart Association Task Force on Clinical Practice Guidelines. *Hypertension.* 2018;71(6):e13–e115.

526. Williams B, Mancia G, Spiering W, et al. 2018 ESC/ESH guidelines for the management of arterial hypertension. *Eur Heart J.* 2018;39(33):3021–3104.

**7.3 Carotid Artery Evaluation**

527. Abbott AL, Paraskevas KI, Kakkos SK, et al. Systematic review of guidelines for the management of asymptomatic and symptomatic carotid stenosis. *Stroke.* 2015;46:3288–3301.

528. Bakri SJ, Luqman A, Pathik B, Chandrasekaran K. Is carotid ultrasound necessary in the clinical evaluation of the asymptomatic Hollenhorst plaque? *Trans Am Ophthalmol Soc.* 2013;111:17–23.

529. Bickley LS, Szilagyi, PG. The cardiovascular system. In: Bickley LS, ed. *Bates' Guide to Physical Examination and History Taking.* 11th

ed. Philadelphia, PA: Lippincott, Williams & Wilkins; 2013:333–404.

530. Casser L, Fingeret M, Woodcome HT. *Atlas of Primary Eyecare Procedures*. 2nd ed. Stamford, CT: Appleton & Lange; 1997:290–295.

531. Huang A, Lee CW, Liu HM. Rolling ball sifting algorithm for the augmented visual inspection of carotid bruit auscultation. *Sci Rep*. 2016;6:30179.

532. Lapum JL, Verkuyl M, Garcia W, St-Amant O, Tan A. *Vital Sign Measurement Across the Lifespan*. 2nd ed. British Columbia: BC Campus; 2021.

533. Lucerna A, Espinosa J. Carotid Bruit. In: *StatPearls*. Treasure Island (FL): StatPearls Publishing; 2022.

534. Morris DR, Ayabe K, Inoue T, et al. Evidence-based carotid interventions for stroke prevention: state-of-the-art review. *J Atheroscler Thromb*. 2017;24:373–387.

535. Mortimer R, Nachiappan S, Howlett DC. Carotid artery stenosis screening: where are we now? *Br J Radiol*. 2018;91:20170380.

536. Naylor AR, Gaines PA, Rothwell PM. Who benefits most from intervention for asymptomatic carotid stenosis: patients or professionals? *Eur J Vasc Endovasc Surg* 2009;37:625–632.

537. Pickett CA, Jackson JL, Hemann BA, Atwood JE. Carotid artery examination, and important tool in patient evaluation. *South Med J*. 2011;104:526–532.

538. Pickett CA, Jackson JL, Hemann BA, Atwood JE. Carotid bruit and cerebrovascular disease risk: a meta-analysis. *Stroke*. 2010;41:2295–2302.

539. Pickett CA, Jackson JL, Hemann BA, Atwood JE. Carotid bruits as a prognostic indicator of cardiovascular death and myocardial infarction: a meta-analysis. *Lancet*. 2008;371:1587–1594.

540. Qaja E, Tadi P, Theetha Kariyanna P. Carotid Artery Stenosis. In: *StatPearls*. Treasure Island (FL): StatPearls Publishing; February 17, 2022.

541. Sandercock PAG, Kavvadia E. The carotid bruit. *Prac Neurol*. 2002;2(4):221–224.

542. Shein DM, Druckenbrod RC. Lipid disorders, atherosclerosis, cardiovascular diseases, and cardiac testing. In: Shein DM, Druckenbrod RC, eds. *Clinical Medicine for Optometrists*. Wolters Kluwer Health/Lippincott Williams & Wilkins; 2021:47–88.

543. Sühn T, Spiller M, Salvi R, et al. Auscultation system for acquisition of vascular sounds - Towards sound-based monitoring of the carotid artery. *Med Devices (Auckl)*. 2020;13:349–364.

544. US Preventive Services Task Force. Screening for asymptomatic carotid artery stenosis. US preventive services task force recommendations statement. *JAMA*. 2021;325(5):476–481.

**7.4 Lymph Node Evaluation**

545. Arjmand P, Yan P, O'Connor MD. Parinaud oculoglandular syndrome 2015: review of the literature and update on diagnosis and management. *J Clin Exp Ophthalmol*. 2015;6:443.

546. Bickley LS, Szilagyi, PG. The head and neck. In: Bickley LS, ed. *Bates' Guide to Physical Examination and History Taking*. 11th ed. Philadelphia, PA: Lippincott, Williams & Wilkins; 2013:205–292.

547. Casser L, Fingeret M, Woodcome HT. *Atlas of Primary Eyecare Procedures*. 2nd ed. Stamford, CT: Appleton & Lange; 1997:274–275.

548. Douglas G, Bevan, J. General clinical examination. In: Douglas G, Nicol F, Robertson C, eds. *Macleod's Clinical Examination*. 13th ed. Edinburgh, Scotland: Churchill Livingtsone; 2013:46–70.

549. Krumholz DM. Patient assessment. In: Thomann KH, Marks ES, Adamczyk DT, eds. *Primary Eyecare in Systemic Disease*. 2nd ed. New York, NY: McGraw-Hill; 2001:1–30.

550. May LA. The physical examination. In: Muchnick BG, ed. *Clinical Medicine in Optometric Practice*. 2nd ed. St Louis, MO: Mosby Yearbook; 2007:9–25.

**7.5 Glucometry**

551. American Diabetes Association. Position statements. *Diabetes Care*. 2014;(suppl 1): S81–S90.

552. Dall TM, Narayan KM, Gillespie KB, et al. Detecting type 2 diabetes and prediabetes among asymptomatic adults in the United States: modeling American Diabetes Association versus US Preventive Services Task Force diabetes screening guidelines. *Popul Health Metr*. 2014;12:1–14.

553. Howse JH, Jones S, Hungin AP. Screening and identifying diabetes in optometric practice: a prospective study. *Br J Gen Pract*. 2011;61(588):436–442.

554. Karter AJ, Ferrara A, Darbinian JA, et al. Self-monitoring of blood glucose—language and financial barriers in a managed care population with diabetes. *Diabetes Care*. 2000;23:477–483.

555. Staff, McMahon T, Philipson L, Tyree J, Gensler L, Glazer M. Diabetes and arthritis and heart disease-oh, my! *Review of Optometry*. Published online; 2020.

556. U.S. Preventive Services Task Force. Screening for type 2 diabetes mellitus in adults: U.S. Preventive Services Task Force recommendation statement. *Ann Int Med*. 2008;148:846–854.

# Chapter 8: Cranial Nerve Screening

## General References

557. Broadway DC, Tufail A, Khaw PT. *Ophthalmology Examination Techniques, Questions, and Answers.* Oxford, England: Butterworth-Heinemann; 1999:19–32.
558. Burde RM, Savino PJ, Trobe JD. *Clinical Decisions in Neuro-ophthalmology.* St Louis, MO: Mosby; 1992.
559. Friedman NJ, Pineda R II, Kaiser PK. *The Massachusetts Eye and Ear Infirmary Illustrated Manual of Ophthalmology.* Philadelphia, PA: Saunders; 1998.
560. Glaser JS. *Neuro-ophthalmology.* Philadelphia, PA: Lippincott; 1990.
561. Hart WM, ed. *Adler's Physiology of the Eye.* 9th ed. St Louis, MO: Mosby; 1992.
562. Miller NR, Newman NJ. *The Essentials: Walsh & Hoyt's Clinical Neuro-ophthalmology.* Philadelphia, PA: Lippincott, Williams & Wilkins; 1999.
563. Newman NM. *Neuro-ophthalmology: A Practical Text.* Norwalk, CT: Appleton & Lange; 1992.
564. Schmitz S, Krummenauer F, Henn S, Dick HB. Comparison of three different technologies for pupil diameter measurement. *Graefes Arch Clin Exp Ophthalmol.* 2003;241:472–477.
565. Skorin L, Muchnick BG. Neuro-ophthalmic disorders. In: Bartlett JD, Jaanus SD, eds. *Clinical Ocular Pharmacology.* 4th ed. Boston, MA: Butterworth-Heinemann; 2001: Chap 22.
566. Walsh TJ. *Clinical Neuro-ophthalmology: Clinical Signs and Symptoms.* Philadelphia, PA: Lea & Febiger; 1992.
567. Willard FH, Perl DP. *Medical Neuroanatomy: A Problem-Oriented Manual with Annotated Atlas.* Philadelphia, PA: Lippincott; 1993.

## Technique-Specific References

### 8.2 Lid and Ptosis Measurements

568. Fante R. Chapter 17: Reconstruction of the eyelids. In: Baker S. *Local Flaps in Facial Reconstruction.* 2nd ed. Mosby; 2007:387–413.
569. Gaddipati RV, Meyer DR. Eyelid retraction, lid lag, lagophthalmos, and von Graefe's sign quantifying the eyelid features of Graves' ophthalmopathy. *Ophthalmology.* 2008;115(6):1083–1088.
570. Lam BL, Lam S, Walls RC. Prevalence of palpebral fissure asymmetry in white persons. *Am J Ophthalmol.* 1995;120(4):518–522.
571. Putterman AM. Margin reflex distance (MRD) 1, 2, and 3. *Ophthalmic Plast Reconstr Surg.* 2012;28(4):308–311.
572. Vasanthakumar P, Kumar P, Rao M. Anthropometric analysis of palpebral fissure dimensions and its position in South Indian ethnic adults. *Oman Med J.* 2013;28(1):26–32.

### 8.3 Levator Function Test

573. Giannoccaro MP, Paolucci M, Zenesini C, Di Stasi V, Donadio V, Avoni P, Liguori R. Comparison of ice pack test and single-fiber EMG diagnostic accuracy in patients referred for myasthenic ptosis. *Neurology.* 2020;95(13):e1800–e1806.
574. Kupersmith MJ, Ying G. Ocular motor dysfunction and ptosis in ocular myasthenia gravis: effects of treatment. *Br J Ophthalmol.* 2005;89:1330–1334.

### 8.4 Near (Accommodative) Pupil Testing

575. Gislén A, Gustafsson J, Kröger RH. The accommodative pupil responses of children and young adults at low and intermediate levels of ambient illumination. *Vision Res.* 2008;48(8):989–993.
576. Kawasaki AK. Diagnostic approach to pupillary abnormalities. *Continuum (Minneap Minn).* 2014;20:1008–1022.

### 8.5 Pharmacological Pupil Testing

577. Alexander LJ, Skorin L Jr, Bartlett JD. Neuro-ophthalmic disorders. In: Bartlett JD, Jaanus SD, eds. *Clinical Ocular Pharmacology.* Boston, MA: Butterworth-Heinemann; 2001;521–532, Chap 23.
578. Friedman NE. The pupil. In: Zadnik K, ed. *The Ocular Examination: Measurements and Findings.* Philadelphia, PA: Saunders; 1997:45–49, Chap 3.
579. Jacobson DM, Vierkant RA. Comparison of cholinergic supersensitivity in third nerve palsy and Adie's syndrome. *J Neuro-ophthalmol.* 1998;18:171–175.
580. Leavitt JA, Wayman LL, Hodge DO, Brubaker RF. Pupillary response to four concentrations of pilocarpine in normal subjects: application to testing for Adie tonic pupil. *Am J Ophthalmol.* 2002;133:333–336.
581. Miller NR, Newman NJ. Examination of the pupils, accommodation, and lacrimation. In: Miller NR, Newman NJ, eds. *Walsh & Hoyt's Clinical Neuro-ophthalmology, The Essentials.* 5th ed. Philadelphia, PA: Lippincott, Williams & Wilkins; 1999:422:Chap 14.
582. Morales J, Brown SM, Abdul-Rahim AX, Crosson CE. Ocular effects of apraclonidine in Horner syndrome. *Arch Ophthalmol.* 2000;118:951–954.

### 8.6 Park's Three-Step Method for a Paretic Vertical Muscle

583. Lira J, Gospe SM 3rd, Bhatti MT, Wynn DP, Warner JEA. Fourth down and five. *Surv Ophthalmol.* 2019;64(5):734–740.

584. Cornblath WT. Diplopia due to ocular motor cranial neuropathies. *Continuum (Minneap Minn).* 2014;20(4 Neuro-ophthalmology):966–980.

585. Fu L, Zhu B, Yan J. Clinical characteristics and surgical outcomes of isolated inferior rectus palsy. *BMC Ophthalmol.* 2021;21(1):422.

**8.7 Red Lens Test for a Paretic Horizontal Muscle**

586. Elder C, Hainline C, Galetta SL, Balcer LJ, Rucker JC. Isolated abducens nerve palsy: update on evaluation and diagnosis. *Curr Neurol Neurosci Rep.* 2016;16(8):69.

587. Peng TJ, Stretz C, Mageid R, et al. Carotid-cavernous fistula presenting with bilateral abducens palsy. *Stroke.* 2020;51(6):e107–e110.

588. Kung NH, Van Stavern GP. Isolated ocular motor nerve palsies. *Semin Neurol.* 2015;35(5):539–548.

**8.8 Trigeminal Nerve Function Test**

589. Gurwood AS, Drake J. Guillain-Barré syndrome. *Optometry.* 2006;77(11):540–546.

590. Kim SJ, Lee HY. Acute peripheral facial palsy: recent guidelines and a systematic review of the literature. *J Korean Med Sci.* 2020;35(30):e245.

591. Lorch M, Teach SJ. Facial nerve palsy: etiology and approach to diagnosis and treatment. *Pediatr Emerg Care.* 2010;26(10):763–769.

592. Muzyka IM, Estephan B. Electrophysiology of cranial nerve testing: trigeminal and facial nerves. *J Clin Neurophysiol.* 2018;35(1):16–24.

593. Owusu JA, Stewart CM, Boahene K. Facial nerve paralysis. *Med Clin North Am.* 2018 Nov;102(6):1135–1143.

594. Posnick JC, Grossman JA. Facial sensibility testing: a clinical update. *Plast Reconstr Surg.* 2000;106:892–894.

**8.9 Facial Nerve Function Test**

595. Gurwood AS, Drake J. Guillain-Barré syndrome. *Optometry.* 2006 Nov;77(11):540–546.

596. Kim SJ, Lee HY. Acute peripheral facial palsy: recent guidelines and a systematic review of the literature. *J Korean Med Sci.* 2020 Aug 3;35(30):e245.

597. Lorch M, Teach SJ. Facial nerve palsy: etiology and approach to diagnosis and treatment. *Pediatr Emerg Care.* 2010;26(10):763–769.

598. Owusu JA, Stewart CM, Boahene K. Facial nerve paralysis. *Med Clin North Am.* 2018;102(6):1135–1143.

**8.10 Screening Tests for Cranial Nerves I, VIII, IX, X, XI, and XII**

599. Davidson TM, Murphy C. Rapid clinical evaluation of anosmia. *Arch Otolaryngol Head Neck Surg.* 1997;123:591–594.

600. Lin HC, Barkhaus PE. Cranial nerve XII: the hypoglossal nerve. *Semin Neurol.* 2009;29(1):45–52.

601. Martinez ARM, Martins MP, Moreira AL, Martins CR Jr, Kimaid PAT, França MC Jr. Electrophysiology of cranial nerve testing: cranial nerves IX and X. *J Clin Neurophysiol.* 2018;35(1):48–58.

602. Stino AM, Smith BE. Electrophysiology of cranial nerve testing: spinal accessory and hypoglossal nerves. *J Clin Neurophysiol.* 2018;35(1):59–64.

## Chapter 9: Ocular Imaging

*Technique-Specific References*

**9.2 Ocular Photography**

603. Bennett TJ. Modes of retinal imaging. An overview of imaging technology on the market. *Ophthalmic Professional.* 2018;7:16–21.

604. Saine PJ, Tyler ME. *Ophthalmic Photography: Retinal Photography, Angiography, and Electronic Imaging.* 2nd ed. Butterworth-Heinemann; 2001.

**9.3 Corneal Topography**

605. Fam HB, Lim KL. Validity of the keratometric index: large population-based study. *J Cataract Refract Surg.* 2007;33:686–691.

606. Oculus. *Oculus Pentacam interpretation manual.* 3rd ed. Oculus, Inc.

607. Olsen T, Arnarsson A, Sasaki H, Sasaki K, Jonasson F. On the ocular refractive components: the Reykjavik Eye Study. *Acta Ophthalmol Scand.* 2007;85:361–366.

**9.4 Optical Coherence Tomography (OCT)**

608. Murthy RK, Haji S, Sambhav K, et al. Clinical applications of spectral domain optical coherence tomography in retinal diseases. *Biomed J.* 2016;39(2):107–120.

609. Kashani A, Chen C-L, Gahm JK, et al. Optical coherence tomography angiography: a comprehensive review of current methods and clinical applications. *Prog Retin Eye Res.* 2017;60:66–100.

610. Zeiss. *Cirrus HD-OCT User Manual – models 500, 5000.* Carl Zeiss Meditec. Inc., 2015.

**9.5 Ocular Biometry**

611. Barrett GD. Understanding intraocular lens calculation and biometry. *J Cataract Refract Surg.* 2021;47(12):1499–1501.

612. Mainster MA, Ham WT Jr, Delori FC. Potential retinal hazards. Instrument and environmental light sources. *Ophthalmology.* 1983;90(8):927–932.

613. Meng W, Butterworth J, Malecaze F. Axial length of myopia: a review of current research. *Ophthalmologica.* 2011;225(3):127–134.

614. Montes-Mico R, Carones F, Buttacchio A, et al. Comparison of immersion ultrasound, partial coherence interferometry, and low coherence

reflectometry for ocular biometry in cataract patients. *J Refractive Surg.* 2011;27(9):1–7.

615. Olsen T. Calculation of intraocular lens power: a review. *Acta Ophthalmol Scand.* 2007;85(5):472–485.

616. Song JS, Yoon DY, Hyon JY. Comparison of ocular biometry and refractive outcomes using IOL Master 500, IOL Master 700, and Lenstar LS900. *Korean J Ophthalmol.* 2020;34(2):126–132.

617. Vera-Diaz F. The importance of measuring axial length. *Review of Myopia Management.* 2019.

618. Zeiss. *IOLMaster 700 user manual.* Carl Zeiss Meditec. 2020.

**9.6 B-Scan Ultrasound**

619. Biffi EZ, Young B, Kane JE Jr., Najafi M. The Use of B-Scan Ultrasound in Primary Eye Care. *Advances in Ophthalmology and Optometry.* 2022;7(1):31-49.

620. Byrne SF, Green RL. *Ultrasound of the Eye and Orbit.* 2nd ed. Philadelphia, PA: Mosby, 2002.

621. Casser L, Fingeret M, Woodcome TH. *Atlas of Primary Eyecare Procedures.* 2nd ed. Stamford, CT: Appleton & Lange; 1997.

622. Coleman DJ, Silverman RH, Chabi A, et al. High-resolution ultrasonic imaging of the posterior segment. *Ophthalmol.* 2004;111(7):1344–1351.

623. Richard L, Hart LJ. Ultrasound diagnosis of the eye and orbit. *Principle Pract Ophthalmol.* 1997;5:98.

624. Silverman RH. High-resolution ultrasound imaging of the eye – a review. *Clin Exp Ophthalmol.* 2009;37(1):54–67.

**9.7 Automated Visual Field**

625. Haag-Streit Diagnostics. *Octopus 600 see the new pulse in perimetry.* Haag-Streit AG. 2014.

626. Haag-Streit Diagnostics. *Octopus 900 flexibility and reliability.* Haag-Streit AG. 2020.

627. Heijl A, Patella VM, Bengtsson B. *The Field Analyzer Primer: Effective Perimetry.* 4th ed. Carl Zeiss Meditec. Inc., 2012.

628. Heijl A, Patella VM, Bengtsson B. *The Field Analyzer Primer: Excellent Perimetry.* 5th ed. Carl Zeiss Meditec. Inc., 2021.

629. Ishiyama Y, Murata H, Asaoka R. The usefulness of gaze tracking as an index of visual field reliability in glaucoma patients. *Invest. Ophthalmol. Vis. Sci.* 2015;56(11):6233–6236.

630. Pham AT, Ramulu PY, Boland MV, Yohannan J. The effect of transitioning from SITA Standard to SITA Faster on visual field performance. *Ophthalmology.* 2021;128(10):1417–1425.

631. Zeiss. *Humphrey Field Analyzer 3 (HFA3) instructions for use – models 830, 840, 850, 860.* Carl Zeiss Meditec. Inc., 2018.

## Chapter 10: Advanced Ocular Procedures

*General References*

632. Casser L, Fingeret M. Woodcome HT. *Atlas of Primary Eyecare Procedures.* 2nd ed. Stamford CT: Appleton and Lange; 1997.

*Technique-Specific References*

**10.2 Punctal Plug Insertion**

633. Baxter SA, Laibson PR. Punctal plugs in the management of dry eyes. *Ocul. Surf.* 2004;2(4):255–265.

634. Chen F, Wang J, Chen W, Shen M, Xu S, Lu F. Upper punctal occlusion versus lower punctal occlusion in dry eye. *Invest Ophthalmol Vis Sci.* 2010;51(11):5571–5577.

635. Donthineni PR, Shanbhag SS, Basu S. An evidence-based strategic approach to prevention and treatment of dry eye disease, a modern global epidemic. *Healthcare (Basel).* 2021;9(1):89.

636. Ervin AM, Law A, Pucker AD. Punctal occlusion for dry eye syndrome. *Cochrane Database Syst Rev.* 2017;6(6):CD006775.

637. Jehangir N, Bever G, Mahmood SM, Moshirfar M. Comprehensive review of the literature on existing punctal plugs for the management of dry eye disease. *J Ophthalmol.* 2016;2016:9312340.

638. Management and therapy of dry eye disease: report of the Management and Therapy Subcommittee of the International Dry Eye WorkShop (DEWS 2007). *Ocul. Surf.* 2007;5(2):163–178.

639. Tong L, Beuerman R, Simonyi S, Hollander DA, Stern ME. Effects of punctal occlusion on clinical signs and symptoms and on tear cytokine levels in patients with dry eye. *Ocul Surf.* 2016;14(2):233–241.

640. Tong L, Lim L, Tan D, et al. Assessment and management of dry eye disease and meibomian gland dysfunction: providing a Singapore framework. *Asia Pac J Ophthalmol (Phila).* 2021;10(6):530–541.

641. Reed KK. Diseases of the Lacrimal System. In: Bartlett JD, et al, eds. *Clinical Ocular Pharmacology.* 5th ed. St Louis, MO: Butterworth-Heinemann; 2008:415–435, Chap 24.

**10.3 Dilation and Irrigation**

642. Casser L, Fingeret M, Woodcome HT. Punctal regurgitation/lacrimal sac palpation and lacrimal dilation and irrigation. In: *Atlas of Primary Eyecare Procedures.* Stamford, CT: Appleton & Lange, 1997:128–133.

643. Hurwitz JJ. The lacrimal drainage system. In: Yanoff M, Duker JS. *Ophthalmology.* 3rd ed. London: Mosby Elsevier; 2009:1482–1487.

644. Kunimoto DY. In: *The Wills Eye Manual,* 4th ed. Philadelphia, PA: Lippincott Williams & Wilkins; 2004:116–117.

645. Zaldívar RA, Bradley EA. Primary canaliculitis. *Ophthal Plast Reconstr Surg.* 2009;25(6):481–484.

**10.4 Intense Pulsed Light (IPL)**

646. Arita R, Fukuoka S, Morishige N. Therapeutic efficacy of intense pulsed light in patients with refractory meibomian gland dysfunction. *The Ocular Surface.* 2019;17(1):104–110.

647. Dell SJ. Intense pulsed light for evaporative dry eye disease. *Clin Ophthalmol.* 2017;11:1167–1173.

648. Fitzpatrick TB. The validity and practicality of sun-reactive skin types I through VI. *Arch Dermatol.* 1988;124(6):869–871.

649. Lumenis. *M22 aesthetic treatment system operator's manual.* Lumenis Ltd. 2011.

650. Toyos R, McGill W, Briscoe D. Intense pulsed light treatment for dry eye disease due to meibomian gland dysfunction: a 3-year retrospective study. *Photomed Laser Surg.* 2015;33(1):41–46.

651. Ullmann Y. The aesthetic applications of intense pulsed light using the Lumenis M-22 device. *Laser Therapy.* 2011;20(1):23–28.

652. Wat H, Wu DC, Rao J, Goldman MP. Application of intense pulsed light in the treatment of dermatologic disease: a systematic review. *Dermatologic Surgery.* 2014;40(4):359–377.

**10.5 Eyelash Epilation**

653. Aumond S, Bitton E. The eyelash follicle features and anomalies: A review. *J Optom.* 2018;11(4):211–222.

654. Burton M, Habtamu E, Ho D, Gower EW. Interventions for trachoma trichiasis. *Cochrane Database Syst Rev.* 2015;2015(11):CD004008.

655. Casser L, Fingeret M. Woodcome HT. In: *Atlas of Primary Eyecare Procedures.* 2nd ed. Stamford CT: Appleton and Lange;1997:100–101.

656. Habtamu E, Rajak SN, Tadesse Z, et al. Epilation for minor trachomatous trichiasis: four-year results of a randomised controlled trial. *PLoS Negl Trop Dis.* 2015;9(3):e0003558.

657. Rajak SN, Habtamu E, Weiss HA, et al. Epilation for trachomatous trichiasis and the risk of corneal opacification. *Ophthalmol.* 2012;119(1):84–89.

658. Thibaut S, De Becker E, Caisey L, et al. Human eyelash characterization. *Br J Dermatol.* 2010;162(2):304–310.

**10.6 Foreign Body (FB) Removal**

659. Casser L, Fingeret M, Woodcome HT. Conjunctival procedures and Corneal procedures. In: *Atlas of Primary Eyecare Procedures.* 2nd ed. Stamford, CT: Appleton & Lange, 1997:152–173.

660. Guier CP, Stokkermans TJ. Cornea foreign body removal. In: *StatPearls.* Treasure Island (FL): StatPearls Publishing; 2021.

661. Gerstenblith AT, Rabinowitz MP. In: *The Wills Eye Manual,* 6th ed. Philadelphia, PA: Wolters Kluwer Health/Lippincott Williams & Wilkins; 2012:13–16.

662. Ozkurt ZG, Yuksel H, Saka G, Guclu H, Evsen S, Balsak S. Metallic corneal foreign bodies: an occupational health hazard. *Arq Bras Oftalmol.* 2014;77(2):81–83.

663. Shelter J, Lighthizer N. Foreign body removal in 12 steps. *Rev Optom.* 2015;152(1):22–29.

664. Sigurdsson H, Hanna I, Lockwood AJ, Longstaff S. Removal of rust rings, comparing electric drill and hypodermic needle. *Eye (Lond).* 1987;1(3):430–432.

**10.7 Chalazion Removal**

665. Alsuhaibani AH, Al-Faky YH. Large anterior orbital cyst as a late complication of chalazion surgical drainage. *Eye (Lond).* 2015 Apr;29(4):585-7.

666. Aycinena A, Achiron A, Paul M, Burgansky-Eliash Z. Incision and curettage versus steroid injection for the treatment of chalazia: A meta-analysis. *Ophthal Plast Reconstr Surg.* 2016;32(3):220–224.

667. Casser L, Fingeret M, Woodcome HT. Chalazion removal: Incision and curettage. In: *Atlas of Primary Eyecare Procedures.* 2nd ed. Stamford, CT: Appleton & Lange, 1997:128–122.

668. Casser L, Fingeret M, Woodcome HT. Periocular injection procedures. In: *Atlas of Primary Eyecare Procedures.* 2nd ed. Stamford, CT: Appleton & Lange, 1997:401–436.

669. Das N, Nasir AS. Comparison of intralesional kenacort injection versus surgical intervention for primary chalazion. *Pakistan Journal of Ophthalmology.* 2019 Jul 1;35(3).

670. Gerstenblith AT, Rabinowitz MP. In: *The Wills Eye Manual,* 6th ed. Philadelphia, PA: Wolters Kluwer Health/Lippincott Williams & Wilkins; 2012:137–138.

671. Nabie R, Soleimani H, Nikniaz L, et al. A prospective randomized study comparing incision and curettage with injection of triamcinolone acetonide for chronic chalazia. *Journal of Current Ophthalmology.* 2019 Sep 1;31(3):323-6.

672. Skorin L, Goemann L. Eyelid inflammation: approach to hordeolum, chalazion, and pyogenic granuloma. *Consultant.* 2017;57(5):282–285.

**10.8 Suturing, Excision, and Biopsy**

673. Carniciu A, Jovanovic N, Kahana A. Eyelid complications associated with surgery for periocular cutaneous malignancies. *Facial Plast Surg.* 2020;36(02):166–175.

674. Casser L, Fingeret M, Woodcome HT. Periocular injection procedures. In: *Atlas of Primary Eyecare Procedures*. 2nd ed. Stamford, CT: Appleton & Lange, 1997:401–436.

675. Casser L, Fingeret M, Woodcome HT. Suture cutting. In: *Atlas of Primary Eyecare Procedures*. 2nd ed. Stamford, CT: Appleton & Lange, 1997:360–367.

676. Chaugule, Sonal S., Santosh G. Honavar, and Paul T. Finger. Surgical ophthalmic oncology: a collaborative open access reference. Springer Nature, 2019.

677. Robinson JK, Hanke CW, Siegel DM, Fratila A, Bhatia A, Rohrer TE. *Surgery of the Skin: Procedural Dermatology*. 3rd ed. London/New York: Elsevier/Saunders; 2015.

678. Rene C. Oculoplastic aspects of ocular oncology. *Eye*. 2013;27:199–207.

679. Rupp J. Ophthalmic Suturing 101. American Academy of Ophthalmology. June 2018. Website. https://www.aao.org/young-ophthalmologists/yo-info/article/ophthalmic-suturing-101. Accessed April 10, 2022.

**10.9 Anterior Segment Lasers**

680. Bhargava R, Kumar P, Phogat H, et al. Neodymium-Yttrium Aluminum garnet laser capsulotomy energy levels for posterior capsule opacification. *J Ophthalmic Vis Res*. 2015;10(1):37–42.

681. Freisberg L, Lighthizer N, Skorin L, Stonecipher K, Zimmerman A. *The Ophthalmic Laser Handbook*. Philadelphia: Wolters Kluwer Health/Lippincott Williams & Wilkins; 2022.

682. Gazzard G, Konstantakopoulou E, Garway-Heath D, et al. Selective laser trabeculoplasty versus eye drops for first-line treatment of ocular hypertension and glaucoma (LiGHT): a multicenter randomized controlled trial. *Lancet*. 2019;393(10180):1505–1516.

683. Groth SL, Albeiruti E, Nunez M. et al. SALT trial: steroids after laser trabeculoplasty: impact of short-term anti-inflammatory treatment on selective laser trabeculoplasty efficacy. *Ophthalmology*. 2019;126(11):1511–1516.

684. Gulati V, Fan S, Gardner BJ, et al. Mechanism of action of selective laser trabeculoplasty and predictors of response. *Invest Ophthalmol Vis Sci*. 2017;58(3):1462–1468.

685. Koucheki B, Hashemi H. Selective laser trabeculoplasty in the treatment of open-angle glaucoma. *J Glaucoma*. 2012;21(1):65–70.

686. Matys J, Dominiak M, Flieger R. Energy and power density: a key factor in lasers studies. *J Clin Diagn Res*. 2015;9(12):ZL01–ZL02.

687. Radhakrishnan S, Chen PP, Junk AK, et al. Laser peripheral iridotomy in primary angle closure: a report by the American Academy of Ophthalmology. *Ophthalmology*. 2018;125(7):1110–1120.

688. Sinha R, Shekhar H, Sharma N, et al. Posterior capsular opacification: A review. *Indian J Ophthalmol*. 2013;61(7):371–376.

689. Spaeth GL, Idowu O, Seligsohn A, et al. The effects of iridotomy size and position on symptoms following laser peripheral iridotomy. *J Glaucoma*. 2005;14(5):364–367.

690. Vera V, Naqi A, Belovay GW, et al. Dysphotopsia after temporal versus superior laser peripheral iridotomy: a prospective randomized paired eye trial. *Am J Ophthalmol*. 2014;157(5):929–935.

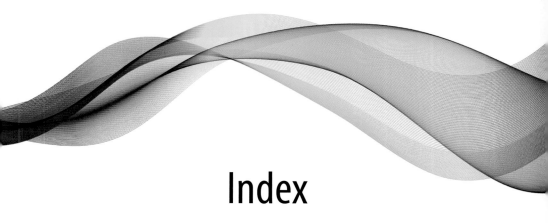

# Index

*Note:* Page locators followed by *f* and *t* indicate figures and tables, respectively.